The Self
in Understanding and Treating
Psychological Disorders

The Self
in Understanding and Treating
Psychological Disorders

Edited by

Michael Kyrios
Research School of Psychology, The Australian National University, Canberra, ACT, Australia

Richard Moulding
School of Psychology, Deakin University, Melbourne, VIC, Australia

Guy Doron
The Baruch Ivcher School of Psychology, Interdisciplinary Center (IDC) Herzliya, Herzliya, Israel

Sunil S. Bhar
Swinburne University of Technology, Melbourne, VIC, Australia

Maja Nedeljkovic
Swinburne University of Technology, Melbourne, VIC, Australia

Mario Mikulincer
Interdisciplinary Center (IDC) Herzliya and Baruch Ivcher School of Psychology, Herzliya, Israel

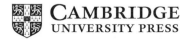

CAMBRIDGE
UNIVERSITY PRESS

University Printing House, Cambridge CB2 8BS, United Kingdom

Cambridge University Press is part of the University of Cambridge.

It furthers the University's mission by disseminating knowledge in the pursuit of
education, learning and research at the highest international levels of excellence.

www.cambridge.org
Information on this title: www.cambridge.org/9781107079144

© Cambridge University Press 2016

First published 2016

Printed in the United Kingdom by TJ International Ltd. Padstow Cornwall

A catalogue record for this publication is available from the British Library

Library of Congress Cataloguing in Publication data
The self in understanding and treating psychological disorders / edited by
Michael Kyrios [and five others].
    p. ; cm.
Includes bibliographical references and index.
ISBN 978-1-107-07914-4 (hardback)
I. Kyrios, Michael, editor.
[DNLM: 1. Mental Disorders–therapy.   2. Self Concept.
3. Evidence-Based Medicine. WM 400]
RC480.5
616.89′1–dc23   2015028162

ISBN 978-1-107-07914-4 Hardback

....

Contents

Section 4   Conclusions and future directions

Contributors

Claire Ahern
Clinical Psychologist & Postdoctoral Researcher, Swinburne University of Technology, Melbourne, VIC, Australia

Christopher Basten
Senior Clinical Psychologist, Basten and Associates, Clinical Psychologists, Westmead, NSW, Australia

Sunil S. Bhar
Associate Professor and Deputy Chair at the Department of Psychological Sciences, Swinburne University of Technology, Melbourne, VIC, Australia

Lisa S. Caddell
Postdoctoral Research Associate, University of Sheffield, Sheffield, UK

Eline Coppens
PhD student, Special Fund FWO, Faculty of Psychology and Educational Sciences, University of Leuven, and Clinical Psychologist at University Hospitals of Leuven, Leuven, Belgium

David A. Clark
Professor Emeritus, University of New Brunswick, NB, Canada

Nicki A. Dowling
Associate Professor of Psychology at the School of Psychology, Deakin University, VIC, Australia

Guy Doron
Associate Professor at the Baruch Ivcher School of Psychology, Interdisciplinary Center (IDC) Herzliya, Herzliya, Israel

Benedetto Farina
Associate Professor of Clinical Psychology, Università Europea (European University) Roma, Rome, Italy

Peter Fonagy
Professor, Research Department of Clinical, Educational and Health Psychology, University College London, London, UK

Bree Gregory
PhD candidate, Centre for Emotional Health, Macquarie University, Sydney, NSW, Australia

Kate Hall
Senior Lecturer of Psychology at the School of Psychology, Deakin University, VIC, Australia, and Senior Clinical Psychologist, Youth Support and Advocacy Service, Fitzroy, VIC, Australia

Mardi J. Horowitz
Distinguished Professor of Psychiatry at the University of California, San Francisco, CA, USA

Stefan Kempke
Postdoctoral Researcher of the Research Foundation Flanders (FWO) at the Faculty of Psychology and Educational Sciences, University of Leuven, Leuven, Belgium

Michael Kyrios
Professor and Director, Research School of Psychology, The Australian National University, Canberra, ACT, Australia

Gal Lazarus
Doctoral Student, Department of Psychology, Bar-Ilan University, Ramat Gan, Israel

Giovanni Liotti
Director of Training, Cognitive Psychology Association (APC) Postgraduate School of Psychotherapy, Rome, Italy

Nuwan D. Leitan
Postdoctoral Research Fellow, Faculty of Health, Arts and Design, Swinburne University of Technology, Melbourne, VIC, Australia

Patrick Luyten

Professor, Faculty of Psychology, University of Leuven, Belgium and Research Department of Clinical, Educational and Health Psychology, University College London, London, UK

Serafino G. Mancuso

Honorary Research Fellow, Department of Psychiatry, Faculty of Medicine, Dentistry and Health Sciences, The University of Melbourne, VIC, Australia

Stephanie Mathews

PhD student at the Faculty of Health, Arts and Design, Swinburne University of Technology, Melbourne, VIC, Australia

Offer Maurer

Psychology Lecturer at the Center for Academic Studies – Or Yehuda, and Head of the New Wave in Psychology Program at the Baruch Ivcher School of Psychology at the Interdisciplinary Center (IDC) Herzliya, Israel

Mario Mikulincer

Professor of Psychology and Provost of the Interdisciplinary Center (IDC) Herzliya and founding Dean of the Baruch Ivcher School of Psychology, Herzliya, Israel

Istvan Molnar-Szakacs

Research Neuroscientist, Tennenbaum Center for the Biology of Creativity, Semel Institute for Neuroscience and Human Behavior, University of California Los Angeles, CA, USA

Richard Moulding

Senior Lecturer, School of Psychology, Deakin University, Melbourne, VIC, Australia

Maja Nedeljkovic

Senior Lecturer in Psychology, Department of Psychological Sciences, Faculty of Health, Arts and Design, Swinburne University of Technology, Melbourne, VIC, Australia

Barnaby Nelson

Associate Professor, Orygen, The National Centre of Excellence in Youth Mental Health, University of Melbourne, VIC, Australia

Josef Parnas

Clinical Professor of Psychiatry and Psychopathology at the University of Copenhagen, Copenhagen, Denmark

Lorna Peters

Senior Lecturer, Centre for Emotional Health, Department of Psychology, Macquarie University, Sydney, NSW, Australia

Eshkol Rafaeli

Associate Professor and Director of (Adult) Clinical Training Program at the Department of Psychology and Gonda Multidisciplinary Brain Research Center of Bar-Ilan University, Ramat-Gan, Israel

Ronald M. Rapee

Distinguished Professor and Director at the Centre for Emotional Health, Macquarie University, Sydney, NSW, Australia

Imogen Rehm

PhD (Clinical Psychology) candidate at the Faculty of Health, Arts and Design, Swinburne University of Technology, Melbourne, VIC, Australia

Simone N. Rodda

Lecturer at the School of Public Health and Psychological Studies, AUT University, Auckland, New Zealand, and Honorary Fellow at the School of Psychology, Deakin University, VIC, Australia

Louis A. Sass

Professor, Department of Clinical Psychology, Graduate School of Applied and Professional Psychology, Rutgers University, Newark, NJ, USA

Moran Schiller

Doctoral student, The Stress, Self and Health Lab (STREALTH), Department of Psychology, Ben-Gurion University of the Negev, Israel

Golan Shahar

Professor of Clinical Health and Developmental Health Psychology, The Stress, Self and Health Lab (STREALTH), Department of Psychology, Ben-Gurion University of the Negev, Israel

Monica A. Sicilia

Doctoral candidate in Clinical Psychology, Long Island University, Brooklyn, NY, USA

Petra K. Staiger
Associate Professor, School of Psychology, Deakin University, Burwood, VIC, Australia

Nathan C. Thoma
Instructor of Psychology, Department of Psychiatry, Weill Cornell Medical College, New York, NY, USA

Stephen Touyz
Professor of Clinical Psychology and Clinical Professor in Psychiatry, University of Sydney, NSW, Australia

Lucina Q. Uddin
Assistant Professor, Department of Psychology, University of Miami, Miami, FL, USA

Boudewijn Van Houdenhove
Emeritus Professor at the Department of Psychiatry, University of Leuven, Leuven, Belgium

Doug P. VanderLaan
Canadian Institutes of Health Research Postdoctoral Fellow, Gender Identity Clinic, Child, Youth, and Family Services, Centre for Addiction and Mental Health, Toronto, ON, Canada

Robert D. Zettle
Professor of Psychology, Department of Psychology, Wichita State University, Wichita, KS, USA

Kenneth J. Zucker
Clinical Lead, Gender Identity Clinic, Child, Youth, and Family Services, Centre for Addiction and Mental Health, Toronto, ON, Canada

Foreword

I have made the self-concept a central feature of my writing and treatment approach for more than five decades – it is a unifying feature in depression, positive and negative symptoms of schizophrenia, and personality disorders, to name a few. The notion that we have something in us that expresses itself in so many ways is puzzling, yet elegant and exciting. Up to now, we have had to dip in and out of the literature to piece together the various perspectives on the self in such disorders.

But now, we have this book. The editors have done an excellent job in providing us with a collection of up-to-date overviews of the existing literature on the concept of self from social, cognitive, philosophical, neuroscientific, and experimental perspectives. They have brought together experts in the field to consider the role of the self in our understanding of psychological disorders and their treatment. The self remains the centerpiece in this book, and is showcased in a diverse array of psychological problems ranging from depression to dementia.

I was very pleased to see that the authors in this book went beyond simply describing the role of self in our understanding of psychological disorders. Across the various chapters, the authors encourage us to consider how the concept of self is addressed in various models of psychological treatment such as cognitive therapy, acceptance and commitment therapy, and psychodynamic therapy. In these chapters, the clinician will find a range of practical techniques for repairing or enhancing the self-concept of individuals in treatment. The message is clear. When psychological disorders are understood as disorders of self, clinicians can apply a fresh perspective towards treatment.

It is my pleasure to provide resounding praise for the team and contributors of this book.

Aaron T. Beck, MD
Emeritus Professor
Department of Psychiatry
University of Pennsylvania

Acknowledgments

The preparation of a book of this scope requires an amazing group effort from contributing authors, the editorial team and our supportive families, additional editorial supports, and our publishers and the production team at Cambridge University Press.

The editors started off as close colleagues and friends and ended up closer than ever before. On a personal note, I have been extremely lucky in my professional life to have been able to work with a group of individuals who started off as students but ended up as friends and colleagues, and who were then able to establish their own successful professional lives, opening up new collaborations and opportunities. While we no longer work in the same workplace or indeed city or country, that hasn't changed the quality of our interactions. It was indeed a privilege to work together on this as we have done from the outset. It was a particular pleasure to have Mario join us on this project, especially as he has been a fantastic support to Guy. At times, we needed some support in editing specialist chapters and it was great to be able to rely on colleagues such as Drs. Ross King and Rachel Shlomit Brezis. Throughout the long road that we took to completing the book, we were sustained by the belief that Richard Marley from Cambridge University Press had in the initial book idea and in our capacity to finish the project.

Most importantly, we were fortunate to have the remarkable focus and organizational support of Dr. Claire Ahern, without whom this book just would not have been possible. Claire was incredible in her positivity, motivational powers, and incomparable competence. When Claire had to take some time off to give birth to gorgeous baby Abigail Rose, we were indeed privileged to have Dr. Daniel Fassnacht fill Claire's role in order to facilitate completion of the book. We'd also like to thank Professor Tim Beck for his very kind words and endorsement and the Cambridge University Press production team for their professionalism and patience.

We are indebted to our contributing authors who did a fantastic job in sharing their ideas and in responding to our invitations and unreasonable timelines. Finally, we are grateful for the support of our families who put up with the late nights, our disengaged selves when concentrating on our chapters, and with the endless talk over the years about "the book." While this has been a long time in the making, we look forward to bringing back the "self" to the language of evidence-based practitioners.

Mike Kyrios on behalf of
Richard Moulding, Guy Doron, Sunil S. Bhar,
Maja Nedeljkovic and Mario Mikulincer

Chapter

1

The self in psychological disorders: an introduction

Michael Kyrios

Evidence-based practice has led to a revolution in how we manage psychological disorders such as anxiety and somatic symptom disorders, mood disorders, bipolar disorder, the obsessive–compulsive spectrum disorders, addictions, schizophrenia and related disorders, eating disorders, borderline personality disorder, fatigue, and other conditions (Hofmann, Asnaani, Vonk, Sawyer, & Fang, 2012; Hunsley, Elliott, & Therrien, 2014; McMain, Newman, Segal, & DeRubeis, 2015). One of the effects of this revolution, as translated by service agencies and organizations, has been an unintended tendency to overly focus on the disorders or problems that we treat rather than on the nature of the individuals who present to clinical practice, individuals who come with rich personal histories that impact on the development of the disorder and its trajectory throughout their lifespan and throughout their treatment.

Of course, a focus on disorder is not necessarily the foundation of evidence-based treatments such as cognitive-behavior therapy (CBT), where research and validated theory based on an essentially phenomenological approach are integrally linked and support the need to target general and idiosyncratic beliefs, as well as behavioral and affective responses to situations or stimuli. Salkovskis (2002) supports the need for scientist-practitioners to utilize Empirically Grounded Clinical Interventions that are based on a mix of "clinical observation, theoretical and experimental development" (p. 8), accounting for the social and cultural milieu. The personal and developmental context of individuals presenting for psychotherapy has long constituted a part of the "clinical observation" to which Salkovskis refers. Case formulations

that ought to guide treatment have traditionally been founded on a broader understanding of individual biological, developmental, intra- and interpersonal and contextual factors or vulnerabilities that underlie the development and maintenance of psychological disorders and problems in specific individuals. However, somewhere along the way, possibly due to the nature of health service funding models and their focus on outcomes and economic efficiencies, clinical psychology has arguably lost "the person" in evidence-based psychotherapy and now treats "the disorder."

A purely evidence-based framework is limited by the very fact that it is based on group analyses, while there is actually little evidence within the literature to help guide clinicians on individual predictors of disorder or treatment outcomes, idiosyncratic treatment processes and longer-term follow-up outcomes. In support of this view, there have been recent calls to identify "predictors, mediators, and moderators of treatment response in order to increase knowledge on how to personalise interventions for each client" (McMain *et al.*, 2015, p. 321). While this tome is not proposing a rejection of the normative framework characteristic of the evidence-based literature in preference for a totally idiographic framework, there are advantages to incorporating a broader range of individual factors in the treatment of psychological disorders.

Numerous studies are now beginning to show that individual factors impact on outcomes, especially personality traits, although this may depend on treatment modality. For instance, Ramos-Grille, Gomà-i-Freixanet, Aragay, Valero, and Vallès (2015)

The Self in Understanding and Treating Psychological Disorders, ed. Michael Kyrios, Richard Moulding, Guy Doron, Sunil S. Bhar, Maja Nedeljkovic, and Mario Mikulincer. Published by Cambridge University Press. © Cambridge University Press, 2016.

reported that problem gamblers were not only characterized by high scores on neuroticism–anxiety relative to controls, but that those in treatment who relapsed or dropped out rated themselves as more impulsive and sensation-seeking, while high impulsivity emerged as a predictor of poorer treatment outcome. Min, Lee, Lee, Lee, and Chae (2012) found that low trait anxiety and positive resilience or emotional regulation predicted treatment response in depressed outpatients. In examining outcomes from either CBT or pharmacotherapy, Bagby et al. (2008) found main effects for the personality traits of openness and neuroticism, and moderating effects of agreeableness. In contrast, in a cohort of inpatients with a mixture of mainly neurotic diagnoses undertaking psychodynamically oriented therapy, no personality traits predicted outcome after accounting for baseline symptoms, although moderate to large effect size magnitude changes were found (Steinert, Klein, Leweke, & Leichsenring, 2015). Nonetheless, such studies do show growing interest in individual predictors of treatment outcome across all psychotherapies.

While identifying individual differences as a way forward, in his introduction to a special feature on the self and identity, Livesley (2006) emphasized that a focus on personality traits misses important components in understanding disorder. Despite a focus on personality disorder, his point about the need to examine more comprehensive aspects of functioning in delineating disorder is well taken.

> The trait system is only one component of the larger system … Other sub-systems include control structures and mechanisms that regulate affects and impulses and coordinate goal-directed action, and the knowledge systems that encode information about the self, others, and the world and guide subsequent action … Research tends to neglect disturbances in the self system that are central to understanding the disorder. These disturbances involve problems with both the contents and the organisation of the self. (Livesley, 2006, p. 541).

In support, research from a variety of theoretical perspectives has demonstrated that individual factors related to cognitions, early schemas and identity also impact on outcomes across a range of disorders. For instance, Quilty, McBride, and Bagby (2008) found a mediational role for general maladaptive cognitions in outcomes for depression following CBT and pharmacotherapy, but not interpersonal therapy. Furthermore, Haaland et al. (2011) explored whether early maladaptive schemas were related to treatment outcome

in outpatients with obsessive–compulsive disorder (OCD) who completed exposure with response prevention. Higher pre-treatment abandonment schema scores were related to poor outcome, while higher pre-treatment scores on the self-sacrifice schema were related to better outcome. During treatment, changes in the failure schema were significantly related to positive outcome at post-treatment. Moreover, one of our own studies has shown that the resolution of self-ambivalence during CBT for OCD predicted better post-treatment outcomes (Bhar, Kyrios, & Hordern, 2015). Specifically, when pre-treatment depression, anxiety and OCD severity were accounted for, pre-to-post changes in self-ambivalence significantly predicted recovery. A one standard deviation change in self-ambivalence was in fact associated with nearly four times the likelihood of recovery in OCD symptoms.

A better understanding of self and related constructs such as early schemas and attachment styles in psychological disorders may offer ways forward in advancing our understanding of psychological disorders and their treatment. That is not to say that existing theoretical frameworks ignore the self. In CBT, for instance, core beliefs about the self, others, and the world are considered to underpin all functioning. However, little work has examined or brought together the literature focusing on specific aspects of the self as they relate to particular disorders. Much work needs to be undertaken to bring together the various strands of the psychological literature on the self, inclusive of social psychological, clinical, personality, cognitive, philosophical, neuroscientific, and experimental research (Gallagher, 2011). This book is an attempt to do exactly that for specific psychological and cognitive disorders, while also exploring implications for psychological treatment.

The concept of the "self" is a complex multidimensional construct, but has long been of interest to researchers of human psychology from developmental and clinical perspectives. Katzko (2003) states: "The term 'self' is used by too many different theorists in too many different ways" (p. 84). Brinthaupt and Lipka (1992) consider that the self is variously defined as schema, prototype, cognitive representation, multidimensional hierarchical construct, narrative sequence, linguistic descriptor, process, and elaborate theory, among other terms. Nonetheless, it is a construct that encapsulates many of the biological, developmental, intra- and interpersonal and contextual factors that we use in case formulations and that are thought to underlie the development and maintenance of psychological disorders and problems.

With respect to psychological disorders, the "self" has been seen as important: (a) to our *understanding* of disorder (e.g., a disturbance of the basic sense of self, i.e., a *pre-reflective*, *tacit* level of selfhood, is seen as a phenotypic trait marker of schizophrenia spectrum disorders; ego dystonic thoughts are core to our understanding and the definition of OCD); (b) the *experience* of those with disorders (e.g., compromised self-esteem across many disorders); (c) in the *etiology* of disorder (e.g., the importance of self-ambivalence in OCD; Guidano & Liotti, 1983); and (d) to *cognitive factors* central to the etiology, maintenance, and treatment of disorder (e.g., the importance of self-oriented perfectionism in depression; Sherry, Richards, Sherry, & Stewart, 2014).

A myriad of self constructs have been studied and variously applied to specific disorders, although there is no reference that brings together the topics of disorder and "self" so as to help academics and practitioners alike summarize the associations through a review of the literature and its inherent issues and applications. While Kircher and David (2003) highlighted the importance of the self from psychiatric and neuroscientific perspectives, focusing on consciousness and self-consciousness, they focused on schizophrenia and related disorders alone. As there is a range of cognitive, affective, behavioral, developmental, organizational, content, and process components that contribute to our understanding of the self in psychopathology across the range of disorders, this tome takes a broader view.

Self processes, complexity, stability, and interactions with experiential or contextual factors all have a role to play in the emergence and maintenance of psychological disorders. This complex interplay of factors differs from disorder to disorder, although some disorders may demonstrate some commonalities, while there are also areas of the literature that are as yet uncharted for some disorders. The different treatment modalities take specific approaches to dealing with these complex self-related factors. Moreover, various approaches to psychotherapy use particular strategies based on specific theoretical frameworks. Despite such differences, one thing remains constant: the study of the self brings with it a rich tapestry of implications and the potential to improve our evidence base with respect to our understanding and treatment of psychological disorders.

Overview of this volume and its structure

The book is divided into three parts. In Section 1 (Chapters 1–3), we present constructs that are important in understanding the construct of the self and factors that influence the development of self. In Section 2 (Chapters 4–7), the authors present ways in which the self is generally dealt with in various treatment frameworks. While not all treatment approaches are represented, the editors have chosen major approaches that have a widespread practitioner base and that have existing or emerging evidence bases. Section 3 (Chapters 8–22) constitutes the major body of the volume and deals with a range of psychological or cognitive disorders representing major groups within diagnostic taxonomies such as the DSM-5 (American Psychiatric Association, 2013). The volume finishes with a concluding chapter (Chapter 23) that sets out some ways to move this area forward, particularly with respect to the integration of self constructs into evidence-based conceptual models of disorders and treatment.

Summary of each main chapter

Bhar and Kyrios (Chapter 2) start by providing an overview of self constructs and the dimensions which can be used to understand the self. They cover self concepts from early Western models of selfhood to current construals seen in research, including those focused on content and structure. Mikulincer and Doron (Chapter 3) go on to outline the importance of an attachment framework to understanding the development of self. This is an important chapter as it emphasizes developmental influences and how they impact on the emergence of self and, in particular, how they lead to a compromised self which is ultimately expressed in idiosyncratic ways, depending on the nature of early experiences and trauma.

The second section of the book focuses on treatment and includes chapters by Shahar, Clark, Zettle and Rafaeli as lead authors on the self in psychodynamic therapy (Chapter 4), cognitive behavioral therapy (Chapter 5), acceptance and commitment therapy (Chapter 6), and schema therapy (Chapter 7), respectively. These therapeutic frameworks were chosen due to the current extent of their dissemination. Psychodynamic theory has a long history of focusing on the self, albeit encompassing a range of perspectives. While acceptance and commitment therapy and schema therapy are considered part of the "third wave" of cognitive and behavioral therapies, they have particular relevance to self-based therapeutic targets. Each chapter explicates how the self is defined and managed generally within the specific therapeutic approach. Many of these issues are then taken up in Section 3, which examines the self with respect to specific disorders.

In Chapter 4, Shahar and Schiller emphasize that, given that the key mechanism of psychodynamic therapy is to *increase self-knowledge*, focusing attention on the self is of particular relevance. The authors integrate a traditional Kleinian approach to object relations, anxieties, and defense mechanisms with social-cognitive and neurocognitive foci on schemas, narratives, affect regulation, and future representations. They go on to describe three ways of working with depressed patients to facilitate a "future orientation." The use of "multiple selves analysis/personal projects analysis" is emphasized. Clark (Chapter 5) provides case studies and outlines several ways in which cognitive-behavioral theories and treatment conceptualize and target the self, inclusive of notions about self-discrepancy, self-schemas, incongruence, and complexity. He emphasizes that CBT would likely profit by further accounting for self-construals. Zettle (Chapter 6) reviews how self and related topics are considered and targeted within acceptance and commitment therapy (ACT), one of the therapies within the third wave of cognitive and behavioral therapies that have emerged in recent decades (Hayes, Strosahl, & Wilson, 1999). In particular, he reviews three distinctive ways in which self-related behaviors are regarded within ACT, and examines therapeutic strategies that deal with maladaptive behaviors, as well as the current evidence base for their efficacy. In Chapter 7, Rafaeli and colleagues adopt a multifaceted view of the self and review the development of the schema therapy approach to treatment, emphasizing the efficacy of working with the multiplicity of selves.

Section 3 starts with chapters on mood disorders. Luyten and Fonagy examine psychodynamic and cognitive-behavioral approaches to the self and self processes in major depression, and integrate these in discussing treatment strategies and processes (Chapter 8). Specifically, they see disruptions in the self as both a cause and an outcome of depression, and consider disturbances in interactions with others and in individuals' capacities to mentalize as generating vulnerability to depression. Leitan expounds on the various approaches to the self in bipolar disorder (BD), opening the way for greater clarity and new research directions in the etiology and treatment of this disabling disorder (Chapter 9). In particular, he emphasizes the importance of self-based cognitive processing and the role of the body and experience in the relationship between self and BD. He concludes by presenting a discourse as to how understanding the self in BD complements current and emerging treatments for BD.

The next section deals with anxiety disorders, showcasing social anxiety (Chapter 10) and trauma (Chapter 11). Gregory and colleagues discuss the importance of self-constructs, particularly self-images, self-beliefs, and self-focused attention in the etiology and treatment of social anxiety. They emphasize that changing self-structures and using imagery rescripting can improve treatment outcomes (Chapter 10). Horowitz and Sicilia (Chapter 11) discuss posttraumatic stress disorder (PTSD) from the perspective of "person schema theory" (Horowitz, 2011). While they consider PTSD as likely to impact negatively on one's sense of self, they also emphasize that pre-existing ruptures in coherence of self-organization make it challenging for individuals to process and integrate traumatic experiences. They use neurobiological and relational or attachment frameworks to understand how the self develops, themes commonly encountered throughout this book.

Chapters 12 and 13 deal with the obsessive-compulsive spectrum disorders. Ahern and Kyrios outline self constructs in OCD with an emphasis on Guidano and Liotti's (1983) earlier theoretical work on self-ambivalence, a construct thought to derive from early attachment patterns. They further elucidate a range of related constructs such as self-contingency, self sensitivity and implicit self processes. Expanding on a similar theoretical perspective, Moulding and colleagues (Chapter 13) focus on hoarding disorder, body dysmorphic disorder, and trichotillomania, and conclude that overidentification with some aspect of the self or its extensions (e.g., possessions, appearance, and hair, respectively) is associated with shame, misperceptions, and compromised emotional regulation strategies to deal with perceived challenges to self. In Chapter 14, Rodda and colleagues expound on self constructs, in particular self regulation associated with impulse control and addictive behaviors which are an important focus in effective treatments.

The chapters that follow examine the self in disorders many consider to be biologically based, specifically autism (Chapter 15) and schizophrenia spectrum disorders (Chapter 16). As the authors demonstrate, psychological constructs play an important role in understanding the emergence of these disorders and their treatment. Molnar-Szakacs and Uddin examine self constructs and related neurocognitive functions in autism and spectrum disorders. They argue that certain features of physical and embodied self-representation are generally functional in autism; however, psychological and evaluative self-related cognition appear to be impaired, especially theory of mind, although many studies point to a lack of differences between representations of self and other. Nonetheless, an examination of self-related processing deficits affords a promising framework for understanding the complex symptomatology in autism spectrum disorders. The authors conclude that bringing together imaging methods and behavioral approaches to studying self-related cognition in autism will lead to a more complete understanding of the self in this baffling disorder. Nelson and colleagues summarize new directions in understanding bidirectional relationships between self construals in schizophrenia and schizotypy, offering exceptional insights into new ways of understanding relevant phenomena. Specifically, they consider schizophrenia to be characterized by the form of experience rather than the content of experience or disturbance in particular modalities. They support the notion that schizophrenia is characterized by instability in the first-person perspective, a diminished sense of presence and a loss of contact with reality, and consider their model as demonstrating a trait disturbance distinctive to the schizophrenia spectrum.

The book then goes on to consider self construals in personality disorders, specifically borderline personality disorder (BPD) and obsessive–compulsive personality disorder (OCPD). In Chapter 17, Liotti and Farina outline an attachment-based model of self in BPD and highlight important elements of a therapeutic framework for managing this complex disorder. They emphasize that self experience emerges from the quality of our relationships and, as such, they take a radically relational approach to the treatment of BPD. Their treatment focus is on the impact of disorganized attachment and the central role that the therapeutic alliance and use of parallel integrated interventions can play, rather than on specific therapeutic techniques which they see as useful in correcting maladaptive

relational information. Integrating a broader range of influences, Nedeljkovic and colleagues examine etiological factors in OCPD and present a research and therapeutic framework for this intriguing disorder (Chapter 18). They propose that individuals with OCPD hold restricted self-views with a focus on work-related competence, extreme perfectionism and need for control. They cite earlier theoretical work by Kyrios (1998), which has implicated ambivalence in self, lack of trust, low self-efficacy, role limitation, and ethical/moral inflexibility in OCPD. They emphasize the need for treatments to target relevant cognitive distortions and limited self conceptualizations.

The next few chapters examine self concepts in disorders where the interface between psychological and physiological factors is central. Chapter 19 by Kempke and colleagues deals with the self in chronic fatigue syndrome as an exemplar of a somatic condition. They emphasize the importance of specific mental representations or cognitive–affective schemas associated with self-criticism or attachment avoidance, along with early negative experiences which impact on the neurobiological stress response system. Basten and Touyz examine self constructs in eating disorders (ED) and highlight the bidirectional relationship between self and EDs (Chapter 20). They consider compromised self as being at the center of the need to change or perfect those aspects of the self considered central to one's sense of identity, a theme that is seen across a range of disorders. In EDs, individuals attempt to manifest control over eating and weight, whether consciously or unconsciously, in order to compensate for their perceived deficiencies. The authors suggest that intrapsychic and behavioral interventions must be tailored to fit the individual's psychological profile and ED symptomatology. In Chapter 21, Caddell examines the variety of self constructs used in research on dementia, an issue of enormous importance to communities experiencing an aging population. A loss of self (or related terms) has been used to characterize dementia, although qualitative studies suggest that much of the sense of self is actually maintained in people with dementia despite some aspects of deterioration. Caddell also reviews interventions in patients with dementia, most of which focus on well-being, but also have implications for identity. Despite limitations in the literature, taking a self perspective on dementia appears to offer a range of opportunities to understand the experience of dementia and to provide novel management strategies. In the final chapter in Section 3, Zucker and VanderLaan examine self constructs in individuals with gender identity disorder (GID) (Chapter 22). There is enormous interest in and understanding of the degree to which gender identity is important to one's sense of self, and that social dynamics play an important role in the adjustment of individuals with GID. As individuals can and do change their gender identity, the influence of gender identity in defining the self may be more fluid in some people; however, the authors identify central developmental issues with a self focus that could be successfully targeted in the understanding of individuals with GID. Treatment issues in GID are somewhat more complex, but fundamental developmental issues and self construals are likely to be an important focus.

In the final chapter (Chapter 23), the editors attempt to briefly summarize and integrate the information presented by the various authors within the book, and discuss ways in which psychopathology and its management can be advanced by examining the self. While not quite constituting the fourth wave of cognitive and behavioral psychotherapies, consideration of the self has enormous potential to change the way in which we conceptualize disorders and our approach to psychotherapy. Consideration of the self offers: (a) constructs that allow us to integrate a developmental framework into evidence-based models of disorder and psychotherapies; (b) a way of integrating psychodynamic frameworks and a range of cognitive-behavioral therapeutic frameworks; (c) research directions for experimental and clinical studies aimed at understanding the development of psychological dysfunction; and (d) a way forward for incorporating the lived experience into our understanding of psychological disorders.

References

American Psychiatric Association. (2013). *Diagnostic and Statistical Manual of Mental Disorders* (5th ed.). Washington, DC: APA.

Bagby, R. M., Quilty, L. C., Segal, Z. V., *et al.* (2008). Personality and differential treatment response in major depression: A randomized controlled trial comparing Cognitive-Behavioural Therapy and Pharmacotherapy. *Canadian Journal of Psychiatry. Revue Canadienne de Psychiatrie*, 53(6), 361–370.

Bhar, S. S., Kyrios, M., & Hordern, C. (2015). Self-ambivalence in the cognitive-behavioral treatment of obsessive–compulsive disorder. *Psychopathology*, 48(5), 349–56. doi: 10.1159/000438676

Brinthaupt, T. M., & Lipka, R. P. (Eds.). (1992). *The Self: Definitional and Methodological Issues.* Albany: State University of New York Press.

Gallagher, S. (Ed.). (2011). *The Oxford Handbook of the Self: Oxford Handbooks.* Oxford: Oxford University Press.

Guidano, V. F., & Liotti, G. (Eds.). (1983). *Cognitive Processes and Emotional Disorders: A Structural Approach to Psychotherapy.* New York, NY: Guilford Press.

Haaland, A. T., Vogel, P. A., Launes, G., *et al.* (2011). The role of early maladaptive schemas in predicting exposure and response prevention outcome for obsessive-compulsive disorder. *Behaviour Research and Therapy*, 49(11), 781–788. doi: 10.1016/j.brat.2011.08.007

Hayes, S. C., Strosahl, K., & Wilson, K. G. (1999). *Acceptance and Commitment Therapy: An Experiential Approach to Behavior Change.* New York, NY: Guilford Press.

Hofmann, S. G., Asnaani, A., Vonk, I. J. J., Sawyer, A. T., & Fang, A. (2012). The efficacy of cognitive behavioral therapy: A review of meta-analyses. *Cognitive Therapy and Research*, 36(5), 427–440. doi: 10.1007/s10608-012-9476-1

Horowitz, M. J. (2011). *Stress Response Syndromes* (5th ed.). Northvale, NJ: Jason Aronson.

Hunsley, J., Elliott, K., & Therrien, Z. (2014). The efficacy and effectiveness of psychological treatments for mood, anxiety, and related disorders. *Canadian Psychology. Psychologie canadienne*, 55(3), 161–176. doi: 10.1037/a0036933

Katzko, M. W. (2003). Unity versus multiplicity: A conceptual analysis of the term "self" and its use in personality theories. *Journal of Personality*, 71(1), 83–114. doi: 10.1111/1467–6494.t01-1-00004

Kircher, T., & David, A. (2003). *The Self in Neuroscience and Psychiatry.* Cambridge: Cambridge University Press.

Kyrios, M. (1998). A cognitive-behavioral approach to the understanding and management of obsessive–compulsive personality disorder. In C. Perris & P. McGorry (Eds.), *Cognitive Psychotherapy of Psychotic and Personality Disorders: Handbook of Theory and Practice* (pp. 351–378). New York, NY: Wiley.

Kyrios, M., Nedeljkovic, M., Moulding, R., & Doron, G. (2007). Problems of employees with personality disorders: The exemplar of obsessive–compulsive personality disorder (OCPD). In J. Langan-Fox, C. L. Cooper, & R. J. Klimoski (Eds.), *Research Companion to the Dysfunctional Workplace: Management Challenges and Symptoms* (pp. 40–57). Cheltenham: Elgar.

Livesley, W. J. (2006). Introduction to special feature on self and identity. *Journal of Personality Disorders*, 20(6), 541–543. doi: 10.1521/pedi.2006.20.6.541

McMain, S., Newman, M. G., Segal, Z. V., & DeRubeis, R. J. (2015). Cognitive behavioral therapy: Current status and future research directions. *Psychotherapy Research*, 25(3), 321–329. doi: 10.1080/10503307.2014.1002440

Min, J.-A., Lee, N.-B., Lee, C.-U., Lee, C., & Chae, J.-H. (2012). Low trait anxiety, high resilience, and their interaction as possible predictors for treatment response in patients with depression. *Journal of Affective Disorders*, 137(1), 61–69. doi: 10.1016/j.jad.2011.12.026

Quilty, L. C., McBride, C., & Bagby, R. M. (2008). Evidence for the cognitive mediational model of cognitive behavioural therapy for depression. *Psychological Medicine*, 38(11), 1531–1541. doi: doi:10.1017/S0033291708003772

Ramos-Grille, I., Gomà-i-Freixanet, M., Aragay, N., Valero, S., & Vallés, V. (2015). Predicting treatment failure in pathological gambling: The role of personality traits. *Addictive Behaviors*, 43, 54–59. doi: http://dx.doi.org/10.1016/j.addbeh.2014.12.010

Salkovskis, P. M. (2002). Empirically grounded clinical interventions: Cognitive-behavioural therapy progresses through a multi-dimensional approach to clinical science. *Behavioural and Cognitive Psychotherapy*, 30, 3–9.

Sherry, S. B., Richards, J. E., Sherry, D. L., & Stewart, S. H. (2014). Self-critical perfectionism is a vulnerability factor for depression but not anxiety: A 12-month, 3-wave longitudinal study. *Journal of Research in Personality*, 52, 1–5. doi: http://dx.doi.org/10.1016/j.jrp.2014.05.004

Steinert, C., Klein, S., Leweke, F., & Leichsenring, F. (2015). Do personality traits predict outcome of psychodynamically oriented psychosomatic inpatient treatment beyond initial symptoms? *British Journal of Clinical Psychology*, 54(1), 109–125. doi: 10.1111/bjc.12064

Chapter 2

The self-concept: theory and research

Sunil S. Bhar and Michael Kyrios

There is a burgeoning literature on the theoretical relevance of self-constructs to maladaptive behavior, cognition, and emotion. Likewise, there is widespread acceptance that the self-concept is a useful explanatory factor in research on psychopathology. Thousands of research publications are produced every year on the self-concept; over 30,000 publications on the self-concept were found between 1974 and 1993 (Ashmore & Jussim, 1997), and more recent estimates suggest that 1 in 7 publications in psychology addresses the self-concept (Tesser, Stapel, & Wood, 2002).

Despite the widespread acceptance of the self-concept as a meaningful construct in psychological theory and research, the term itself remains elusive. The self-concept has been studied through various approaches, and has variously been defined as schema (Taylor & Boggiano, 1987), concept (Rogers, 1961), value (Hermans, 1987), representation (Markus, 1990), narrative (McAdams & McLean, 2013), role (Deaux, 1993), and theory (Epstein, 1973). Terms are sometimes used interchangeably to refer to the same construct, or conversely, different constructs are associated with the same term. For example, terms such as self, self-estimation, self-identity, self-image, self-perception and self-consciousness are used interchangeably with self-concept (Hattie, 2014), which in turn can refer variously to self-esteem as well as descriptions of self-characteristics. The "self", Westen (1992, p. 4) surmises, is a "mushy, muddle-headed construct without empirical referents."

Given the difficulties in defining the self-concept, along with its widespread and inconsistent usage, some theorists have disputed that the self-concept is a viable construct, suggesting that it remains an abstraction, deduced from one's activity. Baumeister (1998, p. 683) suggests one cannot be aware of self "in the same way you are aware of a table or painting," and surrenders to a position that "it is much easier to feel the self than to define the self."

Hence, there is a need for an overview of models for appreciating the diverse ways in which the self-concept is understood and applied in research. The self-concept is theoretically informed, and hence definitions for the term are best understood within the context of theory; otherwise, as suggested, such definitions remain barren (Hattie, 2014). Likewise, the way in which the concept is employed in research can be appreciated in the context of such theory. Therefore, there are two aims of this chapter. First, it provides a starting point for understanding the major theories that have been influential in defining the self-concept. It outlines early western philosophical positions, as well as more recent psychodynamic, cognitive, social, and narrative theories. Second, it offers an overview of the application of the self-concept in psychological research, which in turn illustrates the theories that contextualize the meaning of the term. The self-concept is often used in such research with reference to its content and structural properties. It is hoped the broad overview of theory and applications of the concept provides readers with a framework for appreciating the diverse perspectives on the self-concept, and its utility as a focus in psychological investigations. It is envisaged that such a framework will help integrate the range of perspectives used to understand and treat psychological disorder.

The Self in Understanding and Treating Psychological Disorders, ed. Michael Kyrios, Richard Moulding, Guy Doron, Sunil S. Bhar, Maja Nedeljkovic, and Mario Mikulincer. Published by Cambridge University Press. © Cambridge University Press, 2016.

Theories of the self-concept

Early Western models

The notion of self-concept as distinct from other concepts such as person, memory, soul, thinking, and perception has been debated for centuries. In early Western-based theories, the self has been variously equated with soul, perception, and consciousness (Hattie, 2014). In particular, many theorists have rejected the distinction between the self as the thinker and an object of thought. Descartes' exclamation "I think therefore I am" points to the difficulty of separating the thinker from the object of thought (Descartes, 1967). Likewise, for Locke (1960), the self was equated with the person who was engaged in knowing. Hence, the self, according to such philosophers, was equated with the subject that is the "thing that carries out the action … the thinker of our thoughts, experiences of our experiences, perceiver of our perceptions, feeler of our feelings as well as the initiator of our physical actions …" (Watson, 2014, p. 1). In short, the self was semantically equated with the modern meaning of "I."

The concept of self as a representation rather than as subject emerged in the eighteenth century, when thinkers such as Hume (2014) began to represent the self as distinct from the person, or from a spiritual substance, and more closely aligned to a mental construction. Hume proposed that such a concept was essentially a series of perceptions about the subject.

> For my part, when I enter most intimately into what I call myself, I always stumble on some particular perception or other, of heat or cold, light or shade, love or hatred, pain or pleasure. I never catch myself at any time without a perception and can never observe anything but the perception. (p. 334)

Early writers stressed that such perceptions were provided with thematic unity through the associations with a felt sense of commonality. Mill (1869) claimed that the idea of "myself" was related closely with previous ideas of myself, thus bringing about a sense of temporal cohesion to the nature of self. Spencer (1963) argued that although the self was a series of impressions and ideas, there was a principle of unity and continuity that bound these impressions. For some authors (e.g., Bergson, 1975), memory served the function of a binding agent for blending past and present experiences into a coherent and organic whole. Hence, the mental representation of self as defined through such perspectives was argued to comprise collections of perceptions that were unified within a cohesive frame.

Psychodynamic models

Unlike earlier models of the self-concept that emphasized unity between different aspects of self-experiences, the psychoanalytic perspective of the self-concept focused on the fragmented and conflictual nature of the self-system. Freud (1916) rejected the existence of any viable answer to questions such as "Who am I?" or "What am I?" He argued that major aspects of selfhood were hidden from our awareness in an unconscious domain. This domain comprised desires, wishes, impulses, and ideas that were inaccessible to self-knowledge (reviewed in Elliott, 2013). He argued that human subjectivity was plural – that is, the same person could have conscious and unconscious motivations, knowledge, and impulses that were not unified. Freud envisaged the human mind as a hierarchy of agencies – the ego which regulated impulses; the id, which generated the drive towards satisfying pleasure, impulses, and instincts; and the superego, which operated as a conscience based on learned social standards. The Freudian perspective, as summarized by Watson (2014), was as follows: "We neither are nor contain anything that remains identical over time. Even at one moment of time, we are not one thing. Rather we are a multiplicity of interacting systems and processes" (p. 2).

In his review of the literature on the psychoanalytic view of the self, Westen (1992) suggested that the self-concept was a repertoire of representations that could be contradictory. He noted that one of the most important ideas about the self-representation in psychoanalytic thinking was that such representations could reflect compromised functions – that is, a compromise between opposite or conflicting motives. For example, he cites a patient who strives for success but then avoids such success because of a compromised function – that is, to be great like he imagined his father to be, but also not to betray his father by succeeding where his father had failed. Similarly, conflicts between self-representations were purported to include conscious (explicit) and unconscious (implicit) representations. A narcissistic patient, for example, may insist that he is better than all his superiors because he unconsciously feels weak and inferior. Hence, the self-concept was not assumed to be unitary, but rather an interplay between various motives that occurred at various levels of awareness.

The self as portrayed through these models was also a relational representation, that is, a representation of self in relation to others (Westen, 1992). In object relations theories, the self-concept was said to include a representation of others and one's early relationships with caretakers. Kohut (1971, 1977) forwarded the concept of self as including ambitions and ideals. Ambitions were described as grandiose views of the self as all-knowing and powerful. Ideals were derived from the child's idealized view of his or her parents. Similarly, Klein (1977) described adults as having incorporated early patterns of interpersonal relationships, and contended that such incorporated images or objects become a guide for what to expect from, and how to behave with, others.

Cognitive models

The notion of self-concept as a cognitive representation of information is best associated with cognitive models of the concept. Within such models, the self-concept is viewed as a cognitive construct, comprising descriptions, prescriptions, and expectations about one's attributes, weaknesses, and goals. For example, Epstein (1973) emphasizes that the self-concept was an implicit theory about oneself, and Hattie (2014) refers to the self-concept as cognitive appraisals of self-related attributes.

The self-concept is regarded by many cognitive-oriented theorists not only as a mental representation of one's attributes, but also as a filter for incoming information. In this way, the self-concept operates as a schema, that is, "an organisation of information about who one is, and often who others want one to be, which is stored in long term memory"(Safran, Segal, Hill, & Whiffen, 1990, p. 145), that "guides recall selectively and provide(s) default information to fill in gaps in ongoing processing" (p. 144). Markus (1977) suggests that the self-schema forms a set of beliefs that emerges from one's learning, but then guides the processing of information. Such schemas are said to comprise "cognitive generalizations about the self, derived from past experience that organise and guide the processing of self related information contained in the individual's social experience" (p. 64).

The effects of self-schemas on information-processing resources have been widely researched. Self-schemas have been found to influence cognitive activities such as perception, memory, and inference. For example, researchers have found that individuals are quicker to process information that is congruent with their self-schemas than information that is incongruent (MacDonald & Kuiper, 1985). Further, Markus (1977) found that when people were asked to predict their own behavior, they usually made predictions consistent with their self-schemas. In addition, other researchers have observed that individuals with a low sense of self-worth erroneously predict that others also have congruent beliefs about them (Swann, Wenzlaff, Krull, & Pelham, 1992).

Social models

From a social theory perspective, the self-concept is regarded as a multifaceted concept that is defined and evaluated with reference to a range of social activities, roles, relationships, and memberships. William James (1890) conceptualized the self as having both empirical and agentic quantities, thus drawing upon ideas from Hume and Locke as reviewed above. For James, the self could be regarded as an object of perception or knowledge, and was evaluated on the basis of one's material possessions (including body, clothes, and home), social recognition, and spiritual qualities (e.g., values, ideals, dispositions, thinking). In contrast, the agentic or subjective self was said to refer to the self as a knower and construer of reality. The empirical self and subjective self referred, respectively, to the "me" and "I" of the self-system.

The distinction between self as an object to be known and perceived, and self as the subject doing the knowing and perceiving (i.e., an information-processing structure) has informed many of the empirical approaches within the modern literature on self. The self as an object of perception has most often been the target of empirical studies, and is commonly regarded as the self-concept in modern literature. Many definitions of self-concept in the literature have focused on the set of beliefs that the person holds about himself or herself, which are generally organized into at least a partly coherent system. For example, in her review of research in social cognition, Fiske (1991) described the self-concept as "the person's mental presentation of his or her own personality attributes, social roles, past experience, future goals and the like" (pp. 181–182) and as including facts, beliefs, and memories of the person's past. The self as knower has been less clearly defined in the literature. In current psychological writings about the self, the subjective self is often represented as the reflexive process of representing oneself (Baumeister,

1998). Baumeister calls this aspect of self "executive function," because it "makes choices, initiates, acts and takes responsibility" (p. 682).

Social theorists have extended the definition of self-concept to include societal roles, relationships, and group memberships. Such theorists observe that individuals usually describe themselves according to their roles in society (student, worker, sister, etc.) and in accordance with cultural norms (J. Brown, 1988). Gray (1994) proposed that a person might see himself or herself as authoritative in the role of employer, submissive in the role of daughter or son, but companionable in the role of wife or husband. Fiske (1991) says "We know ourselves by our social roles, such as student, son, or daughter, or spouse, and we have a conceptual sense of ourselves, that is an impression of our own attributes and personal qualities" (p. 180). Accordingly, Harter and Whitesell (2003) found that adolescents gave different ratings to their self-esteem when with teachers, parents, male classmates, and female classmates. Based on factor analysis methods used primarily with children and adolescents, researchers found that the self-concept is best understood not as a global construct, but rather as comprising numerous domains by which individuals judge themselves, such as scholastic competence, athletic competence, peer likeability, physical appearance, and job competence (Harter, 2003).

Mead (1934) emphasizes the role of language in this socialization process. Through the use of language, Mead says that individuals define themselves according to society's constructs and social groups. From a developmental perspective, Sherif (1967) argues that a person matures having a frame of reference that is derived from reference groups – that is, groups serving as guides or standards for the individual's judgment, perception, roles, and behavior. Deaux (1993) refers to identity as social categories in which an individual claims membership coupled with the personal meanings associated with those categories. She argues that "personal identity is defined, at least in part, by group membership and (that) social categories are infused with personal meaning" (p. 5).

Other social theorists (Cooley, 1902/1964; Mead, 1934; Schlenker, 1980) have emphasized the interpersonal aspects of the definition of self-concept. For example, Cooley refers to the self-concept as a "looking glass," implying that self-views are inferences one makes about how others in society regard oneself. Similarly, Schlenker construes identity as a theory constructed about how one is defined and regarded

in social life. As stated by James (1890), "A man has as many social selves as there are individuals who recognise him and carry an image of him in their mind" (p. 179).

The central tenet among theorists within the social framework is that the self-concept involves representations of interpersonal relationships, attachment, social roles, and situational contexts. In particular, the role of caregivers is seen as critical to the development of self-representations. Researchers have suggested that from about two years of age, the child begins to develop an appreciation of parental standards and reactions (Stipek, Recchia, & McClintic, 1992), and that in adolescence, the self-concept increasingly parallels the evaluations of the child's parents (Oosterwegel & Oppenheimer, 1993). Indeed, there is a growing body of evidence revealing that parental approval is critical in determining self-esteem of children. For instance, in reviews of such evidence, parental support in the form of approval and acceptance was found to be highly associated with high self-esteem in children and the sense that one is loveable (Feiring & Taska, 1996). Harter (2003) summarizes this finding, saying:

> … young children who experience their parents as sensitive to their needs and supportive of their mastery efforts will construct a model of self as lovable and competent. In contrast the young child who experiences the parent as rejecting or neglectful will form a model of self as unworthy. (p. 583)

Narrative theory

The self-concept as viewed through the perspective of narrative theory is a story about oneself (McAdams & McLean, 2013; Singer, 2004). From autobiographical memory, a person may construct and internalize an evolving story of their life. Narrative identity is a reconstruction of one's autobiographical past and future, thus creating a coherent account of identity. Through narrative identity, people convey to themselves and to others "who they are now, how they came to be and where they think their lives may be going in the future" (McAdams & McLean, 2013, p. 233). Narrative identity is believed to develop over time as people tell stories about their experiences to and with others. Over time, such stories transition from being accounts of past, current, or expected experiences to a broader and more integrative account of one's values, goals, and priorities that provide the self with a sense of unity and purpose. While initially selves create stories, over time stories create selves (McLean, Pasupathi, & Pals, 2007).

Theories of narrative identity suggest that people use scripts available in their culture for how to think of themselves. For example, when adolescents are asked to recall self-defining memories, their recounts follow familiar plot trajectories of athletic and academic triumphs and failures, relationship beginnings and ends and family disruptions and illness (Singer, 2004). Although such stories reflect personal experiences and insights, they are also informed by the available repertoire of narratives from their cultural context. Hence, it is purported that gender, class, race, ethnicity, sexual orientation, and other social and cultural factors are critical in shaping narrative identity.

The self-concept in research

A plethora of research has been conducted employing cognitive, social, and narrative paradigms of self. The self-concept has been considered important for informing research on psychopathology in two ways – first with reference to its content, and second with reference to its structure. The content of the self-concept refers to the types of beliefs and appraisals that one holds about one's traits, attributes, physical characteristics, and goals. The structure of the self-concept refers to the structural properties of the concept, such as its cohesion, consistency, and clarity. The two approaches are reviewed below, with examples of each in research on psychopathology.

The content of the self-concept

A dominant approach in research on the self-concept in psychopathology has been to investigate the relationship between beliefs about oneself and psychopathology. Research examining the role of self-esteem and beliefs about one's worth, lovability, and importance are exemplars of such an approach. For example, in research on depression, a body of research exists on the role of low self-esteem as not only an aspect of depression, but as also contributing to the onset, maintenance and recurrence of depressive episodes (Roberts & Monroe, 1994; Strauman & Kolden, 1997). In a series of retrospective and prospective surveys, Brown and colleagues demonstrated that chronic low self-esteem was statistically related to vulnerability for depressive episodes (G. W. Brown, Bifulco, Harris, & Bridge, 1986). These researchers found that low self-esteem preceded the onset of an initial depressive episode. In another prospective study, Zuroff, Igreja, and Mongrain (1990) found that after controlling for

initial levels of depression, self-criticism predicted depressive symptoms 12 months later.

Similarly, the notions of self-schema and core beliefs have been widely studied in relation to depression (Strauman & Kolden, 1997). Schemas such as "people who are close to me will disappoint me," "I will never be happy," and "I am not worthy of love" are said to be activated by critical adverse events (e.g., divorce, losing one's job, conflict), and to then exert significant influence on information processing by shaping the individual's expectations and appraisals about ongoing and future events (Strauman & Kolden, 1997). There has been substantial support for the relationship between negative self-schemas, information-processing biases and depressed mood (Segal & Muran, 1993). Research has also suggested that this relationship is reciprocal – that is, negative self-schemas became more elaborate and primed by negative mood states (Davis & Unruh, 1981).

Central to the cognitive model of anxiety disorders is the notion that the self is seen as vulnerable to danger. This model has failed to explicitly address the question of whether some types of self-views confer a specific vulnerability for certain types of anxiety disorders. However, some theorists have begun to identify important differences in self-perceived vulnerabilities across some anxiety disorders. For instance, Beck and Emery (1985) suggest that patients with generalized anxiety disorder view themselves as incompetent across a range of important domains and negatively evaluate their ability to cope with a range of problems and issues concerning finances, health, and relationships. In contrast, they propose that patients with panic disorder, agoraphobia, or social phobia have more restricted views about their vulnerabilities and inadequacies. The patient with panic disorder or agoraphobia is said to be specifically concerned about mental or physical collapse and therefore to construe themselves as "vulnerable to unpredictable and dangerous bodily sensations" (McNally, 1993, p. 84). In contrast, the socially anxious person is depicted as particularly uncertain about his or her acceptability, and sees himself or herself as lacking in resources to meet social demands (Clark & Wells, 1995; Hirsch, Clark, Mathews, & Williams, 2003).

A growing body of research has argued that adverse psychological outcomes following negative or traumatic events can be moderated through the construction of life stories and identities that emphasize redemption, agency, and communion. Individuals who are able construe negative events as leading to positive outcomes, who regard themselves as having high autonomy and control, or who view such events as leading to improved relationships with others, appear to have more resilient outcomes following physical illness, loss, and other hardships (Adler *et al.*, 2015). Similarly, researchers have found that individuals who are primed to think about their lives as unique (Bhar, 2014), or of themselves as having personal attributes useful for solving problems, feel less depressed and hopeless about the future (K. James & Bhar, in press).

Researchers have also begun to attend to the divide between implicit and explicit beliefs about self. Explicit self-beliefs are deliberate and conscious attitudes and representations about oneself, while implicit beliefs are those that occur automatically and are non-conscious. How is explicit self-concept related to implicit schemas about self? Markus and Kunda (1986) provide a framework that helps understand the relationship between implicit and explicit representations of self. They propose that an individual's explicit self-concept at any one time is the result of contextual characteristics (e.g., salient features of the individual's current activity, role, relationships), but also of one's repository of self-concepts. They suggest that the explicit self-concept reflects this repository of stored impressions about the self. Similarly, Guidano (1987) states "…the individual, at any moment and according to particular environmental influences, has a perceived identity that represents … (an) example of his/her range of possible self-images" (p. 86).

Researchers have argued that self-report measures are prone to social desirability biases, and thus are inaccurate devices for measuring how individuals really feel about themselves (Kernis, 2003). For instance, Wilkinson-Ryan and Westen (2000) say that "patients would likely have difficulty providing accurate information about their tendency to hold contradictory beliefs, their overabsorption in particular roles, and so forth" (p. 539). Likewise, Brinthaupt and Erwin (1992) consider that individuals with contradictory beliefs about self may be aware of only some of these beliefs. Hence, a variety of strategies, including word association tasks such as implicit association tasks (Greenwald, McGhee, & Schwartz, 1998), have been used to assess aspects of self-construal that are outside immediate conscious awareness.

Studies using such tasks have found that implicit self-concept may represent a premorbid vulnerability for psychopathology. For example, patients with unipolar and bipolar depression were found to be faster than healthy controls in attributing self-related concepts to depression-related words, suggesting enhanced automatic self-depressive associations (Glashouwer & De Jong, 2010; Jabben *et al.*, 2014). Such an effect was present not only when patients were symptomatic but also when in remission, suggesting that the underlying dysfunctional self-concept may confer vulnerability for further illness episodes. In addition, studies suggest that discordance between implicit and explicit self-concepts is associated with specific types of affective instability and psychopathology profiles. For example, individuals with high explicit self-esteem but low implicit self-esteem (fragile self-esteem pattern) have been linked to narcissistic behavior (Bosson, Swann, & Pennebaker, 2000) and persecutory beliefs (Valiente *et al.*, 2011). Conversely, the opposite pattern – that is, a combination of low explicit and high implicit self-esteem (damaged self-esteem pattern) – has been linked with maladaptive forms of perfectionism (Zeigler-Hill, 2006) and depressive symptoms, suicidal ideation, and loneliness (Creemers, Scholte, Engels, Prinstein, & Wiers, 2012).

The structure of the self-concept

The relationship between the organization of the self-concept and psychopathology has also been a topic of widespread research. Given that the self-concept has been viewed as a multidimensional construct, researchers have been interested in examining the extent to which the cohesion across dimensions, consistency of self-concept over time, and clarity of the construct inform psychopathology. Each structural aspect of the self-concept as applied in research is reviewed in turn.

First, the cohesion of self-structure has been studied in various ways, such as in its complexity, discrepancies, and ambivalence. Self-complexity (Linville, 1987) refers to the number of different and independent dimensions of the self-concept. It describes the number of one's self aspects (e.g., social roles, traits, goals), and the differentiation among them – that is, the extent to which one's appraisals of particular self-aspects do not "spill over" to other self-aspects (p. 664). An individual who is high in self-complexity is said to be more likely to have a wide range of roles in his or her repertoire, and thus, when negative feedback affects one of these self roles, he or she has a wide range of alternative roles to fall back on (Linville, 1987). In contrast, an individual who is low in self-complexity does not have this range of alternative roles available, and so experiences greater swings in affect. Many studies have demonstrated that individuals high in self-complexity are less prone to depression and illness following high levels of stress (Kalthoff & Neimeyer, 1993; Linville, 1987; Niedenthal, Setterlund, & Wherry, 1992). However, in some studies, support for the stress-buffering effect of self-complexity has been equivocal (Hershberger, 1990; Rafaeli-Mor & Steinberg, 2002; Solomon & Haaga, 2003).

Perhaps the best-known theory of discrepancies among views about self is the self-discrepancy theory (Higgins, Klein, & Strauman, 1985). According to this theory, people have various representations of themselves in terms of their actual self (how they currently are), their ideal self (how they would like to be), and their ought self (what they think they should be). Such discrepancies are said to trigger agitation and dejection-related emotions. The presence of such discrepancies can also motivate people to take constructive actions to reduce the discrepancies (Higgins, Strauman, & Klein, 1986). There is some support for the link between self-discrepancies and affective distress. For instance, researchers have found that the wider the discrepancy between different conceptions of self, the higher the level of distress (Higgins *et al.*, 1985; Higgins, Bond, Klein, & Strauman, 1986).

The lack of cohesion among self-views is also illustrated in concepts such as self-ambivalence (Bhar & Kyrios, 2007), contingent self-esteem (Crocker & Wolfe, 2001), and self-sensitivity (Doron, Moulding, Kyrios, & Nedeljkovic, 2008). Self-ambivalence refers to the extent to which the contents of an individual's self-concept are held with uncertainty, contested by conflicting self-knowledge, and constantly under scrutiny for accuracy (Bhar & Kyrios, 2007). As argued by Guidano and Liotti (1983), individuals who are ambivalent about their self-concept may not merely seek knowledge about the self, but rather are anxiously attentive to competing impressions of self. In such individuals, thoughts and behaviors are scanned for their potential to constitute threats to valued notions of self. Research has linked self-ambivalence to symptoms and beliefs associated with OCD (Bhar & Kyrios, 2007; Perera-Delcourt, Nash, & Thorpe, 2014; Tisher, Allen, & Crouch, 2014). Higher levels of ambivalence were predictive of higher levels of OCD severity and linked to the presence of OCD-related beliefs. Bhar and Kyrios found that self-ambivalence was significantly higher in individuals with OCD than in non-clinical groups. Further, changes in self-ambivalence during CBT were predictive of recovery status post treatment for patients with OCD (Bhar, Kyrios, & Hordern, in press). However, no difference was found in levels of ambivalence between an OCD cohort and anxiety disorder controls, suggesting that ambivalence may not constitute a unique vulnerability for, or characteristic of, OCD.

Acknowledging that the self-concept is a non-unitary construct, Crocker and Wolfe (2001) proposed that individuals vary in selecting domains (e.g., work, family, appearance, etc.) that they consider important for self-worth. According to this perspective, people differ in the criteria that must be satisfied to believe that they are a person of worth and to have high self-esteem. In a series of studies, Crocker and colleagues demonstrated support for this model. For example, Crocker, Luhtanen, and Sommers (2004) assessed daily fluctuations in self-esteem within a group of students applying for postgraduate courses. The researchers found that students who based their self-esteem on academic performance were more reactive to the outcomes of their applications than were those participants who did not regard academic performance as essential for self-esteem. Sargent, Crocker, and Luhtanen (2006) found that compared to those who based their self-esteem on internal qualities (e.g., virtue and religious faith), those who invested their self-esteem in in external contingencies (e.g., approval from others, accomplishments on competitive tasks, academic competence, and appearance) were more susceptible to external events, and thus at greater risk of developing depressive symptoms.

Expanding on the model of contingencies for self-worth, Doron *et al.* (2008) investigated the concept of self-sensitivity, which refers to the presence of self-domains that are considered important for self-worth, but in which one feels incompetent. They compared self-sensitivity of various self-domains across individuals with OCD, individuals with other anxiety disorders, and community controls. Sensitivity in moral domains was found to be associated with higher levels of OCD symptoms and to distinguish between the OCD cohort and the other samples, suggesting some specificity of relationships of self-sensitivity to OCD.

While much research has examined the role of consistency across facets of self-concept, other research has focused on the consistency of the concept over time. For example, numerous researchers have suggested that disturbances in the stability of self-views over time may account for psychopathology in a range of conditions such as anxiety disorders and personality disorders. For example, Clark and Wells (1995) suggest that individuals with social anxiety have extremely uncertain views of themselves, and therefore base their sense of self-worth on the reactions of other people. Other authors suggest that patients with posttraumatic stress disorder (PTSD) experience considerable distress because of irreconcilable images of self before and after trauma. McNally (1993) proposes that many of the symptoms in PTSD can be understood as the result of alterations to self-representations following traumatic experiences. In his view, encounters with trauma can destroy a person's illusion of self as secure and invulnerable to threat. He suggests that, following a traumatic incident, the person comes to see themselves as no longer immune to danger. This revision in self-view is purported to underscore many of the symptoms of PTSD such as fears of recurrence of the trauma, chronic anxiety, hypervigilance, and a sense of foreshortened future.

Disturbances in temporal consistency have also been implicated in borderline personality disorder (BPD). With respect to BPD, Westen and Cohen (1993) suggest that this disturbance refers to a range of problems in maintaining consistency in roles and self-representations. These problems include a lack of consistent goals, values, ideals, and relationships, the tendency to make temporary hyperinvestments in roles, value systems, world-views, and relationships that ultimately break down, a sense of emptiness and meaninglessness, and gross inconsistencies in behavior over time and across situations.

A third group of researchers has been primarily interested in the role of self-clarity or certainty in explaining psychopathology. For example, Campbell et al. (1996) coined the term self-clarity to represent the extent to which the contents of the self-concept are clearly and confidently defined, internally consistent and temporally stable. Individuals with poorly developed self views may be more likely than those with certain conceptions of self to make downward revisions of these views when failing to meet social or achievement standards (Pelham & Swann, 1989) and hence more vulnerable for psychopathology.

Conclusions

A wide range of models underpins the definitions of self-concept. Models drawn from early Western philosophical traditions, psychodynamic theory, cognitive theory, social theory, and narrative theory have converged to offer a definition of self-concept that is rich and multifaceted. The self-concept has been variously defined as perceptions, internal representations, mental schema, roles, and reconstructive stories. The beliefs about self as well as the structural aspect of self have been topics of research into depression, anxiety, and personality disorders. While most theorists have focused on the contents of self-concept as important for models of vulnerability, some have also implicated the structural features of the self-concept as central to vulnerability for psychopathology in general and with regard to specific disorders. The self-concept has remained a theoretically rich construct that is widely applied in research on psychopathology. The remainder of this book will cover issues relating to influences on the development of self, as well as examining a broad spectrum of disorders outlining the ways in which the self has been utilized to understand specific disorders and treatment processes.

References

Adler, J. M., Turner, A. F., Brookshier, K. M., et al. (2015). Variation in narrative identity is associated with trajectories of mental health over several years. *Journal of Personality and Social Psychology*, 108(3), 476–496. doi: 10.1037/a0038601

Ashmore, R. D., & Jussim, L. J. (1997). *Self and Identity: Fundamental Issues*. New York, NY: Oxford University Press.

Baumeister, R. (1998). The self. In D. Gilbert & S. Fiske (Eds.), *Handbook of Social Psychology* (pp. 680–740). Boston, MA: McGraw-Hill.

Beck, A., & Emery, G. (1985). *Anxiety Disorders and Phobias: A Cognitive Perspective*. New York, NY: Basic Books.

Bergson, H. (1975). *Creative Evolution*. Westport, CT: Greenwood.

Bhar, S. S. (2014). Reminiscence therapy: A review. In N. A. Pachana & K. Laidlaw (Eds.), *Oxford Handbook of Geropsychology* (pp. 675–690). Oxford: Oxford University Press.

Bhar, S. S., & Kyrios, M. (2007). An investigation of self-ambivalence in obsessive–compulsive disorder. *Behaviour Research and Therapy*, 45(8), 1845–1857.

Bhar, S. S., Kyrios, M., & Hordern, C. (in press). Self-ambivalence in the cognitive-behavioural treatment of obsessive–compulsive disorder. *Psychopathology*.

Bosson, J. K., Swann, W. B., Jr., & Pennebaker, J. W. (2000). Stalking the perfect measure of implicit self-esteem: The blind men and the elephant revisited? *Journal of Personality and Social Psychology*, 79(4), 631–643.

Brinthaupt, T. M., & Erwin, L. J. (1992). Reporting about the self: Issues and implications. In T. M. Brinthaupt & R. P. Lipka (Eds.), *The Self: Definitional and Methodological Issues* (pp. 137–171). Albany: State University of New York Press.

Brown, G. W., Bifulco, A., Harris, T., & Bridge, L. (1986). Life stress, chronic subclinical symptoms and vulnerability to clinical depression. *Journal of Affective Disorders*, 11(1), 1–19.

Brown, J. (1988). *The Self*. Boston, MA: McGraw Hill.

Campbell, J. D., Trapnell, P. D., Heine, S. J., *et al.* (1996). Self-concept clarity: Measurement, personality correlates, and cultural boundaries. *Journal of Personality and Social Psychology*, 70(1), 141–156.

Clark, D. M., & Wells, A. (1995). A cognitive model of social phobia. In R. G. Heimberg & M. R. Liebowitz (Eds.), *Social Phobia: Diagnosis, Assessment, and Treatment* (pp. 69–93). New York, NY: Guilford Press.

Cooley, C. H. (1902/1964). *Human Nature and the Social Order*. New York, NY: Schocken Books.

Creemers, D. H. M., Scholte, R. H. J., Engels, R. C. M. E., Prinstein, M. J., & Wiers, R. W. (2012). Implicit and explicit self-esteem as concurrent predictors of suicidal ideation, depressive symptoms, and loneliness. *Journal of Behavior Therapy and Experimental Psychiatry*, 43(1), 638–646. doi: 10.1016/j.jbtep.2011.09.006

Crocker, J., Luhtanen, R. K., & Sommers, S. R. (2004). Contingencies of self-worth: Progress and prospects. *European Review of Social Psychology*, 15, 133–181. doi: 10.1080/10463280440000017

Crocker, J., & Wolfe, C. T. (2001). Contingencies of self-worth. *Psychological Review*, 108(3), 593–623. doi: 10.1037//0033-295X.108.3.593

Davis, H., & Unruh, W. R. (1981). The development of the self-schema in adult depression. *Journal of Abnormal Psychology*, 90(2), 125–133.

Deaux, K. (1993). Reconstructing social identity. *Personality and Social Psychology*, 19(1), 3–12.

Descartes, R. (1967). *The Philososophical Works of Descartes* (Vol. 1). Cambridge: Cambridge University Press.

Doron, G., Moulding, R., Kyrios, M., & Nedeljkovic, M. (2008). Sensitivity of self-beliefs in obsessive compulsive disorder. *Depression and Anxiety*, 25(10), 874–884. doi: 10.1002/da.20369

Elliott, A. (2013). *Concepts of the Self* (3rd ed.). Hoboken, NJ; Wiley.

Epstein, S. (1973). The self concept revisited: Or a theory of a theory. *American Psychologist*, May, 404–414.

Feiring, C., & Taska, L. S. (1996). Family self-concept: Ideas on its meaning. In B. A. Bracken (Ed.), *Handbook of Self-concept: Developmental, Social, and Clinical Considerations* (pp. 317–373). Oxford: John Wiley & Sons.

Fiske, S. (1991). *Social Cognition*. New York, NY: McGraw Hill.

Freud, S. (1916). Introductory lectures on psychoanalysis. In J. Strachey (Ed.), *Standard Edition* (Vols. 15–16).

Glashouwer, K. A., & De Jong, P. J. (2010). Disorder-specific automatic self-associations in depression and anxiety: Results of the Netherlands study of depression and anxiety. *Psychological Medicine*, 40(7), 1101–1111. doi: 10.1017/S0033291709991371

Gray, P. (1994). *Psychology* (2nd ed.). New York, NY: North Publishers.

Greenwald, A. G., McGhee, D. E., & Schwartz, J. L. K. (1998). Measuring individual differences in implicit cognition: The implicit association test. *Journal of Personality and Social Psychology*, 74(6), 1464–1480.

Guidano, V. (1987). *Complexity of the Self*. New York, NY: The Guilford Press.

Guidano, V., & Liotti, G. (1983). *Cognitive Processes and Emotional Disorders*. New York, NY: Guilford Press.

Harter, S. (2003). The development of self-representations during childhood and adolescence. In M. R. Leary & J. P. Tangney (Eds.), *Handbook of Self and Identity* (pp. 610–642). New York, NY: Guilford Press.

Harter, S., & Whitesell, N. R. (2003). Beyond the debate: Why some adolescents report stable self-worth over time and situation, whereas others report changes in self-worth. *Journal of Personality*, 71(6), 1027–1058.

Hattie, J. (2014). *Self-Concept*. Hoboken, NJ: Taylor and Francis.

Hermans, H. J. (1987). Self as an organized system of valuations: Toward a dialogue with the person. *Journal of Counseling Psychology*, 34(1), 10–19.

Hershberger, P. J. (1990). Self-complexity and health promotion: Promising but premature. *Psychological Reports*, 66(3, Pt 2), 1207–1216.

Higgins, E. T., Bond, R. N., Klein, R., & Strauman, T. (1986). Self-discrepancies and emotional vulnerability: How magnitude, accessibility, and type of discrepancy influence affect. *Journal of Personality and Social Psychology*, 51(1), 5–15.

Higgins, E. T., Klein, R., & Strauman, T. (1985). Self-concept discrepancy theory: A psychological model for distinguishing among different aspects of depression and anxiety. *Social Cognition. Special Issue: Depression*, 3(1), 51–76.

Higgins, E. T., Strauman, T., & Klein, R. (1986). Standards and the process of self-evaluation: Multiple affects from multiple stages. In R. M. Sorrentino & E. T.

Higgins (Eds.), *Handbook of Motivation and Cognition: Foundations of Social Behavior* (pp. 23–63). New York, NY: Guilford Press.

Hirsch, C. R., Clark, D. M., Mathews, A., & Williams, R. (2003). Self-images play a causal role in social phobia. *Behaviour Research and Therapy*, 41(8), 909–921.

Hume, D. (2014). *A Treatise of Human Nature*. Lanham, MD: Lanham Start Classics.

Jabben, N., de Jong, P. J., Kupka, R. W., *et al.* (2014). Implicit and explicit self-associations in bipolar disorder: A comparison with healthy controls and unipolar depressive disorder. *Psychiatry Research*, 215(2), 329–334. doi: 10.1016/j.psychres.2013.11.030

James, K., & Bhar, S. S. (in press). Brief reminiscence intervention improves affect and pessimism in non-clinical individuals: A pilot study. *Clinical Psychologist*.

James, W. (1890). *The Principles of Psychology*. Oxford: Holt.

Kalthoff, R. A., & Neimeyer, R. A. (1993). Self-complexity and psychological distress: A test of the buffering model. *International Journal of Personal Construct Psychology*, 6(4), 327–349.

Kernis, M. H. (2003). Toward a conceptualization of optimal self-esteem. *Psychological Inquiry*, 14(1), 1–26.

Klein, M. (1977). *Envy and Gratitude and Other Works 1946–1963*. New York, NY: Dell Publishing Co.

Kohut, H. (1971). *The Analysis of Self. A Systematic Approach to the Psychoanalytic Treatment of Narcissistic Personality Disorders*. New York, NY: International Universities Press.

Kohut, H. (1977). *The Restoration of the Self*. New York, NY: International Universities Press.

Linville, P. W. (1987). Self-complexity as a cognitive buffer against stress-related illness and depression. *Journal of Personality and Social Psychology*, 52(4), 663–676.

Locke, J. (1960). *Essay Concerning Human Understanding*. Oxford: Clarendon.

MacDonald, M. R., & Kuiper, N. A. (1985). Efficiency and automaticity of self-schema processing in clinical depressives. *Motivation & Emotion*, 9(2), 171–184.

Markus, H. (1977). Self-schemata and processing information about the self. *Journal of Personality and Social Psychology*, 35(2), 63–78.

Markus, H. (1990). Unresolved issues of self-representation. *Cognitive Therapy and Research*, 14(2), 241–253.

Markus, H., & Kunda, Z. (1986). Stability and malleability of the self-concept. *Journal of Personality and Social Psychology*, 51(4), 858–866. doi: 10.1037/0022-3514.51.4.858

McAdams, D. P., & McLean, K. C. (2013). Narrative identity. *Current Directions in Psychological Science*, 22(3), 233–238. doi: 10.1177/0963721413475622

McLean, K. C., Pasupathi, M., & Pals, J. L. (2007). Selves creating stories creating Selves: A process model of self-development. *Personality and Social Psychology Review*, 11(3), 262–278. doi: 10.1177/1088868307301034

McNally, R. J. (1993). Self-representation in post-traumatic stress disorder: A cognitive perspective. In Z. V. Segal & S. J. Blatt (Eds.), *The Self in Emotional Distress: Cognitive and Psychodynamic Perspectives* (pp. 71–99). New York, NY: Guilford Press.

Mead, G. H. (1934). *Mind, Self and Society: From the Standpoint of a Social Behaviorist* (Ed. with intro by C. W. Morris.). Chicago, IL: University of Chicago Press.

Mill, J. (1869). *Analysis of the Phenomena of the Human Mind*. London: Longmans.

Niedenthal, P., Setterlund, M., & Wherry, M. (1992). Possible self complexity and affective reactions to goal-relevant evaluation. *Journal of Personality and Social Psychology*, 63(1), 5–16.

Oosterwegel, A., & Oppenheimer, L. (1993). *The Self-system: Developmental Changes Between and Within Self-concepts*. Hillsdale, NJ: Lawrence Erlbaum Associates, Inc.

Pelham, B. & Swann, W. (1989). From self conceptions to self-worth: On the sources and structure of global self-esteem. *Journal of Personality and Social Psychology*, 57, 672–680.

Perera-Delcourt, R., Nash, R. A., & Thorpe, S. J. (2014). Priming moral self-ambivalence heightens deliberative behaviour in self-ambivalent individuals. *Behavioural and Cognitive Psychotherapy*, 42(6), 682–692. doi: 10.1017/S1352465813000507

Rafaeli-Mor, E., & Steinberg, J. (2002). Self-complexity and well-being: A review and research synthesis. *Personality and Social Psychology Review*, 6(1), 31–58.

Roberts, J. E., & Monroe, S. M. (1994). A multidimensional model of self-esteem in depression. *Clinical Psychology Review*, 14(3), 161–181.

Rogers, C. R. (1961). *On Becoming a Person*. Boston, MA: Houghton Mifflin

Safran, J., Segal, Z., Hill, C., & Whiffen, V. (1990). Refining strategies for research on self-representations in emotional disorders. *Cognitive Therapy and Research*, 14(2), 143–160.

Sargent, J. T., Crocker, J., & Luhtanen, R. K. (2006). Contingencies of self-worth and depressive symptoms in college students. *Journal of Social and Clinical Psychology*, 25(6), 628–646.

Schlenker, B. R. (1980). *Impression Management*. Pacific Grove, CA: Brooks/Cole.

Segal, Z. V., & Muran, J. C. (1993). A cognitive perspective on self-representation in depression. In Z. V. Segal &

S. J. Blatt (Eds.), *The Self in Emotional Distress: Cognitive and Psychodynamic Perspectives* (pp. 131–170). New York, NY: Guilford Press.

Sherif, M. (1967). *Social Interaction: Process and Products*. Oxford: Aldine.

Singer, J. A. (2004). Narrative identity and meaning making across the adult lifespan: An introduction. *Journal of Personality*, 72(3), 437–460. doi: 10.1111/j.0022-3506.2004.00268.x

Solomon, A., & Haaga, D. A. F. (2003). Reconsideration of self-complexity as a buffer against depression. *Cognitive Therapy and Research*, 27(5), 579–591.

Spencer, H. (1963). *Education: Intellectual, Moral and Physical*. Patterson, NJ: Littelfield.

Stipek, D., Recchia, S., & McClintic, S. (1992). Self-evaluation in young children. *Monographs of the Society for Research in Child Development*, 57(1), 100.

Strauman, T., & Kolden, G. (1997). The self in depression: Research trends and clinical implications. *In Session: Psychotherapy in Practice*, 3(3), 5–21.

Swann, W. B., Wenzlaff, R. M., Krull, D. S., & Pelham, B. W. (1992). Allure of negative feedback: Self-verification strivings among depressed persons. *Journal of Abnormal Psychology*, 101(2), 293–306.

Taylor, J., & Boggiano, A. K. (1987). The effects of task-specific self-schemata on attributions for success and failure. *Journal of Research in Personality*, 21(3), 375–388.

Tesser, A., Stapel, D., & Wood, J. (2002). Preface. In A. Tesser, D. Stapel & J. Wood (Eds.), *Self and Motivation: Emerging Psychological Perspectives* (pp. ix–x). Washington, DC: American Psychological Association.

Tisher, R., Allen, J. S., & Crouch, W. (2014). The self-ambivalence measure: A psychometric investigation. *Australian Journal of Psychology*, 66(3), 197–206. doi: 10.1111/ajpy.12046

Valiente, C., Cantero, D., Vázquez, C., *et al.* (2011). Implicit and explicit self-esteem discrepancies in paranoia and depression. *Journal of Abnormal Psychology*, 120(3), 691–699. doi: 10.1037/a0022856

Watson, A. (2014). Who am I? The self/subject according to psychoanalytic theory. *SAGE Open*, 4(3). doi: 10.1177/2158244014545971

Westen, D. (1992). The cognitive self and the psychoanalytic self: Can we put our selves together? *Psychological Inquiry*, 3(1), 1–13.

Westen, D., & Cohen, R. (1993). The self in borderline personality disorder: A psychodynamic perspective. In Z. Segal & S. Blatt (Eds.), *The Self in Emotional Distress: Cognitive and Psychodynamic Perspectives* (pp. 334–360).

Wilkinson-Ryan, T., & Westen, D. (2000). Identity disturbance in borderline personality disorder: An empirical investigation. *American Journal of Psychiatry*, 157(4), 528–541.

Zeigler-Hill, V. (2006). Discrepancies between implicit and explicit self-esteem: Implications for narcissism and self-esteem instability. *Journal of Personality*, 74(1), 119–143. doi: 10.1111/j.1467-6494.2005.00371.x

Zuroff, D. C., Igreja, I., & Mongrain, M. (1990). Dysfunctional attitudes, dependency, and self-criticism as predictors of depressive mood states: A 12-month longitudinal study. *Cognitive Therapy and Research*, 14(3), 315–326.

Chapter 3

Adult attachment and self-related processes

Mario Mikulincer and Guy Doron

Attachment theory (Bowlby, 1973, 1980, 1982) has become one of the leading approaches to conceptualizing interpersonal cognitions and behaviors, social adjustment, and mental health. In this chapter we explore the relevance of attachment theory for understanding individual differences in mental representations of the self, and we propose specific attachment-relevant cognitive and behavioral mechanisms that can explain these differences. We begin with a brief summary of attachment theory and an account of the two major dimensions of adult attachment orientations, attachment anxiety, and avoidance. We then propose a theoretical framework for understanding how attachment experiences and the resulting attachment orientations can shape the ways people regard their selves. Next we review studies of the ways in which attachment orientations contribute to a person's self-perceptions, self-evaluation, and other self-related processes during adolescence and adulthood.

Basic concepts of attachment theory and research

One of the core tenets of attachment theory (Bowlby, 1973, 1980, 1982) is that human beings are born with a psychobiological system (the *attachment behavioral system*) that motivates them to seek proximity to significant others (*attachment figures*) in times of need. According to Bowlby (1982), the goal of this system is to maintain adequate protection and support, which is accompanied by a subjective sense of safety and security. This goal is made salient when people encounter actual or symbolic threats and notice that an attachment figure is not sufficiently near, interested, or responsive (Bowlby, 1982). In such cases, a person's attachment system is upregulated and the person is motivated to increase or re-establish proximity to an attachment figure so that a sense of security is attained. Bowlby (1988) assumed that, although age and development increase a person's ability to gain comfort from internal, symbolic representations of attachment figures, no one at any age is completely free from reliance on actual others.

Bowlby (1973) devoted a great deal of attention to individual differences in attachment-system functioning that arise as a result of the availability, responsiveness, and supportiveness of a person's key attachment figures, especially in times of need. Interactions with attachment figures who are available, sensitive, and supportive in times of need promote a sense of connectedness and security and strengthen positive mental representations (*working models*) of self and others. In contrast, when attachment figures are not reliably available and supportive, a sense of security is not attained, worries about one's social value and others' intentions become ingrained, and strategies of affect regulation other than proximity-seeking are developed (*secondary attachment strategies*, characterized by *anxiety* and *avoidance*).

When studying individual differences in attachment-system functioning in adults, attachment research has focused primarily on *attachment orientations* (or *styles*) – patterns of relational expectations, emotions, and behaviors that result from internalizing a particular history of attachment experiences (Mikulincer & Shaver, 2007). Research, beginning with Ainsworth, Blehar, Waters, and Wall (1978) and continuing through scores of recent studies by social and personality psychologists (reviewed by Mikulincer & Shaver, 2007), indicates that attachment

The Self in Understanding and Treating Psychological Disorders, ed. Michael Kyrios, Richard Moulding, Guy Doron, Sunil S. Bhar, Maja Nedeljkovic, and Mario Mikulincer. Published by Cambridge University Press. © Cambridge University Press, 2016.

styles are conceptually located in a two-dimensional space defined by two roughly orthogonal dimensions, attachment anxiety and attachment-related avoidance (Brennan, Clark, & Shaver, 1998). The avoidance dimension reflects the extent to which a person distrusts relationship partners' good will and defensively strives to maintain behavioral independence and emotional distance. The anxiety dimension reflects the extent to which a person worries that a partner will not be available in times of need, partly because of the person's self-doubts about his or her own love-worthiness. A person's location in the two-dimensional space can be measured with reliable and valid self-report scales (e.g., the Experiences in Close Relationships scale, or ECR; Brennan et al., 1998), and this location is associated in theoretically predictable ways with a wide variety of measures of relationship quality and psychological adjustment.

Mikulincer and Shaver (2007) proposed that a person's location in the two-dimensional anxiety-by-avoidance space reflects both his or her sense of attachment security and the ways in which he or she deals with threats and stressors. People who score low on these dimensions are generally secure, hold positive working models of self and others, and tend to employ constructive and effective affect-regulation strategies. Those who score high on either attachment anxiety or avoidance, or both (a condition called fearful avoidance), suffer from attachment insecurities, self-related worries, and distrust of others' goodwill and responsiveness in times of need. Moreover, such insecure people tend to use secondary attachment strategies, which Mikulincer and Shaver (2007) conceptualize as attachment-system "hyperactivating" or "deactivating" to cope with threats, frustrations, rejections, and losses.

People who score high on attachment anxiety rely on hyperactivating strategies – energetic attempts to achieve support and love combined with a lack of confidence that these resources will be provided and with feelings of anger and despair when they are not provided (Cassidy & Kobak, 1988). These reactions occur in relationships in which an attachment figure is sometimes responsive but unreliably so, placing the needy person on a partial reinforcement schedule that rewards exaggeration and persistence in proximity-seeking attempts because these efforts sometimes succeed. In contrast, people who score high on attachment-related avoidance tend to use deactivating strategies: trying not to seek proximity to others

when threatened, denying vulnerability and the need for other people, and avoiding closeness and interdependence in relationships. These strategies develop in relationships with attachment figures that disapprove of and punish frequent expressions of need and bids for closeness (Ainsworth et al., 1978).

Both anxious hyperactivation and avoidant deactivation are defenses against the psychological pain induced by the unresponsiveness of attachment figures (Mikulincer & Shaver, 2007). Although these strategies are initially adaptive, in the sense that they adjust a child's behavior to the requirements of an inconsistently available, or consistently distant, attachment figure, they prove maladaptive when used in later relationships where proximity-seeking and collaborative interdependence could be productive and rewarding. They also foster the continued use of non-optimal affect-regulation strategies that interfere with psychological adjustment and mental health (Ein-Dor & Doron, 2015). Hundreds of studies, summarized in Mikulincer and Shaver (2007) and substantiated by ongoing research, confirm that attachment insecurities place a person at risk for emotional difficulties and psychopathology including depression (e.g., Catanzaro & Wei, 2010), general anxiety disorder (e.g., Marganska, Gallagher, & Miranda, 2013), obsessive–compulsive disorder (e.g., Doron et al., 2012), posttraumatic stress disorder (e.g., Ein-Dor, Doron, Solomon, Mikulincer, & Shaver, 2010), eating disorders (e.g., Illing, Tasca, Balfour, & Bissada, 2010), and suicide ideation (e.g., Davaji, Valizadeh, & Nikamal, 2010). In the following section, we review evidence concerning the detrimental effects that attachment insecurities have on a person's mental representations of the self.

Attachment and self-representations

In our model of the attachment behavioral system in adulthood, repeated interactions with available, sensitive, and supportive attachment figures result in positive representations of oneself as worthy and competent. During such positive interactions, people find it easy to perceive themselves as valuable and loveable thanks to being valued and loved by responsive others. Moreover, they learn to view themselves as active, strong, and competent because they can effectively mobilize others' support and manage distress. In this way, interactions with responsive attachment figures become natural building blocks of what Rogers (1961) called the "real self." These building blocks are genuine, non-defensive, positive self-perceptions derived from one's own accomplishments and from receipt of others' love and encouragement.

Attachment research on infants indicates that interactions with responsive attachment figures and the resulting sense of attachment security during the first years of life allows children to distance themselves more easily from attachment figures to explore the world and learn about both it and themselves. This kind of learning enriches competencies and strengthens self-regulatory skills, allowing secure children to do things on their own without continuous help from others (see Thompson, 2008, for a review). In middle childhood, the sense of attachment security allows children to engage effectively in affiliative play with peers (Zeifman & Hazan, 2008), which provides an increasing range of social options for developing skills and broadening one's sense of self-worth and efficacy. During adolescence and adulthood, secure individuals are able to form reciprocal and mutually satisfying couple relationships, relationships in which they provide comfort to their partners, as well as receiving support, and act as co-regulators of their own and their partners' occasional distress (see Mikulincer & Shaver, 2015, for a review). These abilities strengthen a secure person's sense of value and mastery and bolster confidence in being able to form satisfying relationships and provide comfort to others when needed.

According to Mikulincer and Shaver (2004), the link between secure attachment and positive self-representations is also sustained by including attachment figures' traits and capacities within mental representations of self. Through identification with sensitive and responsive attachment figures, a child develops implicit beliefs that he or she embodies the goodness, strength, and wisdom of what Bowlby (1982) called "stronger and wiser" others. Moreover, a well-treated child internalizes the soothing, approving, encouraging, and coaching functions originally performed by a responsive attachment figure into his or her own self representations. As a result, people become sensitive and responsive to their own selves and take a caring, loving, and accepting attitude toward themselves in the same way attachment figures treated them. Moreover, they can be relatively immune to harsh self-criticism and they can retain a sense of self-worth while recognizing their normal weaknesses, and shortcomings. This is partly a matter of internal composure and ability to soothe oneself,

but it is sustained by expectations that others will value and accept oneself even if one makes mistakes or has faults. On this basis, Mikulincer and Shaver (2004) contended that attachment security facilitates what Kohut (1984) called "healthy narcissism," which allows a person to establish a cohesive and comfortable self-structure.

Mikulincer and Shaver (2004) also suggested that a lack of attachment figures' responsiveness contributes to disorders of the self, characterized by a lack of self-cohesion, doubts about one's coherence and continuity over time, and vulnerable or unstable self-esteem. This is the condition of insecurely attached people, whose frustrating, frightening, and disappointing interactions with unavailable and rejecting attachment figures raised doubts about the degree to which one is esteemed and loved by others. During negative interactions with attachment figures, insecure people gradually incorporate degrading and disapproving messages, making it likely that they will regard and treat themselves with disapproval and disdain. Thus, insecure people are likely to suffer from self-criticism and painful self-doubts, or erect distorting defenses to counter feelings of worthlessness and hopelessness.

Although both anxious and avoidant people have difficulty constructing an authentic, positive, and stable sense of self-worth, their reliance on different secondary attachment strategies can result in different self-configurations (Mikulincer & Shaver, 2004). Attachment-anxious people, who hope to gain a partner's love and approval, tend to take some of the blame for a partner's unreliable care and to ruminate about why they are so worthless that others don't want to provide the love and approval they need. These thought processes reinforce negative self-representations and doubts about one's social value. Attachment-system activation also interferes with the construction of a sense of self-efficacy. Anxiously attached people prefer to rely on their partner rather than engage in challenging activities alone, thereby preventing them from exploring and learning new information and skills. In addition, deliberate attempts to gain an attachment figure's love and care can reinforce a negative self-image, because anxious people often present themselves in incompetent, childish, or excessively needy ways in an effort to elicit others' compassion, sympathy, and help.

In the case of avoidant people, Mikulincer and Shaver (2004) proposed that they attempt to prop up their self-image through unconscious defenses and narcissistic behavior (defensive self-enhancement). Avoidant people's defensive efforts to dismiss attachment needs are accompanied by attempts to deny vulnerability, negative self-aspects, and memories of personal failures while trying to focus on and display traits and feelings compatible with their need for self-reliance. Avoidant people often entertain fantasies of perfection and power, exaggerate their achievements and talents, and avoid situations that challenge their defenses and threaten their grandiosity. They can become quite annoyed, however, when someone asks them to alter their behavior, be more considerate, soften their defenses, or admit their mistakes.

With these theoretical ideas in mind, in the next sections we review empirical evidence on attachment-style differences in feelings of self-worth and self-competence and defensive self-enhancement, as well as the psychological processes that sustain the link between attachment insecurities and people's self-related vulnerabilities.

Attachment-related differences in self-esteem and perceived self-competence

In support of attachment theory, dozens of studies have found that attachment anxiety is associated with lower self-esteem (e.g., Felton & Jowett, 2013; Lee & Hankin, 2009; McWilliams & Holmberg, 2010). For example, in a study conducted in 53 nations, Schmitt and Allik (2005) found a significant negative association between attachment anxiety and self-esteem in 49 countries. With regard to avoidant attachment, the findings are less consistent and about half of the studies have found a significant negative association with self-esteem. Although attachment theory does not necessarily predict self-esteem deficits in avoidant individuals, because of their defensive tendency to exclude thoughts of vulnerability and deficiency from consciousness, research suggests that these defenses are not always successful in preventing self-doubts and mental pain. In fact, Schmitt and Allik (2005) found a significant negative association between avoidance and self-esteem in 18 of the 53 countries they sampled.

In order to overcome the limitations of explicit self-report measures of self-esteem, Dewitte, De Houwer, and Buysse (2008) examined associations between attachment orientations and an implicit measure of self-esteem – the Implicit Association Test (IAT; Greenwald, McGhee, & Schwartz, 1998). Findings revealed that more anxiously attached individuals had less positive implicit self-concepts on the IAT. In contrast, attachment-related avoidance was not significantly associated with implicit self-concept.

Several studies examined correlations between attachment measures and scales measuring self-efficacy (e.g., Caldwell, Shaver, & Minzenberg, 2011; Jenkins-Guarnieri, Wright, & Hudiburgh, 2012; Wei & Ku, 2007). The results show that attachment anxiety is associated with more negative evaluations of competence across all life domains studied and that avoidant attachment is associated with more negative evaluations only in social and interpersonal domains but not in non-social domains. Similar findings have been reported in longitudinal, prospective studies (e.g., Doyle & Markiewicz, 2009; Lopez & Gormley, 2002). For example, Doyle and Markiewicz (2009) found that avoidant attachment with fathers as assessed in early adolescence predicted lower self-perceived peer competence two years later.

Defensive self-enhancement

According to attachment theory, defensive self-enhancement is a core characteristic of avoidant attachment. More specifically, avoidant people's self-reliance and reluctance to rely on other people encourages them to inflate their positive self-views and deny or suppress negative information about themselves (Mikulincer & Shaver, 2007). In support of this view, Gjerde, Onishi, and Carlson (2004) found that avoidant people's descriptions of their traits were more favorable than descriptions provided by trained observers. Moreover, Dentale, Vecchione, De Coro, and Barbaranelli (2012) found that avoidant attachment was associated with higher levels of implicit–explicit self-esteem discordance. That is, the higher the avoidance, the higher the positivity bias of explicit self-esteem (as assessed in a self-report scale) in comparison to an implicit measure of self-esteem (IAT). Mikulincer (1995) also found clear-cut signs of defensive organizations of self-traits: avoidant individuals had quick access to positive but not negative self-attributes and their different self-aspects were poorly integrated.

There is also evidence that avoidant people react to threatening events with defensive self-inflation (Mikulincer, 1998; Hart, Shaver, & Goldenberg,

2005). In these studies, participants scoring higher in avoidant attachment appraised themselves more positively (in both explicit and implicit measures of self-esteem) following a threatening as compared with a neutral context. Interestingly, secure individuals' self-appraisals did not differ much across neutral and threatening conditions. That is, secure people made relatively stable and unbiased self-appraisals even when coping with threats. Mikulincer (1998) also found, using procedures that discourage defensive self-enhancement (a "bogus pipeline" device that purportedly measures "true feelings about things" or the presence of a knowledgeable friend), that surveillance diminished avoidant individuals' otherwise positively distorted self-views under threatening conditions. In addition, Mikulincer (1998) found that avoidant individuals' tendency to report more positive self-views under threatening conditions was inhibited by a message that broke the link between a positive self-view and self-reliance. This finding implies that avoidant people's positive self-appraisals are strategic attempts to convince others of their admirable (and perhaps enviable) qualities.

Two experimental studies have shown that a contextual priming of attachment security tends to reduce activation of defensive self-inflation maneuvers (Arndt, Schimel, Greenberg, & Pyszczynski, 2002; Schimel, Arndt, Pyszczynski, & Greenberg, 2001). In these studies, participants were asked to think about attachment-figure availability (e.g., thinking about an accepting and loving other) or neutral topics, and their use of particular self-enhancement strategies was assessed. Schimel et al. (2001) assessed defensive biases in social comparison – searching for more social-comparison information when it was likely to suggest that one has performed better than other people. Arndt et al. (2002) assessed defensive self-handicapping – emphasizing factors that impair one's performance in an effort to protect against the damage to self-esteem that might result from attributing negative outcomes to one's lack of ability. In both studies, momentary strengthening of mental representations of attachment-figure availability weakened the tendency to make self-enhancing social comparisons or self-handicapping attributions.

Along similar lines, Kumashiro and Sedikides (2005) asked participants to perform a difficult cognitive task and then asked them to visualize either a responsive close friend or a distant or negative partner. Following the priming procedure, all participants received negative feedback about their performance and were asked about their interest in obtaining further information about the task and the underlying cognitive ability it tapped. Findings indicated that participants who were primed with a responsive close relationship partner expressed more interest in receiving information about their newly discovered liability than participants in other conditions. That is, being infused with a sense of security, participants seemed to be so confident of their self-worth that they were willing to explore and learn about potential personal weaknesses.

In all of the above studies, anxiously attached individuals failed to exhibit defensive self-enhancement. Rather, they tended to suffer from negative self-views and to exaggerate their already negative self-appraisals. Mikulincer (1995) also found that attachment-anxious people had ready mental access to negative self-attributes, and exhibited pervasive negative affect when sorting through these attributes. Moreover, anxiously attached people tended to make more negative self-appraisals in threatening as compared with neutral conditions (Mikulincer, 1998). Interestingly, this tendency was reduced by a message that broke the likely connection between self-devaluation and others' supportive responses (Mikulincer, 1998), implying that anxious people devalue themselves overtly at least partly to gain other people's approval and compassion. Such self-devaluation has also been noted in anxiously attached people's admittedly self-derogating, Woody Allen-like forms of humor (Kazarian & Martin, 2004; Saroglou & Scariot, 2002).

These attachment-related biases in self-perceptions, either positive or negative, tend to fuel pathological forms of narcissism (e.g., Dickinson & Pincus, 2003). In particular, avoidance is thought to contribute to *overt* narcissism or grandiosity, which includes both self-praise and denial of weaknesses. Attachment anxiety, in contrast, seems to contribute to *covert* narcissism, which is characterized by self-focused attention, hypersensitivity to other people's evaluation of oneself, and a sense of entitlement. Indeed, Rothman and Steil (2012), and Tolmacz and Mikulincer (2011) found that both attachment anxiety and avoidance were positively associated with a global sense of psychological entitlement as well as strong entitlement urges in close relationships. In addition, Rohmann, Neumann, Herner, and Bierhoff (2012) found associations between avoidant attachment and measures of overt, grandiose narcissism and between anxious attachment and measures of covert, vulnerable narcissism.

Psychological processes that sustain insecure people's self-related vulnerabilities

Adult attachment researchers have identified psychological processes that sustain and exacerbate insecure people's self-related vulnerabilities. Studies have focused on insecure people's interpretations of negative life events, their search for negative information about themselves, their reliance on unstable, external sources of self-worth, and their tendency to suffer from painful self-criticism and perfectionism. These processes, in turn, have been lined with increase vulnerability to psychopathology such as depression (e.g., Wei, Heppner, Russell, & Young, 2006) and OCD (e.g., Doron, Moulding, Kyrios, Nedeljkovic & Mikulincer, 2009). In the following sections we review evidence concerning attachment-related variations in these self-destructive processes.

Hopeless cognitive style

Attachment researchers have shown that attachment anxiety is associated with a hopeless cognitive style – taking responsibility for achievement-related failures and interpersonal rejections and attributing these unpleasant experiences to a stable lack of ability, skill, or personal value (e.g., Gamble & Roberts, 2005; Sumer & Cozzarelli, 2004; Wei & Ku, 2007). With regard to avoidant attachment, some studies have found that avoidant individuals also display a "hopeless" cognitive style (e.g., Gamble & Roberts, 2005; Sumer & Cozzarelli, 2004), but other studies have found that avoidant people display a more defensive pattern of attributions (Man & Hamid, 1998).

Patterns of feedback-seeking

According to attachment theory, anxiously attached people's core sense of unlovability and weakness may lead them to seek confirmatory negative information about themselves (Mikulincer & Shaver, 2004). Such negative feedback, although offering the solace of belief validation, is still a cause of mental pain and suffering and can aggravate doubts about self-worth and self-competence. In support of this view, several studies have found that more anxiously attached people are more likely to seek for negative feedback from the relationship partner (e.g., Brennan & Morris, 1997; Cassidy, Ziv, Mehta, & Feeney, 2003; Hepper & Carnelley, 2010). These studies have also found

that avoidant attachment was associated with preference for negative feedback. It is possible that avoidant people may be less certain about their positive self-views, and this uncertainty may inhibit the search for self-verifying feedback. This explanation fits well with the findings we reviewed earlier indicating that avoidant individuals' self-representations lack clarity, coherence, and integration.

Bases of self-esteem

According to attachment theory, anxiously attached people tend to perceive partners as their major source of value and esteem rather than rooting self-worth on inner standards of value and competence (Mikulincer & Shaver, 2007). This stance causes them to become dependent on continual validation from relationship partners and overly susceptible to a partner's reactions. As a result, they are unable to maintain a stable sense of self-esteem, because relationship partners cannot always be ideal attachment figures. Moreover, even minimal signs of a partner's disapproval, criticism, or disinterest can remind anxious people of their worthlessness, thereby validating and strengthening their low self-esteem.

There is correlational evidence that anxious people's self-worth is especially dependent on others' approval and love (e.g., Cheng & Kwan, 2008; Knee, Canevello, Bush, & Cook, 2008; Park, Crocker, & Mickelson, 2004). In contrast, more avoidant individuals are less dependent on interpersonal sources of self-esteem (e.g., Park et al., 2004). In fact, avoidant people tend to care more about their general public image than about close relationship partners' approval of them (e.g., Cheng & Kwan, 2008; Schachner & Shaver, 2004). Anxious people's tendency to derive self-worth from others' reactions has been further documented in naturalistic and experimental settings (e.g., Broemer & Blumle, 2003; Carnelley, Israel, and Brennan, 2007; Srivastava & Beer, 2006).

Further evidence of the overdependence of anxious people on others' approval as a source of self-worth was provided by diary studies that examined the impact of different kinds of real-life, transient feedback on state self-esteem. For example, Hepper and Carnelley (2012) conducted a 14-day diary study and found that the daily self-esteem of more anxiously attached participants fluctuated more with daily interpersonal feedback conveying a romantic partner's rejection or approval. Similarly,

Foster, Kernis, and Goldman (2007) found positive associations between attachment anxiety and higher fluctuations in appraisals of self that were assessed twice daily for one week. These fluctuations were associated with high responsiveness to momentary signs of others' rejection and approval. This kind of "rollercoaster-like" experience is also manifested in the extent to which a person's sense of self is malleable in relational contexts. For example, Slotter and Gardner (2012) found that attachment anxiety was associated with participants' appraisals of self being more malleable in the context of romantic relationships and being more susceptible to change and confusion during and after relationship termination. Doron, Szepsenwol, Karp, and Gal (2013) found attachment anxiety coinciding with relationship-contingent self worth increased vulnerability to relationship obsessions.

Self-standards, self-criticism, and perfectionism

Adult attachment researchers have considered the negative effects that self-criticism and highly demanding self-standards have on insecure people's self-representations. Self-criticism and demanding self standards can come about through two interrelated processes. First, insecure people can incorporate their attachment figures' negative qualities into their own self-representations and then evaluate and treat themselves in the same critical and disapproving manner in which they were treated by inadequate attachment figures. Second, they can set overly demanding, unrealistic self-standards and strive for perfection as a way of coping with their insecurity. Whereas anxious people's hyperactivating strategies can motivate them to be "perfect" and to pursue high self-ideals to gain others' love and esteem, avoidant people's deactivating strategies can incline them toward perfectionism as a way to hide imperfections, self-enhance, and justify self-reliance. In support of this view, several studies have found positive associations between higher scores in anxious or avoidant attachment and self-criticism (e.g., Davila, 2001; Wiseman, Mayseless, & Sharabany, 2005; Zuroff & Fitzpatrick, 1995). Neff and McGehee (2010) also found that both forms of attachment insecurity interfere with self-compassion – another sign of a critical attitude toward oneself.

There is also evidence linking attachment anxiety and avoidance to measures of maladaptive perfectionism (e.g., Gamble & Roberts, 2005; Gnilka, Ashby, & Noble, 2013; Ulu & Tezer, 2010). Furthermore, Chen et al. (2012) found that more securely attached adolescents were less likely to be focused on actively promoting their supposed "perfection" and did not have problems in revealing their perceived imperfections. In contrast, more avoidant adolescents scored higher on the tendency to avoid disclosing imperfections.

Concluding remarks

The reviewed findings clearly show that for both anxious and avoidant people, a history of painful and frustrating interactions with unavailable, cold, or rejecting attachment figures interferes with the formation of a solid, stable sense of personal esteem. Anxious people's desire to gain a partner's love, esteem, and protection keeps them from "owning" their anger toward this person and causes them to take responsibility for the frustration and pain, thereby reinforcing their sense of worthlessness and weakness. This negative self-view is then sustained and aggravated by a hopeless cognitive style, openness to negative information about the self, reliance on others' approval as a source of self-worth, self-criticism, and adoption of unrealistic high self-standards. These processes also encourage attachment-system hyperactivation, because a helpless person cannot live without constant care, love, and protection provided by other people. This is a self-exacerbating cycle in which attachment-system hyperactivation and lack of self-esteem contribute to covert narcissism.

Avoidant people's commitment to self-reliance leads them to push negative self-representations out of awareness and defensively inflate their self-image. As a result, they often report high levels of explicit self-esteem and describe themselves in positive terms. However, their positive models of self seem to be less stable and authentic than the positive self-representations of secure individuals. Avoidant people's self-enhancement is accompanied by unrealistically high self-standards, which leads to reliance on external sources of validation combined with self-criticism, perfectionism, and a renewal of self-doubts. These dynamic processes create a self-exacerbating cycle in which self-criticism and defensive self-inflation contribute to grandiose narcissism.

In the present chapter we have attempted to show how attachment theory characterizes and explains individual variations in representations of the self. Future research should attempt to examine the interplay of attachment insecurities and other developmental sources of self-esteem (e.g., failure in achievement settings) in promoting poor or distorted self-esteem. More systematic studies should be conducted attempting to understand how attachment injuries and resulting distortions in self-representations contribute to personality disorders and other forms of psychopathology. Longitudinal research should also examine how the link between attachment security and self-esteem emerges from understandable developmental processes and the familial context. Finally, research should also attempt to examine the ways by which attachment security can protect a person from injuries to the self and how attachment-related processes in clinical or counseling settings can contribute to the healing of these injuries.

References

Ainsworth, M. D. S., Blehar, M. C., Waters, E., & Wall, S. (1978). *Patterns of Attachment: Assessed in the Strange Situation and At Home.* Hillsdale, NJ: Erlbaum.

Arndt, J., Schimel, J., Greenberg, J., & Pyszczynski, T. (2002). The intrinsic self and defensiveness: Evidence that activating the intrinsic self reduces self-handicapping and conformity. *Personality and Social Psychology Bulletin, 28,* 671–683.

Bowlby, J. (1973). *Attachment and Loss: Vol. 2. Separation: Anxiety and Anger.* New York, NY: Basic Books.

Bowlby, J. (1980). *Attachment and Loss: Vol. 3. Sadness and Depression.* New York, NY: Basic Books.

Bowlby, J. (1982). *Attachment and Loss: Vol. 1. Attachment* (2nd ed.). New York, NY: Basic Books. (Orig. ed. 1969.)

Bowlby, J. (1988). *A Secure Base: Clinical Applications of Attachment Theory.* London: Routledge.

Brennan, K. A., Clark, C. L., & Shaver, P. R. (1998). Self-report measurement of adult romantic attachment: An integrative overview. In J. A. Simpson & W. S. Rholes (Eds.), *Attachment Theory and Close Relationships* (pp. 46–76). New York, NY: Guilford Press.

Brennan, K. A., & Morris, K. A. (1997). Attachment styles, self-esteem, and patterns of seeking feedback from romantic partners. *Personality and Social Psychology Bulletin, 23,* 23–31.

Broemer, P., & Blumle, M. (2003). Self-views in close relationships: The influence of attachment styles. *British Journal of Social Psychology, 42,* 445–460.

Caldwell, J. G., Shaver, P. R., Li, C., & Minzenberg, M. J. (2011). Childhood maltreatment, adult attachment, and depression as predictors of parental self-efficacy in at-risk mothers. *Journal of Aggression, Maltreatment & Trauma, 20,* 595–616.

Carnelley, K. B., Israel, S., & Brennan, K. (2007). The role of attachment in influencing reactions to manipulated feedback from romantic partners. *European Journal of Social Psychology, 37,* 968–986.

Cassidy, J., & Kobak, R. R. (1988). Avoidance and its relationship with other defensive processes. In J. Belsky & T. Nezworski (Eds.), *Clinical Implications of Attachment* (pp. 300–323). Hillsdale, NJ: Erlbaum.

Cassidy, J., Ziv, Y., Mehta, T. G., & Feeney, B. C. (2003). Feedback seeking in children and adolescents: Associations with self-perceptions, attachment representations, and depression. *Child Development, 74,* 612–628.

Catanzaro, A., & Wei, M. (2010). Adult attachment, dependence, self-criticism, and depressive symptoms: A test of a mediational model. *Journal of Personality, 78,* 1135–1162.

Chen, C., Hewitt, P. L., Flett, G. L., *et al.* (2012). Insecure attachment, perfectionistic self-presentation, and social disconnection. *Personality and Individual Differences, 52,* 936–941.

Cheng, S. T., & Kwan, K. W. (2008). Attachment dimensions and contingencies of self-worth: The moderating role of culture. *Personality and Individual Differences, 45,* 509–514.

Davaji, R. B. O., Valizadeh, S., & Nikamal, M. (2010). The relationship between attachment styles and suicide ideation: The study of Turkmen students, Iran. *Procedia – Social and Behavioral Sciences, 5,* 1190–1194.

Davila, J. (2001). Refining the association between excessive reassurance seeking and depressive symptoms: The role of related interpersonal constructs. *Journal of Social and Clinical Psychology, 20,* 538–559.

Dentale, F., Vecchione, M., De Coro, A., & Barbaranelli, C. (2012). On the relationship between implicit and explicit self-esteem: The moderating role of dismissing attachment. *Personality and Individual Differences, 52,* 173–177.

Dewitte, M., De Houwer, J., & Buysse, A. (2008). On the role of the implicit self-concept in adult attachment. *European Journal of Psychological Assessment, 24,* 282–289.

Dickinson, K. A., & Pincus, A. L. (2003). Interpersonal analysis of grandiose and vulnerable narcissism. *Journal of Personality Disorders, 17,* 188–207.

Doron, G., Moulding, R., Kyrios, M., Nedeljkovic, M., & Mikulincer, M. (2009). Adult attachment insecurities are related to obsessive compulsive phenomena. *Journal of Social and Clinical Psychology, 28,* 1022–1049.

Doron, G., Moulding, R., Nedeljkovic, M., *et al.* (2012). Adult attachment insecurities are associated with obsessive compulsive disorder. *Psychology and Psychotherapy: Theory, Research and Practice*, 85(2), 163–178.

Doron, G., Szepsenwol, O., Karp, E., & Gal, N. (2013). Obsessing about intimate-relationships: Testing the double relationship-vulnerability hypothesis. *Journal of Behavior Therapy and Experimental Psychiatry*, 44(4), 433–440.

Doyle, A. B., & Markiewicz, D. (2009). Attachment style with father and mother in early adolescence: Gender differences and perceived peer competence. *European Journal of Developmental Science*, 3, 80–93.

Ein-Dor, T., & Doron, G. (2015). Attachment and psychopathology. In J. A. Simpson & W. S. Rholes (Eds.), *Attachment Theory and Research: New Directions and Emerging Themes* (pp. 346–373). New York, NY: Guilford Press.

Ein-Dor, T., Doron, G., Solomon, Z., Mikulincer, M., & Shaver, P. R. (2010). Together in pain: Attachment-related dyadic processes and posttraumatic stress disorder. *Journal of Counseling Psychology*, 57(3), 317–327.

Felton, L., & Jowett, S. (2013). Attachment and well-being: The mediating effects of psychological needs satisfaction within the coach–athlete and parent–athlete relational contexts. *Psychology of Sport and Exercise*, 14, 57–65.

Foster, J. D., Kernis, M. H., & Goldman, B. M. (2007). Linking adult attachment to self-esteem stability. *Self and Identity*, 6, 64–73.

Gamble, S. A., & Roberts, J. E. (2005). Adolescents' perceptions of primary caregivers and cognitive style: The roles of attachment security and gender. *Cognitive Therapy and Research*, 29, 123–141.

Gjerde, P. F., Onishi, M., & Carlson, K. S. (2004). Personality characteristics associated with romantic attachment: A comparison of interview and self-report methodologies. *Personality and Social Psychology Bulletin*, 30, 1402–1415.

Gnilka, P. B., Ashby, J. S., & Noble, C. M. (2013). Adaptive and maladaptive perfectionism as mediators of adult attachment styles and depression, hopelessness, and life satisfaction. *Journal of Counseling & Development*, 91, 78–86.

Greenwald, A. G., McGhee, D. E., & Schwartz, J. L. K. (1998). Measuring individual differences in implicit cognition: The Implicit Association Test. *Journal of Personality and Social Psychology*, 74, 1464–1480.

Hart, J. J., Shaver, P. R., & Goldenberg, J. L. (2005). Attachment, self-esteem, worldviews, and terror management: Evidence for a tripartite security system. *Journal of Personality and Social Psychology*, 88, 999–1013.

Hepper, E. G., & Carnelley, K. B. (2010). Adult attachment and feedback-seeking patterns in relationships and work. *European Journal of Social Psychology*, 40, 448–464.

Hepper, E. G., & Carnelley, K. B. (2012). The self-esteem roller coaster: Adult attachment moderates the impact of daily feedback. *Personal Relationships*, 19, 504–520.

Illing, V., Tasca, G. A., Balfour, L., & Bissada, H. (2010). Attachment insecurity predicts eating disorder symptoms and treatment outcomes in a clinical sample of women. *The Journal of Nervous and Mental Disease*, 198, 653–659.

Jenkins-Guarnieri, M. A., Wright, S. L., & Hudiburgh, L. M. (2012). The relationships among attachment style, personality traits, interpersonal competency, and Facebook use. *Journal of Applied Developmental Psychology*, 33, 294–301.

Kazarian, S. S., & Martin, R. A. (2004). Humor styles, personality, and well-being among Lebanese university students. *European Journal of Personality*, 18, 209–219.

Knee, C. R., Canevello, A., Bush, A. L., & Cook, A. (2008). Relationship-contingent self-esteem and the ups and downs of romantic relationships. *Journal of Personality and Social Psychology*, 95, 608–627.

Kohut, H. (1984). *How Does Analysis Cure?* Chicago, IL: University of Chicago Press.

Kumashiro, M., & Sedikides, C. (2005). Taking on board liability-focused information: Close positive relationships as a self-bolstering resource. *Psychological Science*, 16, 732–739.

Lee, A., & Hankin, B. L. (2009). Non-secure attachment, dysfunctional attitudes, and low self-esteem predicting prospective symptoms of depression and anxiety during adolescence. *Journal of Clinical Child and Adolescent Psychology*, 38, 219–231.

Lopez, F. G., & Gormley, B. (2002). Stability and change in adult attachment style over the first-year college transition: Relations to self-confidence, coping, and distress patterns. *Journal of Counseling Psychology*, 49, 355–364.

Man, K. O., & Hamid, P. (1998). The relationship between attachment prototypes, self-esteem, loneliness, and causal attributions in Chinese trainee teachers. *Personality and Individual Differences*, 24, 357–371.

Marganska, A., Gallagher, M., & Miranda, R. (2013). Adult attachment, emotion dysregulation, and symptoms of depression and generalized anxiety disorder. *American Journal of Orthopsychiatry*, 83, 131–141.

McWilliams, L. A., & Holmberg, D. (2010). Adult attachment and pain catastrophizing for self and significant other. *Pain*, 149, 278–283.

Mikulincer, M. (1995). Attachment style and the mental representation of the self. *Journal of Personality and Social Psychology*, 69, 1203–1215.

Mikulincer, M. (1998). Adult attachment style and affect regulation: Strategic variations in self-appraisals. *Journal of Personality and Social Psychology*, 75, 420–435.

Mikulincer, M., & Shaver, P. R. (2004). Security-based self-representations in adulthood: Contents and processes. In W. S. Rholes & J. A. Simpson (Eds.), *Adult Attachment: Theory, Research, and Clinical Implications* (pp. 159–195). New York, NY: Guilford Press.

Mikulincer, M., & Shaver, P. R. (2007). *Attachment Patterns in Adulthood: Structure, Dynamics, and Change*. New York, NY: Guilford Press.

Mikulincer, M., & Shaver, P. R. (2015). An attachment perspective on prosocial attitudes and behavior. In D. A. Schroeder & W. Graziano (Eds.), *The Oxford Handbook of Prosocial Behavior*. New York, NY: Oxford University Press.

Neff, K. D., & McGehee, P. (2010). Self-compassion and psychological resilience among adolescents and young adults. *Self and Identity*, 9, 225–240.

Park, L. E., Crocker, J., & Mickelson, K. D. (2004). Attachment styles and contingencies of self-worth. *Personality and Social Psychology Bulletin*, 30, 1243–1254.

Rogers, C. R. (1961). *On Becoming A Person*. Boston, MA: Houghton Mifflin.

Rohmann, E., Neumann, E., Herner, M. J., & Bierhoff, M. H. W. (2012). Grandiose and vulnerable narcissism: Self-construal, attachment, and love in romantic relationship. *European Psychologist*, 17, 279–290.

Rothman, A. M., & Steil, J. M. (2012). Adolescent attachment and entitlement in a world of wealth. *Journal of Infant, Child & Adolescent Psychotherapy*, 11, 53–65.

Saroglou, V., & Scariot, C. (2002). Humor Styles Questionnaire: Personality and educational correlates in Belgian high school and college students. *European Journal of Personality*, 16, 43–54.

Schachner, D. A., & Shaver, P. R. (2004). Attachment dimensions and sexual motives. *Personal Relationships*, 11, 179–195.

Schimel, J., Arndt, J., Pyszczynski, T., & Greenberg, J. (2001). Being accepted for who we are: Evidence that social validation of the intrinsic self reduces general defensiveness. *Journal of Personality and Social Psychology*, 80, 35–52.

Schmitt, D. P., & Allik, J. (2005). Simultaneous administration of the Rosenberg Self-Esteem Scale in 53 nations: Exploring the universal and culture-specific features of global self-esteem. *Journal of Personality and Social Psychology*, 89, 623–642.

Slotter, E. B., & Gardner, W. L. (2012). How needing you changes me: The influence of attachment anxiety on self-concept malleability in romantic relationships. *Self and Identity*, 11, 386–408.

Srivastava, S., & Beer, J. S. (2005). How self-evaluations relate to being liked by others: Integrating sociometer and attachment perspectives. *Journal of Personality and Social Psychology*, 89, 966–977.

Sumer, N., & Cozzarelli, C. (2004). The impact of adult attachment on partner and self-attributions and relationship quality. *Personal Relationships*, 11, 355–371.

Thompson, R. A. (2008). Early attachment and later development: Familiar questions, new answers. In J. Cassidy & P. R. Shaver (Eds.), *Handbook of Attachment: Theory, Research, and Clinical Applications* (2nd ed., pp. 348–365). New York, NY: Guilford Press.

Tolmacz, R., & Mikulincer, M. (2011). The sense of entitlement in romantic relationships: Scale construction, factor structure, construct validity, and its associations with attachment orientations. *Psychoanalytic Psychology*, 28, 75–94.

Ulu, I. P., & Tezer, E. (2010). Adaptive and maladaptive perfectionism, adult attachment, and big five personality traits. *Journal of Psychology*, 144, 327–340.

Wei, M., Heppner, P. P., Russell, D. W., & Young, S. K. (2006). Maladaptive perfectionism and ineffective coping as mediators between attachment and future depression: A prospective analysis. *Journal of Counseling Psychology*, 53(1), 67.

Wei, M., & Ku, T. (2007). Testing a conceptual model of working through self-defeating patterns. *Journal of Counseling Psychology*, 54, 295–305.

Wiseman, H., Mayseless, O., & Sharabany, R. (2005). Why are they lonely? Perceived quality of early relationships with parents, attachment, personality predispositions, and loneliness in first-year university students. *Personality and Individual Differences*, 40, 237–248.

Zeifman, D., & Hazan, C. (2008). Pair bonds as attachments: Reevaluating the evidence. In J. Cassidy & P. R. Shaver (Eds.), *Handbook of Attachment: Theory, Research, and Clinical Applications* (2nd ed., pp. 436–455). New York, NY: Guilford Press.

Zuroff, D. C., & Fitzpatrick, D. K. (1995). Depressive personality styles: Implications for adult attachment. *Personality and Individual Differences*, 18, 253–365.

Chapter

4

Working with the future: a psychodynamic–integrative approach to treatment

Golan Shahar and Moran Schiller

Recent empirical research provides considerable support for the efficacy, effectiveness, and cost-effectiveness of psychodynamic psychotherapy for a host of psychopathologies (Abbass, Rabung, Leichsenring, Refseth, & Midgley, 2013; Gibbons, Crits-Christoph, & Hearon, 2008; Leichsenring & Rabung, 2008; Leichsenring, Leweke, Klein, & Steinert, 2015; Shedler, 2010), inclusive of unipolar depression (e.g., Leichsenring & Schauenburg, 2014; Luyten & Blatt, 2012). The key mechanism of psychodynamic therapy appears to be *an increase in self-understanding* (Barber, Muran, McCarthy, & Keefe, 2013; Kivlighan, Multon, & Patton, 2000). Hence, a focus on the self, in the context of this form of therapy, appears to be of particular relevance to this edited volume. This chapter uses the exemplar of depression to illustrate the utility of integrating self-constructs in our understanding of psychodynamic treatment.

Despite the purported effectiveness of psychodynamic therapy and its assumed mechanisms, research characteristically suffers from a noxious methodological problem labeled "The Construct Validity of the Cause." In their classic methodological treatise, D. T. Campbell and J. C. Stanley (1963) described five types of validity of findings obtained in the context of intervention research. These are:

Internal validity (IV): pertaining to the causal status of X (e.g., psychodynamic therapy) in relation to Y (e.g., a reduction in depression). Threats to IV question the extent to which a certain study really eliminated alternative explanations for the presumably causal effect of X. A classic threat is *maturation*, or when the mere passage of time changes a certain outcome, constituting an alternative explanation for an effect of treatment.

Obviously, maturation is eliminated as a threat via the inclusion of a control group, and a random allocation of participants to treatment groups. Arguably, we are now at a point where extant research on psychodynamic psychotherapy provides reasonable evidence for the successful elimination of maturation and other threats to IV (e.g., Leichsenring & Rabung, 2008).

External validity (EV): also labeled "Ecological Validity," EV refers to the generalizability of the causal effect of X on Y across various conditions. In psychotherapy research, EV is questioned only after at least some evidence consistent with IV has been accumulated. Here too, it seems that extant research demonstrates a reasonable EV for psychodynamic psychotherapy (Gibbons *et al.*, 2008).

Statistical conclusion validity (SCV): relates to the extent to which the statistical conditions applied in a study are adequate for drawing valid conclusions. There is a huge debate around this issue in psychotherapy research in general, but it lies outside the scope of this book chapter.

Construct validity of the effect (CVE): addresses the identity of Y (e.g., depression) and whether it is measured appropriately. This is of no concern here.

Construct validity of the cause (CVC): concerns *the identity of X*, namely, the treatment (in our case, psychodynamic psychotherapy). Specifically, CVC pertains to the extent in which various studies examining the effect of psychodynamic psychotherapy on clinical outcomes *converge into a coherent view of what "psychodynamic" is and what differentiates it from other types of treatment (e.g., interpersonal, experiential).*

The Self in Understanding and Treating Psychological Disorders, ed. Michael Kyrios, Richard Moulding, Guy Doron, Sunil S. Bhar, Maja Nedeljkovic, and Mario Mikulincer. Published by Cambridge University Press. © Cambridge University Press, 2016.

Originally, the term psychodynamic was coined to address the unique way in which psychoanalysis, psychodynamic psychotherapy's parent, construes unconscious processes. In psychoanalysis, mental contents (urges, thoughts, and emotions) that are anxiety-provoking are actively pushed out of awareness by the mind – through the operation of defense mechanisms – but are constantly aiming at returning to awareness. The task of psychoanalytic (psychodynamic) therapy is to help patients become aware of these mental contents, so as to gain control over them (see Mitchell & Black, 1995). However, there are huge differences between the psychoanalytic perspective of Melanie Klein and her followers (i.e., "The Kleinians") and that of Heinz Kohut and his followers (i.e., "The Self Psychologists"). "The Kleinians" emphasize the presence of deep-seated anxieties (persecutory, depressive) in the psyche, powerfully concealed by primitive, dissociative-like defense mechanisms (splitting, idealization, projective identification; see Ogden, 1991). These anxieties may only be extracted by bold, penetrating interpretations that get to the core of what makes the patient terrified. In contrast, for "The Self-Psychologists," the unconscious contains mainly affect-related self-states which are narcissistically injuring. These self-states lie right beneath the surface of awareness, and they may be extracted by therapists' empathic attunement to the unfolding *of the here-and-now* in patients' discourse. Consistent with these marked theoretical differences, psychodynamic therapy guided by a Kleinian persuasion would be quite different from a psychodynamic psychotherapy guided by a Kohutian one. No wonder, therefore, that psychoanalysis itself is highly preoccupied (some would say obsessed) with what does – and what does not – constitute psychoanalysis (e.g., Blass, 2010).

As a way around this problem, Blagys and Hilsenroth (2000) identified seven features that distinguish psychodynamic psychotherapy from other forms of therapy. These include:

(1) encouraging emotional insight;
(2) exploring attempts to avoid troubling feelings;
(3) identifying vicious, maladaptive cycles;
(4) exploring past experiences that are painfully relived in the present;
(5) focusing on the self, in context of interpersonal relationships;
(6) working with repetitive interpersonal themes that emerge also in the therapy relationship; and
(7) exploring fantasy life.

As cogent as these criteria appear to be, many psychodynamic therapies might fulfill only a part of the list of criteria, and very different treatments might fulfill most (consider, for instance, mentalization-based therapy [MBT; Allen, Fonagy, & Bateman, 2008] and transference-focused psychotherapy [TFP; Clarkin, Yeomans, & Kernberg, 2007] for borderline personality disorder).

Back to the theoretical drawing board

The only way out of this quagmire is theoretical: one has to go back to the original meaning of the term "psychodynamic," examine it closely, and then: (a) retain what appears coherent and in line with extant basic psychological research; (b) discard what has not withstood extant research; (c) add conceptual aspects that emerge from basic psychological research as central to the understanding of psychodynamic processes; and (d) align what remains with (i) psychoanalytic theory, and (ii) the evolving social-cognitive nomenclature, the latter constituting a consensual academic-psychological discourse (see Blatt, Auerbach, & Levy, 1997; Shahar, 2015a; Shahar, Cross, & Henrich, 2004; Westen, 1991, 1998).

Going through the above process, this is our definition of "psychodynamic":

> The term "psychodynamic" refers to constellations of (a) schemas and scripts pertaining to the self-in-relationships, which are (b) colored by specific emotional and affect regulation tendencies, and are (c) directed to the past, present, and – most revealingly – the future. The three components, (a), (b), and (c), operate in concert to maintain a sense of identity which is as clear as possible. For each individual, the various constellations compete over maximum awareness, and hence some are actively – but not necessarily permanently – pushed outside of awareness, so as to increase self-clarity. All constellations are manifested in interpersonal behavior, in turn impacting individuals' well-being.

The above definition is faithful to the psychoanalytic tradition that describes the psyche as self-protecting, actively pushing material outside awareness (Cramer, 2006; Westen, 1991, 1998). However, by noting that material pushed outside of awareness is not necessarily permanently unconscious, we eschew the Freudian/Lacanian notion of a clear, repressive line (Billig, 1999; Fink, 2009) strictly distinguishing between what is conscious and what is not, and adopt a phenomenological–experiential–humanistic approach that construes consciousness as a continuum

(Stolorow, Brandshaft, & Atwood, 1987). This is highly consistent with Freud's (1895) early notion of disavowal as an alternative to unconscious denial, the former process pertaining to the person deliberately dimming his/her consciousness with respect to known facts, or what Zepf (2013) labels as "a type of laying that is not consciously intended" (p. 36).

The psychoanalytically astute reader will notice that our notion of the constellations comprising the psychodynamic unconscious is extremely consistent with Melanie Klein's notion of the "Positions" (Klein, 1928). The term refers to a developmental phase that is characterized by specific anxieties, defense mechanisms, impulses, and object relations (Spillius, Milton, Garvey, Couve, & Steiner, 2011). Markedly distinguished from the notion of "stages," the idea of positions offers an observation of development as an ongoing, spiral process that occurs throughout life and is very much influenced by relationships.

With the original notion of Positions, we have translated obscure Kleinian terms (object relationships, good and bad breast, projective identification, etc.) into a social-cognitive language. Specifically, object relations are now deemed *self-in-relationships schemas and scripts*, the paranoid/depressive anxieties are replaced with "emotional tendencies," allowing for other emotions besides anxiety, and "defense mechanisms" are replaced with "*affect regulation*," again placing it within the context of social-cognitive research (Gross, 1998). In line with our above-described liberal approach towards "the unconscious," we make no distinction between "defense mechanisms" and "coping strategies," rendering both to be attempts at regulating affect related to self-knowledge, and conducted via variable levels of awareness.

As well, we have also included an existentially informed time dimension, pertaining to self-in-relationships schemas (and related emotional styles), and affective regulatory tendencies – located in individuals' past, present, and future. We are particularly interested in individuals' *future representations*. Here we draw from the psychoanalytic works of Harry Stack Sullivan (1953) and, more recently, of Frank Summers (2003), which attempt to correct psychoanalysis' relative disregard of the future-oriented nature of the psyche. The growing attention placed on the future, labeled as the nexus of mental activity (e.g., Seligman, Railton, Baumeister, & Sripada, 2013; Shahar & Davidson, 2009), has led to a profusion of goal-oriented constructs in the field of personality psychology (Austin

& Vancouver, 1996). Further pushing the envelope, Shahar (2010, 2011) argues that individuals' attempts to launch themselves into the future and become what they might (labeled "projectuality") occurs primarily in relationships. Specifically, individuals attempt to create themselves by acting upon other people (see also Buss, 1987; Strenger, 1998). To maintain the active, goal-oriented, and future-related nature of interpersonal behavior, Shahar proposes that the term "agent-in-relationships" (AIR) should replace "object relations" (Shahar, 2010).

Yet another important aspect of our definition of "psychodynamic" is that it strongly links internal processes to interpersonal behavior. Here we rely on the now-formidable impact of interpersonal psychoanalysis on contemporary clinical thought, with the latter's focus on conflict and defense as *externalized* via behavior with others (Horney, 1937; Sullivan, 1953; Wachtel, 1977, 1994, 1997, 2014; see also Shahar, 2011), in turn leading to various forms of psychopathology, most notably, to unipolar depression.

Psychodynamic treatment of the self: the case of depression

An application of our notion of "Psychodynamic" to depression is summarized in Table 4.1. An additional approach integrating psychodynamic and cognitive-behavioral frameworks to understanding and treating depression can be found in Chapter 8 of this book, by Luyten and Fonagy. Both approaches agree that decades of robust, empirical research implicate self-criticism as a formidable dimension of vulnerability to depression and related psychopathology (Blatt, 1995, 2004; Shahar, 2001, 2013, 2015b; Shahar & Henrich, 2013). Defined as the tendency to set unrealistically high self-standards, and to adopt a punitive stance towards the self once these standards are not met, self-criticism actively produces "depressogenic" interpersonal conditions that lead to depression. Specifically, self-critics generate life stress and "de-generate" (failure to generate) both positive life events and social support (Shahar, 2001, 2013, 2015b; Shahar & Priel, 2003). This "active vulnerability" also occurs in the context of treatment for depression: self-critical depressed patients derail the therapeutic alliance, and also erode relationships with significant others, in turn impeding their own response to treatment (Blatt & Zuroff, 2005; Shahar, Blatt, Zuroff, and Pilkonis, 2003). Building on the above-described

Table 4.1 The depressive psychodynamics.

	The depressive psychodynamics
Schemas/scripts	A critical self-stance in relation to a representation of others as harsh and punitive
Emotions	A flood of negative affect, including "interpersonal" negative emotions (i.e., contempt, shame, disgust), coupled with a dearth of positive affect
Affect regulation	Maladaptive: • defense mechanisms (e.g., acting out, undoing, projection, devaluation, denial, isolation and splitting, turning against self and others) • coping strategies (e.g., venting distress to others without attempting to solve the putative problem) • motivational regulative endeavors (suppressing authentic interest in activities; fostering motivations for non-authentic pursuits)
Future representations	Gloomy future representations, experiencing their future goals as largely outside their reach

definition of "psychodynamics," we would like to propose that self-criticism is the most salient factor in a conglomeration of psychological variables underlying unipolar depressive conditions.

Self-criticism is consistently associated with malevolent representations of significant others, both parents and peers (e.g., Mongrain, 1998; Parker & Macnair, 1979; Sadeh, Rubin, & Berman, 1993; Whiffen, Parker, Wilhelm, Mitchell, & Malhi, 2003). These representations emanate either from actual victimization (e.g., Enns, Cox, & Larsen, 2000; Koestner, Zuroff, & Powers, 1991; Lassri & Shahar, 2012), or from self-critics ultra-sensitivity to even mild forms of disapproval (as theorized by Shahar, 2015b). Regardless of the particular source of these "object representations," however, self-critics view close people as critical, harsh, controlling, and affectionless (Blatt, 1995; Shahar, 2001).

Empirical research consistently points out self-critics' dire emotional style, characterized not only by marked negative affect and improvised positive affect (as would be expected from a depressive personality dimension, see Fichman, Koestner, Zuroff, & Gordon, 1999; Gilbert et al., 2008), but also by painful "interpersonal" emotions such as contempt, disgust,

and shame (Gilbert et al., 2010; Whelton & Greenberg, 2005), and even paranoid sentiments (Mills, Gilbert, Bellew, McEwan, & Gale, 2007). Self-critics exhibit severe difficulties in affective regulation, and the nature of these difficulties further attests to the interpersonal nature of their distress. Thus, self-critics appear to use maladaptive defense mechanisms (e.g., acting out, undoing, projection, devaluation, denial, isolation and splitting, turning against self and others; Besser, 2004; Campos, Besser, & Blatt, 2013; Zuroff, Moskowitz, Wielgus, Powers, & Franko, 1983), maladaptive coping strategies, such as venting distress to others without attempting to solve the putative problem (Dunkley & Blankstein, 2000; Dunkley, Zuroff, & Blankstein, 2003; Fichman et al., 1999), and highly maladaptive motivational regulative endeavors, namely, attempting to suppress authentic interest in activities (Shahar, Henrich, Blatt, Ryan, & Little, 2003; Shahar, Kalnitzki, Shulman, & Blatt, 2006), and fostering motivations for non-authentic pursuits (e.g., Powers, Koestner, & Zuroff, 2007; Shahar, Henrich, et al., 2003). Finally, self-critics also exhibit incredibly gloomy future representations, experiencing their future goals and projects as largely outside their reach (Powers et al., 2007; Shahar et al., 2006; Thompson & Zuroff, 2010).

Locating self-criticism research in the context of our reconceptualization of "psychodynamics," we propose that individuals experience themselves as fundamentally flawed in light of what they perceive to be a critical, harsh, and affectionless attitude from others towards them. These representations of self-in-relationships suppress joy and curiosity, and evoke intense sadness, shame, and contempt, but also anger, devaluation of others, and, in extreme cases, even some forms of paranoia. Attempts made to ward off these painful emotions – possibly so as to maintain a level of functioning that will secure approval from self and others – ultimately fail because of the use of maladaptive defense mechanisms, coping strategies, and other forms of affect regulatory maneuvers. These maladaptive attempts create interpersonal ruptures and derail attempts at generating positive experiences (positive life events) and enlisting support. Over time, individuals accumulate enough interpersonal and functional failure to understandably doubt that they may lead a different kind of life. Put differently, they develop gloomy future expectations (i.e., "hopelessness"). This, of course, further amalgamates emotional distress, particularly depressive symptoms, which – as research attests – further exacerbates self-criticism, particularly during adolescence (Shahar, Blatt, Zuroff, Kuperminc, & Leadbeater, 2004).

As pessimistic as this dynamic might (justifiably) sound, it does include good news. This is actually reflected in individuals' active creation of the social context which – in the case of self-critics – pertains to the generation of interpersonal stress and "de-generation" of positive events and social support. From the point of view advanced here, the fact that self-critics repeatedly generate interpersonal havoc, despite years of doing so at their own peril, suggests that they still have hope for a different type of interpersonal experience. Of course, this hope is likely to be frustrated due to self-critics' inept interpersonal conduct which is likely to beget more rejections, confrontations, and ruptures. The latter serves to increase self-critics' frustration and to further illuminate the tragic nature of psychopathology (Wachtel, 1994). And yet, there is one interpersonal context in which this need not – must not – be the case: the therapeutic arena.

Working with the future

Because of the co-dependence of schemas/scripts of self, schemas/scripts of other people, emotional and affective regulative styles, and time-based representations (particularly malignant future representations), effective treatment is bound to be multilayered. As well, because individuals with depressive psychodynamics actively – if inadvertently – generate the very social conditions that maintain/exacerbate their depression, psychotherapy must focus on both internal and interpersonal arenas. Fortunately, Wachtel's *cyclical psychodynamic approach* provides a general, integrative, psychotherapeutic umbrella that bridges the inner world and outer (interpersonal) context (Wachtel, 1977, 1994, 1997, 2014). Wachtel posits that (a) psychopathology emerges from and is maintained by the generation of negative social relations, and (b) individuals create the very conditions they dread. He advocates both insight-oriented work aimed at understanding patients' anxieties, and active, primarily behavioral, techniques designed to short-circuit the vicious interpersonal cycles these prompt (Wachtel, 1977). Recently, Wachtel has become more tolerant towards acceptance and mindfulness-based interventions aimed at increasing present-moment awareness and cognitive flexibility (Wachtel, 2011, 2014).

Extending this approach, Shahar and colleagues (Shahar, 2004, 2013, 2015b; Shahar, Cross, & Henrich, 2004; Shahar & Davidson, 2009) have stipulated that human beings actively create the things they dread in order to ensure that they may eventually become what they wish to be. They argue that an emphasis on a *patient's future representations* as they are tied to the self should accompany any and all interventions with depressed patients (see Shahar, 2013). The remaining part of this chapter will focus on the therapeutic work with future representations of individuals characterized by the above-described depressive psychodynamic. Before we explicate this, however, we must provide some context for the entire treatment process (for details, see Shahar, 2013, 2015b).

Treatment begins with actively instilling warmth, so as to challenge mental representations of others ("objects") as harsh and punitive. Psycho-education regarding the hazard of self-criticism and criticism-based interpersonal exchanges follows. Next, a series of active and clearly delineated interventions are introduced. The first is Multiple Selves Analysis/Personal Project Analysis (MSA/PPA), which will be described below. The remaining interventions are (1) mindfulness-based techniques, and (2) "participatory" interventions such as behavioral activation, dereflection, analyses of daily routines, a detailed inquiry into interpersonal exchanges, and trail-based cognitive restructuring. Through these techniques, patients learn to identify the self-criticism, tie it to the way they view others (i.e., as harsh and punitive), link their self-in-relationships representations to the way they experience and regulate painful affect, and preempt their tendency to generate stress and derail positive events and social support. Importantly, the active interventions are carried out flexibly, patiently, *and on an iterative basis*, namely, time and time again, without pressure to "maintain schedule" or an expectation that a single round would "do the job." In between, there are potentially long stretches of what would seem to the outsider as a standard psychodynamic psychotherapy closer to the Winnicotian/Kohutian traditions, that is, coloured with an empathic immersion of the therapist to patients' painful affect, an "experience-near" focus of the "here and now," and an active encouragement of a curious, playful state of mind in both parties of the therapeutic dyad (Shahar, 2015b).

Turning now to a particular focus of working with depressed patients' futures, we emphasize the following three clinical issues.

Fighting for the future

It goes without saying that depressed individuals are pessimistic, indeed frequently hopeless (Abramson, Metalsky, & Alloy, 1989). The link between schemas and scripts of self-in-relationships and this pessimism and hopelessness has been noted above (e.g., Powers *et al.*, 2007; Shahar *et al.*, 2006), and has been construed as a central component of the depressive psychodynamics. Moreover, from our psychodynamic (-integrative) point of view, such pessimism/hopelessness is bound to infiltrate the therapeutic relationships: patients will convey considerable disbelief about therapists' abilities to help them, and are likely to even extract this very disbelief from therapists themselves. The challenge for therapists in this respect is to (a) withstand these attacks on the future of the therapy, and (b) once the future of therapy appears to survive, actively work with patients to generalize this fortitude to other realms of patients' lives.

Elsewhere, the first author of this chapter (GS) described a patient whose self-criticism propelled an attack on the future of the therapy, in turn confirming his negative future representation (Kelly, Zuroff, & Shahar, 2014; chapters 4 and 6 in Shahar, 2015b). Ilan, a bright, 20-year-old undergraduate with a history of success, experienced child neglect, which led him to suffer from depression throughout all of his life. Underlying his double depression (low-level depression with acute suicidal depressive episodes) lay a malignant self-criticism manifested in his self-deprecation. Relying on an integrative psychotherapeutic approach, the therapist's "first line of defense" was administering a slightly modified version of cognitive-behavioral therapy for depression. After gaining a sense of some progress in the first few sessions, the therapist was dumbfounded by Ilan's scornful approach. Ilan felt the sessions weren't helpful and that the therapist was arrogant and inaccessible. Insulted and affected by the patient's skepticism, the therapist began to doubt his own ability to help Ilan. Disclosing this uncertainty in front of Ilan only made it worse, as Ilan protested that the therapist readily "gives up on him." This made it clear for the therapist that his own dejection and pessimism resulted from Ilan's maladaptive inquisitive action (IA; Shahar, 2015b), an inept form of self-exploration, whereby Ilan, who sought to answer the question of "Can people survive my depression and suspiciousness?" actually pressured other people to provide a negative answer. When confronted as to this possibility, Ilan confirmed that he was testing his therapist. This paved the way to an enhanced therapeutic alliance, as well as to an increased understanding, on the part of the therapeutic dyad, as to the ways Ilan propelled others to provide responses consistent with his (Ilan's) gloomy depiction of his future. Moreover, throughout the relatively long treatment process (lasting about two years), whenever Ilan found himself stuck in frustrating interpersonal relationships, he was able to rely on this successful resolution of this rupture so as to summon hope for resolving other difficult interpersonal exchanges. In Winnicottian terms, the therapist and therapy were thus "holding Ilan's future" for him (Winnicott, 1955), first within treatment, and then – by way of a gradually increasing generalization – in other life domains.

Explicating the future

Expanding awareness to the existence of various aspects of one's self is pivotal to self-knowledge, leading to greater self-acceptance and well-being (see Shahar, 2015b). Shahar (2013, 2015b) developed MSA/PPA as a focal technique that aims to increase self-knowledge.

In the context of treating self-criticism, MSA/PPA purports to enable patients to discover benign self-aspects and to put them into action in everyday life. The step in MSA/PPA is attending to patients' language as they express their inner critic. For instance, when a patient says, "I'm good for nothing," the therapist – rather than dismissing this statement – will say, "There is a part of you that feels he is good for nothing." The main purpose of this phase is to evoke patients' curiosity as to their multiplicity, and enable them to begin speaking in terms of multiple selves.

Next, the therapist encourages patients to identify other, more beneficial and supportive self-aspects. Objections made by patients to the effect that they actually do not possess such "sides" are met with gentle encouragements regarding moments in their lives during which they were able to withstand stress and connecting these moments to benevolent "sides." Another way to circumvent resistance to the exploration of non-self-critical self-aspects is therapeutic self-disclosure (Ziv-Beiman, 2013). For instance, the therapist could reveal the fact that he also struggled in some points in his life, and talk about his own personal journey, inviting the patient to take his journey with him. To the extent that objections are adequately addressed, and patients begin to identify both self-critical and benevolent "sides," the therapist also encourages patients to personify these sides (e.g., give names to the various self-aspects) and to examine the presence and absence of these sides (names) in patients' biographies.

When patients' key self-aspects have been identified, personified, and situated within the patients' life biographies, they are invited to identify the future projects associated with *benevolent self-aspects*. Here, we follow Irvin D. Yalom's general dictum, whereby "Memory ('the organ of the past') is concerned with *objects*; the will is concerned with *projects*. ... Effective psychotherapy must focus on patients' *project relationships* as well as on their *object relationships*" (Yalom, 1980, p. 291 [original italics]). This is the PPA segment of the intervention. Moreover, patients are encouraged to put benevolent PPAs into action by immersing themselves in activities consistent with the future goals of their non-self-critical "sides." For instance, with Ilan, the aforementioned patient, this entailed encouraging him to pursue vegan activity and advocacy, which was very close to his heart (i.e., "enabling the growth of the vegan self-aspect"). With other patients, this might entail identifying/encouraging other activities, or other forms of relationships (e.g., forming new friendships).

When actual activities consistent with personal projects and benevolent self-aspects have been launched, we examine patients' experiences and relate these to the way they experience their self and other people ("object relationships" or "agents-in-relations"), as well as the emotions and affect regulatory procedures that patients experienced/employed throughout these activities. In essence, this enables patients to realize that they can experience self-and-world that is different from the "depressive position" that usually haunts them.

Playing with the future

Panksepp, who developed the field of affective neuroscience, argues that playfulness is an intrinsic brain function which promotes maturation of the prefrontal cortex and facilitates development (e.g., Panksepp, 2007). This idea strongly tallies with Winnicott's (1971) notion of play as paramount to self-development and mental health. From the perspective advanced here, encouraging patients to play – in their own lives – might serve as a powerful vehicle, not only to their self-discovery in the present, but also to their identification of pertinent personal projects, and even for

preparing for these projects in the future while the latter are still unknown.

Luck, a remarkably brilliant 24-year-old law student, sought treatment for depression. The depression was so crippling that Luck found himself unable to get out of bed for weeks. Instead, he used to surf the Internet aimlessly almost all day long, much to his own dismay. Through a slow and arduous treatment process, however, his depression finally began to improve. When this happened, Luck was mainly directing his renewed energies to playing with his PlayStation. His parents, following the treatment process closely, were horrified by this development, construing it either as testimony to a treatment-resistant depression or as a manifestation of sheer indulgence. I (GS), on the other hand, experienced Luck's interest in his PlayStation as an essential phase of coming back to life. Listening to Luck's description of his PlayStation activities, I easily discerned a rejuvenated ingenuity, reflected by some clever military moves he had made in the course of battling imaginary enemies (echoing, parenthetically, his exemplary military former service in the Israel Defense Forces), leadership (evinced via his ability to form, and command, a group of like-minded PlayStation fans of various ages in locations worldwide) and, most importantly, a growing stream of curiosity and enthusiasm. I, therefore, conveyed to Luck's parents my unequivocal support for his PlayStation activities, recommending that they not only tolerate it, but actually encourage it. Although Luck's parents found my recommendations difficult to absorb, they did follow them. As expected, Luck's recovery proceeded, and the PlayStation was forsaken on behalf of very different activities, albeit with the same ingenuity, leadership, curiosity and enthusiasm.

Summary and conclusion

Various forms of "psychodynamic" psychotherapy have been shown to be effective and efficacious in alleviating various psychopathological constellations, including unipolar depression. Self-understanding emerges as the key mechanism accounting for the beneficial effect of psychodynamic psychotherapy. Nevertheless, the field is threatened by a weak construct validity of the cause (CVC). Namely, it is not clear what "psychodynamic" means.

Herein, we propose a definition that is consistent with traditional, Kleinian conceptualizations of *Positions*, as reflecting object relations, anxieties, and defense mechanisms. However, we have reformulated the *Positions* by using social-cognition terms emanating from empirical psychological science (e.g., schemas and scripts, affect regulation), and linking it to neurocognitive research attesting to the centrality of the future in the psyche. Specifically, we posit that Positions refers to constellations of schemas and scripts of self-in-relations reflecting mutual influences (agents-in-relationships), linked with particular emotions and their regulations, and with various representations of a person's past, present, and – most pronouncedly – his/her future.

We then postulate the *Depressive Position* as comprised of a critical self-stance operating upon harsh and punitive others, in the context of failure to regulate negative affect, including interpersonal emotions such as contempt and shame, and a gloomy representation of the self as projected into the future. Such a position activates a depressogenic social environment marred with negative events (stress) and replete with positive events and social support. The inevitable depression that ensues from this active vulnerability further amalgamates the Depressive Position. Arguably, all four components of the depressive position – schemas/scripts of self and others, emotions, their regulation, and future representations – must be addressed in treatment. However, the latter component – representations of the future – must be targeted more vigorously. Without being able to represent their own future, patients will not be able to work constructively in any kind of therapy.

Consequently, we recommend that psychodynamic therapists will "fight for the future" of depressed patients, both within and outside treatment. We proffer three ways of working with depressed patients' futures: (1) withstanding patients' attempts to terminate the future of the therapy by generating ruptures ("holding the future"), (2) assisting patients to identify future goals and plans ("projects") of non-self-critical self-aspects ("explicating the future" using MSA/PPA), and (3) encouraging patients to engage in "playful" activities – not necessarily explicitly tied to personal projects – so as to identify hitherto unexamined future plans, and to prepare themselves for future tasks.

References

Abbass, A. A., Rabung, S., Leichsenring, F., Refseth, J. S., & Midgley, N. (2013). Psychodynamic psychotherapy for children and adolescents: A meta-analysis of short-term psychodynamic models. *Journal of the American Academy of Child & Adolescent Psychiatry*, 52(8), 863–875.

Abramson, L. Y., Metalsky, G. I., & Alloy, L. B. (1989). Hopelessness depression: A theory-based subtype of depression. *Psychological Review*, 96(2), 358–372.

Allen, J. G., Fonagy, P., & Bateman, A. W. (2008). *Mentalizing in Clinical Practice*. Arlington, VA: American Psychiatric Publishing.

Austin, J. T., & Vancouver, J. B. (1996). Goal constructs in psychology: Structure, process, and content. *Psychological Bulletin*, 120, 338–375.

Barber, J. P., Muran, J. C., McCarthy, K. S., & Keefe, R. J. (2013). Research on psychodynamic therapies. In M. J. Lambert (Ed.). *Bergin and Garfield's Handbook of Psychotherapy and Behavior Change* (pp. 443–494). New York, NY: John Wiley & Sons, Inc.

Besser, A. (2004). Self- and best friend assessments of personality vulnerability and defenses in the prediction of depression. *Social Behavior and Personality*, 32, 559–594.

Billig, M. (1999). *Freudian Repression: Conversation Creating the Unconscious*. Cambridge: Cambridge University Press.

Blagys, M. D., & Hilsenroth, M. J. (2000). Distinctive activities of short-term psychodynamic-interpersonal psychotherapy: A review of the comparative psychotherapy process literature. *Clinical Psychology: Science and Practice*, 7, 167–188.

Blass, R. B. (2010). Affirming 'That's not psycho-analysis!' On the value of the politically incorrect act of attempting to define the limits of our field. *The International Journal of Psychoanalysis*, 91(1), 81–89.

Blatt, S. J. (1995). The destructiveness of perfectionism. *American Psychologist*, 50, 1003–1020.

Blatt, S. J. (2004). *Experiences of Depression: Theoretical, Clinical and Research Perspectives*. Washington, DC: American Psychological Association.

Blatt, S. J., Auerbach, J. S., & Levy, K. N. (1997). Mental representations in personality development, psychopathology, and the therapeutic process. *Review of General Psychology*, 1(4), 351.

Blatt, S. J., & Zuroff, D. C. (2005). Empirical evaluation of the assumptions in identifying evidence based treatments in mental health. *Clinical Psychology Review*, 25(4), 459–486.

Buss, D. M. (1987). Selection, evocation, and manipulation. *Journal of Personality and Social Psychology*, 53, 1214–1221.

Campbell, D. T., Stanley, J. C., & Gage, N. L. (1963). *Experimental and Quasi-experimental Designs for Research* (pp. 171–246). Boston, MA: Houghton Mifflin.

Campos, R. C., Besser, A., & Blatt, S. J. (2013). Recollections of parental rejection, self-criticism and depression in suicidality. *Archives of Suicide Research*, 17(1), 58–74.

Clarkin, J. F., Yeomans, F. E., & Kernberg, O. F. (2007). *Psychotherapy for Borderline Personality: Focusing on Object Relations*. Arlington, VA: American Psychiatric Publishers.

Cramer, P. (2006). *Protecting the Self: Defense Mechanisms in Action*. New York, NY: Guilford Press.

Dunkley, D. M., & Blankstein, K. R. (2000). Self-critical perfectionism, coping, hassles, and current distress: A structural equation modeling approach. *Cognitive Therapy and Research*, 24(6), 713–730.

Dunkley, D. M., Zuroff, D. C., & Blankstein, K. R. (2003). Self-critical perfectionism and daily affect: Dispositional and situational influences on stress and coping. *Journal of Personality and Social Psychology*, 84(1), 234.

Enns, M. W., Cox, B. J., & Larsen, D. K. (2000). Perceptions of parental bonding and symptom severity in adults with depression: Mediation by personality dimensions. *Canadian Journal of Psychiatry*, 45(3), 263–268.

Fichman, L., Koestner, R., Zuroff, D. C., & Gordon, L. (1999). Depressive styles and the regulation of negative affect: A daily experience study. *Cognitive Therapy and Research*, 23(5), 483–495.

Fink, B. (2009). *A Clinical Introduction to Lacanian Psychoanalysis: Theory and Technique*. Harvard, MA: Harvard University Press.

Freud, S. (1895). *Studies on Hysteria*. S.E. 2, pp. 1–305.

Gibbons, M. B., Crits-Christoph, P., & Hearon, B. (2008). The empirical status of psychodynamic therapies. *Annual Review of Clinical Psychology*, 4, 93–108.

Gilbert, P., McEwan, K., Irons, C., et al. (2010). Self-harm in a mixed clinical population: The roles of self-criticism, shame, and social rank. *British Journal of Clinical Psychology*, 49, 563–576.

Gilbert, P., McEwan, K., Mitra, P., et al. (2008). Feeling safe and content: A specific affect regulation system? Relationship to depression, anxiety, stress, and self-criticism. *Journal of Positive Psychology*, 3(3), 182–191.

Gross, J. J. (1998). The emerging field of emotion regulation: An integrative review. *Review of General Psychology*, 2(3), 271.

Horney, K. (1937). *The Neurotic Personality of Our Time*. New York, NY: W. W. Norton.

Kelly, A. C., Zuroff, D. C., & Shahar, G. (2014). Perfectionism. In L. Grossman & S. Walfish (Eds.), *Translating Psychological Research into Practice* (pp. 233–240). New York, NY: Springer.

Kivlighan Jr, D. M., Multon, K. D., & Patton, M. J. (2000). Insight and symptom reduction in time-limited psychoanalytic counseling. *Journal of Counseling Psychology*, 47(1), 50.

Klein, M. (1928). Early stages of the Oedipus conflict. *International Journal of Psychoanalysis*, 9, 167–180.

Koestner, R., Zuroff, D. C., & Powers, T. A. (1991). Family origins of adolescent self-criticism and its continuity into adulthood. *Journal of Abnormal Psychology*, 100(2), 191.

Lassri, D., & Shahar, G. (2012). Self-criticism mediates the link between childhood emotional maltreatment and young adults' romantic relationships. *Journal of Social and Clinical Psychology*, 31(3), 289–311.

Leichsenring, F., Leweke, F., Klein, S., & Steinert, C. (2015). The empirical status of psychodynamic psychotherapy – An update: Bambi's alive and kicking. *Psychotherapy and Psychosomatics*, 84(3), 129–148.

Leichsenring, F., & Rabung, S. (2008). Effectiveness of long-term psychodynamic psychotherapy: A meta-analysis. *Journal of the American Medical Association*, 300(13), 1551–1565.

Leichsenring, F., & Schauenburg, H. (2014). Empirically supported methods of short-term psychodynamic therapy in depression – Towards an evidence-based unified protocol. *Journal of Affective Disorders*, 169, 128–143.

Luyten, P., & Blatt, S. J. (2012). Psychodynamic treatment of depression. *Psychiatric Clinics of North America*, 35(1), 111–129.

Mills, A., Gilbert, P., Bellew, R., McEwan, K., & Gale, C. (2007). Paranoid beliefs and self-criticism in students. *Clinical Psychology & Psychotherapy*, 14(5), 358–364.

Mitchell, S., & Black, M. (1995). *Freud and Beyond*. New York, NY: Basic Books.

Mongrain, M. (1998). Parental representations and support-seeking behaviors related to dependency and self-criticism. *Journal of Personality*, 66, 151–173.

Ogden, T. (1991). *The Primitive Edge of Experience*. Northvale, NJ: Aronson.

Panksepp, J. (2007). Can play diminish ADHD and facilitate the construction of the social brain? *Journal of the Canadian Academy of Child and Adolescent Psychiatry*, 16, 57–66.

Parker, G. A., & Macnair, M. R. (1979). Models of parent–offspring conflict. IV. Suppression: Evolutionary retaliation by the parent. *Animal Behaviour*, 27, 1210–1235.

Powers, T. A., Koestner, R., & Zuroff, D. C. (2007). Self-criticism, goal motivation, and goal progress. *Journal of Social and Clinical Psychology*, 26(7), 826–840.

Sadeh, A., Rubin, S. S., & Berman, E. (1993). Parental and relationship representations and experiences of depression in college students. *Journal of Personality Assessment*, 60(1), 192–204.

Seligman, M. E. P., Railton, P., Baumeister, R. F., & Sripada, C. (2013). Navigating into the future or driven by the past. *Perspectives in Psychological Science*, 8, 119–141.

Shahar, G. (2001). Personality, shame, and the breakdown of social bonds: The voice of quantitative depression research. *Psychiatry*, 64, 228–239.

Shahar, G. (2004). Transference–countertransference: Where the (political) action is. *Journal of Psychotherapy Integration*, 14, 371–396.

Shahar, G. (2010). Poetics, pragmatics, schematics, and the psychoanalysis-research dialogue (rift). *Psychoanalytic Psychotherapy*, 24, 315–328.

Shahar, G. (2011). Projectuality vs. eventuality: Sullivan, the (ambivalent) intentionalist. *Journal of Psychotherapy Integration*, 21, 211–220.

Shahar, G. (2013). An integrative psychotherapist's account of his focus when treating self-critical patients. *Psychotherapy*, 50(3), 322–325.

Shahar, G. (2015a). Object relations theory. In *The Encyclopedia of Clinical Psychology*. New York, NY: Wiley.

Shahar, G. (2015b). *Erosion: The Psychopathology of Self-criticism*. New York, NY: Oxford University Press.

Shahar, G., Blatt, S. J., Zuroff, D. C., Kuperminc, G. P., & Leadbeater, B. J. (2004). Reciprocal relations between depressive symptoms and self-criticism (but not dependency) among early adolescent girls (but not boys). *Cognitive Therapy and Research*, 28(1), 85–103.

Shahar, G., Blatt, S. J., Zuroff, D. C., & Pilkonis, P. (2003). Role of perfectionism and personality disorder features in response to brief treatment for depression. *Journal of Consulting and Clinical Psychology*, 71, 629–633.

Shahar, G., Cross, L. W., & Henrich, C. C. (2004). Representations in action (Or: action models of development meet psychoanalytic conceptualizations of mental representations). *The Psychoanalytic Study of the Child*, 59, 261–293.

Shahar, G., & Davidson, L. (2009). Participation-engagement: A philosophically-based heuristic for prioritizing interventions in the treatment of comorbid, complex, and chronic psychiatric conditions. *Psychiatry: Interpersonal and Biological Processes*, 72, 154–176.

Shahar, G., & Henrich, C. C. (2013). Axis of criticism model (ACRIM): An integrative conceptualization of person-context exchanges in vulnerability to adolescent psychopathology. *Journal of Psychotherapy Integration*, 23, 236–249.

Shahar, G., Henrich, C. C., Blatt, S. J., Ryan, R., & Little, T. D. (2003). Interpersonal relatedness, self-definition, and their motivational orientation during adolescence: A theoretical and empirical integration. *Developmental Psychology*, 39(3), 470.

Shahar, G., Kalnitzki, E., Shulman, S., & Blatt, S. J. (2006). Personality, motivation, and the construction of goals during the transition to adulthood. *Personality & Individual Differences*, 40(1), 53–63.

Shahar, G., & Priel, B. (2003). Active vulnerability, adolescent distress, and the mediating/suppressing role of life events. *Personality and Individual Differences*, 35, 199–218.

Shedler, J. (2010). The efficacy of psychodynamic psychotherapy. *American Psychologist*, 65(2), 98–109.

Spillius, E. B., Milton, J., Garvey, P., Couve, C., & Steiner, D. (2011). *The New Dictionary of Kleinian Thought*. Hove: Taylor & Francis.

Strenger, C. (1998). The desire for self-creation. *Psychoanalytic Dialogues*, 8, 625–655.

Stolorow, R. D., Brandshaft, B., & Atwood, G. E. (1987). *Psychoanalytic Treatment: An Intersubjective Approach*. Hillsdale, NJ: Analytic Press.

Sullivan, H. S. (1953). *The Interpersonal Theory of Psychiatry*. New York, NY: Norton.

Summers, F. (2003). The future as intrinsic to the psyche and psychoanalytic therapy. *Contemporary Psychoanalysis*, 39, 135–153.

Thompson, R., & Zuroff, D. C. (2010). My future self and me: Depressive styles and future expectations. *Personality and Individual Differences*, 48(2), 190–195.

Wachtel, P. L. (1977). *Psychoanalysis and Behavior Therapy: Toward an Integration*. New York, NY: Basic.

Wachtel, P. L. (1994). Cyclical processes in personality and psychopathology. *Journal of Abnormal Psychology*, 103, 51–66.

Wachtel, P. L. (1997). *Psychoanalysis, Behavior Therapy, and the Relational World*. Washington, DC: American Psychological Association.

Wachtel, P. L. (2011). *Therapeutic Communication: Knowing What To Say When* (2nd ed.). New York, NY: Guilford.

Wachtel, P. L. (2014). *Cyclical Psychodynamics and the Contextual Self: The Inner World, the Intimate World, and the World of Culture and Society*. New York, NY: Routledge.

Westen, D. (1991). Social cognition and object relations. *Psychological Bulletin*, 109(3), 429.

Westen, D. (1998). The scientific legacy of Sigmund Freud: Toward a psychodynamically informed psychological science. *Psychological Bulletin*, 124(3), 333.

Whelton, W. J., & Greenberg, L. S. (2005). Emotion in self-criticism. *Personality & Individual Differences*, 38(7), 1583–1595.

Whiffen, V. E., Parker, G. B., Wilhelm, K., Mitchell, P. B., & Malhi, G. (2003). Parental care and personality in melancholic and nonmelancholic depression. *The Journal of Nervous and Mental Disease*, 191(6), 358–364.

Winnicott, D. W. (1955). Group influences and the maladjusted child: The school aspect. In *The Family and Individual Development* (pp. 146–155). London: Tavistock.

Winnicott, D. W. (1971). *Playing and Reality*. London: Routledge.

Yalom, I. D. (1980). *Existential Psychotherapy*. New York, NY: Basic.

Zepf, S. (2013). Where are we when we listen to music? *Canadian Journal of Psychoanalysis*, 21(2), 2013, 326–350.

Ziv-Beiman, S. (2013). Therapist self-disclosure as an integrative intervention. *Journal of Psychotherapy Integration*, 23, 59–74.

Zuroff, D. C., Moskowitz, D. S., Wielgus, M. S., Powers, T. A., & Franko, D. L. (1983). Construct validation of the dependency and self-criticism scales of the Depressive Experiences Questionnaire. *Journal of Research in Personality*, 17, 226–241.

Chapter

Finding the self in a cognitive behavioral perspective

David A. Clark

Introduction

Derek, a 33-year-old single man, employed in sales at a technology retailer, feels lost. He has struggled with feelings of depression and anxiety since early adolescence, and now, 20 years later, he seems to have made little progress with his life. He has suffered two episodes of major depression, one after his first year of university and the other five years ago. The first episode remitted with a trial of pharmacotherapy and the second with a combined treatment of antidepressant medication and cognitive behavior therapy (CBT). However, the effectiveness of the CBT was minimal, and Derek prematurely terminated treatment after 11 sessions. It seemed like the sessions were going nowhere, the treatment goals felt lofty and unattainable, and Derek repeatedly failed to follow through with his homework assignments. The therapy became a mirror reflection of Derek's approach to life: drifting, aimless, with no real purpose or meaning.

From a diagnostic perspective, Derek's symptom presentation is consistent with depressive personality disorder (see Clark & Hilchey, 2015). Although not an official diagnostic disorder in the ICD-10 (World Health Organization, 2013) or the DSM-5 (American Psychiatric Association, 2013), Derek's personality constellation was characterized by persistent unhappiness, belief in his own inadequacy and insignificance, heightened pessimism, lack of interest and goal-directedness, and negativity towards others. He had difficulty forming close, stable relationships with others, and had no real goals, ambitions or meaning. He was chronically underemployed and spent much of his free time gaming or binge-watching online movies. He had a nihilistic outlook on life, and often concluded

"why bother?" when it came to taking initiative. He actually felt sluggish much of the time, complaining that he often felt bored and disinterested.

The self is a critical construct in cognitive behavioral formulations. For individuals like Derek, who enter therapy with major personality problems, selfhood issues will be a major focus of the therapeutic enterprise. In fact treatment effectiveness will hinge on an ability to achieve change in biased and dysfunctional self-representation. And yet, work on the self is not only critical for CBT of personality disorders, but it is considered the key change process in CBT for a range of clinical disorders such as major depression, generalized anxiety disorder, eating disorders, and even obsessive–compulsive disorder. For Derek to move beyond his chronic depression, therapy must address his core self-beliefs of worthlessness, insignificance, criticalness, and ineffectiveness. If these fundamental issues of the self are left intact, Derek's treatment will never provide more than temporary symptomatic improvement.

This chapter focuses on the role of the self in cognitive therapy and CBT of the emotional disorders. Much of the research and theoretical development in CBT has focused on anxiety and depression, so it is reasonable to confine our review to these disorders. In this chapter the term *self-concept* or *self-representation* refers to characteristics or attributes that form meaning-based memory for oneself (i.e., self-knowledge), are subject to reflective processing, can be consciously acknowledged through language, and are integral to the regulation of thought, feeling, and behavior (Harter, 1999; Kihlstrom, Beer, & Klein, 2003; Leary & Tangney, 2003). Although self-concept is a multidimensional construct with a multiplicity of corresponding terms, it will be seen

The Self in Understanding and Treating Psychological Disorders, ed. Michael Kyrios, Richard Moulding, Guy Doron, Sunil S. Bhar, Maja Nedeljkovic, and Mario Mikulincer. Published by Cambridge University Press. © Cambridge University Press, 2016.

that CBT theory and treatment has mainly focused on self-concept content, that is, one's self-beliefs and self-evaluations, rather than self-concept structure, which is how self-concept is organized in terms of unity, pluralism, complexity, discrepancies, and the like (Campbell, Assanand, & Di Paula, 2003).

The chapter begins with a brief historical review of the role of the self in early theories of CBT. This is followed by a discussion of the self in contemporary CBT models of anxiety and depression. The chapter concludes by speculating on how a greater appreciation of the self might direct cognitive behavioral treatment of difficult emotional disorders, such as that described in the case of Derek with a depressive personality.

The self in early CBT

The self has always been recognized as an integral concept – even in the earliest versions of CBT. Ellis, for example, does not directly mention the self in rational-emotive therapy (RET), but the basic premise of RET, that psychological disturbance is the result of irrational thinking (Ellis, 1962), is predicated on the notion of a self as object. Most of the irrational beliefs identified in RET are beliefs that concern the self as it interacts with the social and even physical world. There is a strong sense of self-evaluation in the irrational beliefs of RET, but again this is not elaborated in the theory. Rather, RET is much more focused on self-relevant belief content, and how modification of these "irrational beliefs" can correct emotional disturbances like anxiety and depression (Ellis, 1962, 1977). Furthermore, RET is silent on how these negative construals of the self might lead to emotional disturbance. It is assumed their very existence and dominance in self-regulation will lead to excessive negative emotion and maladaptive behavior. Of course, the solution promoted in early RET was the adoption of more rational, realistic beliefs about the self and the personal world.

The publication of Michael Mahoney's *Cognitive and Behaviour Modification* in 1974 was a major contributor to the "cognitive revolution" that was emerging in behavior therapy. The main thesis of this work was an impassioned, empirically based argument for the importance of cognitive mediation in understanding the etiology and treatment of psychological disorders. Of course, an argument for cognitive mediation in the context of emotional disturbance is also an acknowledgment of the importance of the self in understanding psychopathology. Later in this publication, Mahoney provides an eloquent critical analysis of the construct of belief, concluding that concepts like beliefs, counter-control and choice do have a place in a scientific theory of human change. All of these constructs require a notion of self as both the knower (self as subject; I-self) and the object of being known (Me-self; James, 1890). Mahoney concludes by proposing a therapeutic orientation he called the personal scientist paradigm. One of the critical components of this approach is the acquisition of adaptive self-evaluative skills. Mahoney argues that evaluative self-reactions are predominant in the life of individuals, but unfortunately much of this self-evaluation is negative or dysfunctional. We see here an explicit recognition of the importance of self-representations in emotional disturbance, but the discussion is narrowly focused on the evaluative aspect of the self. Twenty years later, Mahoney (1995) embraced the constructivist perspective. In delineating future directions for constructivism psychotherapy, he noted that a greater appreciation of the centrality of the self is needed with recognition that psychotherapy is a participation in "selving processes" and that development of the self occurs through our most intimate relationships.

The original cognitive theory of emotional disorders formulated by Aaron T. Beck makes explicit reference to the importance of self-concept in depression. In his pioneering book *Depression: Causes and Treatment* (1967), Beck refers to a 1960 experiment in which he found that depressed patients endorsed more socially undesirable traits and fewer positive traits. He then proposed that a constellation of negative generalizations about the self constituted a specific vulnerability to depression, along with negative attitudes about the world and future. He further emphasized the importance of self-evaluation, noting that the depressogenic self not only possesses negative self-descriptions but also places high value or judgment on these traits. Thus, the belief "I am stupid" is only pathogenic if the person places high value on being intelligent. As well, Beck argued that self-blame is a key component of the depressogenic self, such that the person holds herself responsible for her deficiencies. In *Cognitive Therapy and the Emotional Disorders* (1976), he appears to again emphasize the self-evaluative aspect of the pathogenic self, noting that low self-esteem and self-criticalness derive from a tendency to compare oneself with others. Beck's seminal treatment manual on depression coined the term "cognitive triad" to refer to the three major negative cognitive patterns in depression: negative views of the self, the personal world, and the future (Beck, Rush, Shaw, & Emery, 1979). Once again, negative self-evaluation was emphasized as both a predisposition to, and characterization of, depression.

Publication of the cognitive therapy manual for anxiety disorders revealed that Beck also considered a pathogenic self to be applicable to generalized anxiety (Beck & Emery, 1985). Here the notion of "self" vulnerability to anxiety involved ideas of inadequacy, helplessness, and weakness so that individuals are susceptible to fears of negative evaluation and rejection by others. This belief that one is incompetent in dealing with problematic situations results in lowered self-confidence and increased likelihood of anxiety in relevant situations. Beck also noted that the self-view of the anxious person fluctuates with the degree of risk or danger perceived in a situation. The lowered self-confidence and self-criticism in anxiety is selective, activated only in anxious situations, whereas in depression the negative self-view is more global and pervasive.

Of the early cognitive clinical theories, Guidano and Liotti (1983) provided the most extensive elaboration of the role of the self or personal identity in psychological disorders. Drawing on both attachment and cognitive theories, Guidano and Liotto discuss how the development of a distorted self-knowledge structure (i.e., personal identity) will result in a rigid and defensive attitude toward oneself, and problems interacting with the real world. This disparity will cause a failure to distance and decenter from the negative, distorted ideas that constitute the self-concept. The failed distancing leads to an emotional self-knowledge that is undifferentiated and poorly controlled, which is evident in the dogmatic thinking often seen in emotional disorders.

Guidano and Liotto (1983) viewed personal identity in terms of the development of a complex cognitive structure that begins as a primitive, undifferentiated, largely intuitive self-conceptualization, and becomes progressively more elaborated through play, fantasy, and early attachment relationships. They noted two key aspects of personal identity relevant to psychopathology. The first, *self-identity*, refers to the traits and attitudes that individuals utilize to define the self. It is the interrelated beliefs one has about the self across various domains like attachments, duty, values, attributions of causality, and the like. *Self-esteem* is the second component of personal identity and refers to our tendency to engage in self-evaluation. The degree of congruence between beliefs about one's value and estimates of one's behavior and emotions will determine level of self-acceptance and self-esteem. In sum, representations of the self in the form of self-identity and self-esteem interact and influence how we perceive or understand our experience. To understand psychological disturbance, like obsessive compulsive disorders (OCD), one had to determine the aberrant personal identity and distorted self-evaluative component (Guidano & Liotto, 1983). In OCD, an ambivalent or contradictory self-identity leads to a form of interaction with the external world in which one feels forced to search for certainty and the perfect solution in order to rectify a state of indecision caused by the ambivalent self (see Chapter 12 by Ahern and Kyrios in this volume).

Early cognitive theories readily recognized the importance of a negative and biased self-view in the etiology and maintenance of emotional disturbance. However, with the exception of Guidano and Liotto (1983), there was little consideration of the development of biased self-representation or the mediating processes responsible for its influence on psychopathology. Also, there was a rather simplistic view of the self that overemphasized self-evaluation or self-esteem as the chief progenitor of psychological disturbance. Other aspects of the self, such as aberration in structure, organization, function, access, and change, were rarely mentioned.

The self in current CBT theories

Theory, research, and treatment have continued to evolve since those early years of the "cognitive revolution." The self has continued to play an important role in the cognitive-behavioral perspective, but it has not taken center stage in our conceptualizations. Advances in psychological theories about the self have had minimal impact on more contemporary cognitive behavioral theories. Despite some apparent "shunning" of the self by cognitive behavioral researchers, there are some glimmers of progress. The first is the continued development of Beck's cognitive theory, the concept of mode and the centrality of the self-schema. Second, certain selfhood theories have been mentioned in the CBT literature, notably Markus' self-schema research, Higgins' self-discrepancy theory, Linville's concept of self-complexity, and the influence of contradictory or feared elements of the self. We now examine a selection of these self-related topics in current CBT formulations.

The elaborated cognitive theory

The schema construct is central to Beck's (1996) cognitive model. Schemas are relatively enduring internal structures of stored information that guide and organize the processing of new information in a manner that determines how phenomena are perceived and interpreted (Clark & Beck, 1999). The critical schemas in the emotional disorders are biased in content and distorted in their structure and organization (Beck, 1967, 1987). In depression, schematic content is excessively focused on negative self-referent material, whereas in anxiety the schemas are oriented around threat, danger, and helplessness. Beck (1996) noted that there are different types of schemas, with the cognitive-conceptual schemas being most relevant to the current discussion. According to Beck, these schemas are critical to the selection, storage, retrieval, and interpretation of information. The cognitive-conceptual schemas provide an internal representation of the self, or self-concept, which constitutes our self-identity, personal goals and values (Clark & Beck, 1999). Together with other schema types, an interrelated schematic array or mode is constituted that relates to particular demands placed on the organism (Beck, 1996). In depression, a *loss mode* predominates, whereas in anxiety the *threat mode* is activated.

In their elaboration of the cognitive model of depression, Clark and Beck (1999) proposed that the cognitive-conceptual schemas of self-knowledge form an interrelated array of schemas we call the self-concept. They identified a number of characteristics that may be important to consider in the dysfunctional self such as (a) the importance or centrality of specific self-representations, (b) whether beliefs represent actual or idealized aspects of the self, (c) the temporal orientation of the beliefs, (d) the valence of the beliefs, (e) the degree of certainty or efficiency associated with the schema, (f) the self-schema's basis in few or varied external referents, (g) the degree of self-belief accessibility, (h) the level of self-schema complexity, and (i) the extent of the interpersonal orientation of self-beliefs. However, as cognitive clinical researchers have tended to focus on schematic content and valence, the importance of these other self-schema characteristics still remains speculative at this time.

Two self-report measures especially important to the measurement of self-schema content are the Beck Self-Concept Test (BSCT; Beck, Steer, Epstein, & Brown, 1990) and the Dysfunctional Attitudes Scale (DAS; Weissman & Beck, 1978). The BSCT was developed to assess characteristics of self-concept relevant to Beck's cognitive triad. Individuals rate themselves on 25 self-relevant domains (e.g., appearance, knowledge, popularity, personality, etc.) in comparison to other people they know, with high scores indicating a more positive self-view. As expected, the BSCT evidenced significant negative correlations with measures of depressive but not anxious symptoms, and depressed patients scored significantly lower than non-depressed individuals. Unfortunately, the BSCT has not been widely used in CBT research, so not much is known about the specific selfhood elements assessed by this measure.

The DAS is a widely researched measure of cognitive vulnerability for depression. Because most, but not all, of the DAS belief statements have a self-referent orientation, the questionnaire can be viewed as a proxy measure of self-concept ("Who I think I am"), although the items reflect an extreme and maladaptive perspective on the self. Some items are highly self-referent (e.g., "I do not need other people's approval for me to be happy," "I should set higher standards for myself than other people"), whereas others are more generalized beliefs about life (e.g., "People will reject you if they know your weaknesses," "If a person is not a success, then his life is meaningless"). Given this ambiguity and complexity in item structure (i.e., use of "if–then" propositional statements), the DAS can be considered only a retrospective self-report measure of some relevance to the self-concept.

A large research literature has shown that clinically depressed individuals have higher DAS scores, that high pre-treatment scores predict poorer response to treatment, that dysfunctional attitudes can be primed by negative mood state in those vulnerable to depression, and that dysfunctional attitudes interact with negative life events as causal factors in depression onset (for reviews see Brown & Beck, 2002; Clark & Beck, 1999). However, there has been little research into the actual selfhood pathology tapped by the DAS. For example, are some DAS self-beliefs more pathological than others, or are some of these beliefs more central to the self-concept than others? Currently respondents rate their level of agreement or disagreement with each statement, but does this metric accurately capture the level of belief or the centrality of the belief to the person's self-concept? In sum there is a greater need for item-level analysis of the DAS in order to disentangle the selfhood aspects of the measure.

One of the best examples of selfhood research within CBT is work published on self-schema organization in depression by Dozois and colleagues. Dozois and Dobson (2001a) utilized a procedure called the Psychological Distance Scaling Task (PDST) where individuals position positive and negative trait adjectives within a two-dimensional space defined by a self-descriptiveness x-axis and a valence y-axis. The coordinate point (x- and y-axis) for each adjective is calculated and the average interstimulus distance among the positive schematic adjectives and negative schematic adjectives is determined. These averages reflect the degree of interconnectedness among the schematic adjectives, with lower average values reflecting greater interconnectedness. The PBST negative stimulus distance was correlated with depressive symptoms, and other indices of self-referent processing such as endorsement and recall on the Self-Referent Encoding Task (Dozois & Dobson, 2001a). In their first study, Dozois and Dobson (2001a) found that depressed patients had fewer interconnected positive schema adjectives than anxious patients, but both clinical groups had greater interconnectedness for negative adjectives than the non-clinical controls. A later study found that negative cognitive structure may persist even when depressive symptoms remit, whereas remitted depressed individuals showed an increase in positive self-schema interconnectedness (Dozois & Dobson, 2001b).

More recent research has indicated that stronger interconnectedness of negative self-schema may be particularly prominent in the interpersonal domain, that negative self-schema organization interacts with negative life event occurrence to predict increase in depressive symptoms, and negative interpersonal self-schema organization remains stable beyond symptom amelioration (Dozois, 2007; Seeds & Dozois, 2010). Furthermore, in a treatment outcome study, only the cognitive therapy plus medication group showed significant improvement in positive and negative interpersonal self-schema connectedness compared to a medication-only group (Dozois et al., 2009).

The PDST research is an excellent example of the deeper understanding and clinical utility associated with selfhood research within a CBT framework. This research provides important new insights into cognitive vulnerability for depression as well as influences on response to treatment. At the very least, it demonstrates that an exclusive focus on self-view content or the self-evaluative process might miss important features of the role that selfhood pathology plays in psychological disorders. And yet, it also reminds us that the role of the self can be complex. For example, should CBT therapists be more concerned about the dominance of negative self-beliefs or the coherence of the negative self-structure? Regardless of depression status, self-concept will comprise an array of negative and positive self-beliefs. Possibly clinicians should be more concerned with the presence of a well-structured negative self-system than the nature of the depressed person's self-beliefs. Likewise, researchers have still not determined the relative functional significance of highly dominant negative self-beliefs versus a poorly developed positive self-system. From a clinical perspective, should therapists be more concerned with weakening negative self-beliefs or strengthening a positive self-view? The core treatment elements of CBT, such as cognitive restructuring, were developed to modify negative self-beliefs. There is considerable research evidence that the interpersonal domain is especially important in depression. Consequently, mastery or achievement may be less important, although it is possible that other self-relevant domains are key constructs in other disorders. For example, appearance would be more central to eating disorders and control might be more critical in the anxiety disorders. Clearly, what is needed is a greater degree of content-specificity in selfhood research because of the congruence between specific selfhood domains and particular disorders. Although many key questions remain, the fundamental importance of self-schema organization has been established.

Self-schemas, complexity and incongruence

While selfhood theory and research has not been well-integrated into cognitive behavioral models and treatment of emotional disorders, one can certainly find cognitive behavioral research that is well-informed by self-system conceptualizations. For instance, Higgins' (1987) self-discrepancy theory has had some recognition within the CBT literature. In this section we focus on three other selfhood influences that can be found in CBT models: self-schemas, self-complexity, and self-incongruence. Additional discussion about important dimensions and constructs of self used in psychopathology research can be found in Bhar and Kyrios (this volume).

Self-schemas

Markus (1977) defined self-schemas as "cognitive generalisations about the self, derived from past experience, that organise and guide the processing of self-related information contained in the individual's social experience" (p. 64). She noted that self-schematic structures facilitate the processing of schema-congruent information, retrieve relevant behavioral evidence, predict future behavior, and resist incongruent self-schema information. Clearly, the concept of self-schema converges easily with Beck's schema-based cognitive theory of emotional disorders. In her introduction to a special issue of *Cognitive Therapy and Research* on self-schema in psychopathology, Markus (1990) noted that most of the self-schema research has focused on differences in schematic content across various domains, such that the self-schemas in depression focus on personal loss or failure, those in anxiety deal with threat and vulnerability, those in the eating disorders body appearance and size, and the like.

Over the years there has been considerable evidence that differences in self-schematic content are important in characterizing the pathogenesis of various psychological disorders. However, Markus (1990) and others have noted that self-schema structural differences may also play a critical role in defining the role of the self in psychopathology. Issues such as degree of connectedness or elaboration within disorder-relevant aspects of the self-system (see discussion of Dozois and colleagues' work above), the centrality of disorder-relevant schemas within the self-system, the degree of differentiation or complexity, and the types of beliefs within the self-schema (i.e., conditional beliefs, generalized assumptions, etc.) have not been adequately researched from a cognitive behavioral perspective. Valence has always been an important attribute of emotion-related schemas, but the actual role and function of positive and negative self-schemas has not been clearly articulated. For example, is it the number of negative self-schemas that is critical or the relative importance (i.e., centrality) of certain core negative schemas that determines their influence in emotional disturbance? On the other hand, can the presence of well-elaborated positive self-schemas offset the impact of negative self-schemas, or might this only occur within a particular situational context? To illustrate, an individual with a depressive personality disorder has well-elaborated negative self-schemas of loss, failure, criticalness, and rejection (Clark & Hilchey, 2015).

Might there be a threshold of positive experience (e.g., an unexpected salary increase) that would cause less-elaborated positive self-schemas to override the more dominant negative self-schema? Indeed, there is much to be learned about the dynamic interplay between negative and positive self-schemas, activating situations and the generation of negative emotion.

Self-complexity

Linville (1985, 1987) states that knowledge about the self consists of multiple cognitive structures called self-aspects that form an associative network. Self-representation differs in terms of the number of self-aspects or structures and their distinctiveness. Greater self-complexity consists of having a greater number of self-aspects and greater distinctiveness among the self-aspects. Linville (1987) predicted that lower self-complexity is associated with more negative change in affect and self-evaluation following a negative event, and a more positive change in affect and self-appraisal following a positive event. In sum, low self-complexity predisposes to greater reactivity to life experiences, whereas higher self-complexity acts as a buffer against stress-related illness and depression. In the original study, Linville (1987) assessed 106 undergraduates for life events, self-complexity, illnesses, and physical and depressive symptoms on two occasions separated by a two-week interval. Regression analyses indicated that students with higher self-complexity had less depression and fewer physical symptoms at Time 2 following self-reported stressful events. Linville (1987) concluded that greater self-complexity acted as a protective buffer against the negative physical and emotional consequences of stressful events.

Initially, self-complexity garnered considerable interest among clinical researchers because the construct was formulated as a predictor of resilience to emotional disturbance. It also fit nicely into a diathesis–stress framework, which has been the dominant etiological perspective in CBT models (see Ingram & Price, 2010 for discussion). However, subsequent research has produced mixed findings that often have not shown a relationship between self-complexity and psychological adjustment. In their meta-analysis, Rafaeli-Mor and Steinberg (2002) concluded there was little support for the mood-buffering effect of high self-complexity, and, in fact, high self-complexity may have a mild depressogenic effect by moderating the positive effects of uplifting events. In discussing this rather contrary conclusion, Rafaeli-Mor and Steinberg (2002) wondered whether a more highly differentiated self (i.e., high self-complexity) might actually reflect fragmentation or lack of a core identity, and so represent a pathological feature of the self.

It is possible that the discouraging findings could be due to methodological and measurement variance across studies. More recently, Brown and Rafaeli (2007) deconstructed self-complexity into two components: number of self-aspects (i.e., differentiation) and degree of overlap among self-aspects (i.e, integration). In one study, fewer self-aspects predicted increased dysphoria under high stress and decreased dysphoria under low stress. In the second study, more self-aspects and greater overlap interacted with severe but not mundane stressors to predict less depression. This latter finding is consistent with self-complexity as a buffer against stress. Nevertheless, these findings indicate that it might be more advantageous for clinical researchers to focus on the differentiation (number of self-aspects) rather than integration (degree of overlap) component of self-complexity. As well, the nature of the stressor, whether a daily hassle or major life event, may be critical in determining whether high self-complexity is a protective or vulnerability factor in emotional disturbance.

Self-incongruence

The term "self-incongruence" is used to describe recent research that investigates the influence of unwanted, feared, or inconsistent aspects of the self. This research attempts to understand the etiology of anxiety, especially OCD, in terms of an incongruent self. Bhar and Kyrios (2007) proposed that the problem in obsessional disorders is an ambivalent self-view. Based on Guidano and Liotti's (1983) concept of self-ambivalence, Bhar and Kyrios argued that individuals with OCD may be especially prone to interpret ego-dystonic intrusions as meaningful threats to valued aspects of the self, whereas non-obsessional individuals with a more established self-view would reject such self-recriminating or contradictory thinking in order to protect their positive sense of self-worth. Moreover, self-ambivalent individuals are thought to hold contradictory and opposing self-views so an unwanted intrusion becomes evidence for the negative as opposed to positive self-view. In a study of self-ambivalence in clinical and nonclinical samples, Bhar and Kyrios (2007) found

that both self-worth ambivalence and moral ambivalence were related to OCD symptoms and beliefs but both were also elevated in anxious controls. This suggests that self-ambivalence may be evident in a range of psychological disorders and not just OCD.

Doron and Kyrios (2005) proposed that OCD is characterized by a self-concept that involves relatively few domains of competence. Unwanted thoughts that signify failure in these "sensitive domains" threaten an individual's self-worth and so have processing priority in terms of heightened attention, evaluation, and associated distress (Moulding, Aardema, & O'Connor, 2014). Doron, Kyrios, and Moulding (2007) found that sensitivity in the moral and job-competence domains was related to obsessive–compulsive symptoms and beliefs in a non-clinical sample. A subsequent clinical study found that sensitivity in the moral, and to a lesser extent, job-competence domains was specific to OCD (Doron, Moulding, Kyrios, & Nedeljkovic, 2008). Furthermore, an experimental study in which students were primed to perceive incompetence in the moral self-domain found that the induction of negative moral self-perceptions increased self-rated urges to engage in neutralization-like responses to hypothetical contamination-relevant scenarios (Doron, Sar-El, & Mikulincer, 2012). In sum, there is emerging evidence that low moral self-perception may be especially relevant in the etiology of OCD. It would be interesting to know whether elevated sensitivity to perceived deficiencies in specific self-worth domains of competence characterize other disorders as well.

Finally, Aardema and O'Connor (2007) offered a perspective on selfhood themes in obsessions that is linked to their inference-based theory of OCD. They begin by noting that obsessional concerns center on a possible cognitive or mental state in which the person with obsessions makes an inferential error that assumes the cognitive intrusion (obsession) is an accurate reflection of the self. It is noted that we all construct a narrative about ourselves that is an attempt to explain our behavior and the non-conscious processes that operate outside conscious awareness. However, what is unique in obsessional states is that discordant self-representations play an integral role in self-representation. This occurs because individuals with OCD commit a number of reasoning errors that attribute a greater degree of reality to thoughts of a possible self. A negative self-representation that involves a possibility (e.g., "What if I lose control and harm my children?") becomes confused with a reality (e.g., "Because I am thinking this way, I must be capable of harming my children") so the individual acts as if the possible were a real probability. The individual then becomes immersed in "a fear of who they could be or might become" (Aardema & O'Connor, 2007, p. 191). In the obsessional sense of self, the individual is heavily invested in the "self-as-could-be" and less invested in the self-as-is. The end result is a strong sense of self-doubt and a distrust of the self-as-is (i.e., the actual or real self). In sum, the obsession is always objectively discordant with the actual self (i.e., ego-dystonic) because it is based on a faulty inference involving a fear of a nonexistent self (Aardema & O'Connor, 2007). Recently, a Fear of Self Questionnaire was developed that showed strong correlations with obsessive–compulsive symptoms, beliefs, and inferential confusion in non-clinical samples (Aardema *et al.*, 2013). As well, fear of self emerged as a significant unique predictor of unacceptable or repugnant obsessions in an OCD sample (Melli, Aardema, & Moulding, 2015). In an inference-induction experiment, feared self-beliefs were related to levels of doubt associated with hypothetical contamination and checking vignettes, especially when the vignette was associated with a possibility-based inference (Nikodijevic, Moulding, Anglim, Aardema, & Nedeljkovic, in press). Clearly, what we fear becoming is an aspect of self-definition that holds promise in understanding vulnerability to obsessions. We can assume that the same perspective might hold true for other clinical disorders such as panic or eating disorders where, for example, a self that lacks control might be a particularly horrifying prospect.

Although the research on self-schemas and self-complexity is well-established, its application to clinical problems has been relatively scant. The few CBT studies that have been conducted suggest that the preoccupation with self-view content and evaluation may be limiting our insights into the role of the self in the psychopathology and treatment of anxiety and depression. However, as the self-complexity research indicates, finer-grained analysis of self structure and function may not always produce a clearer picture of the self in emotional disorders. Nevertheless, a more concentrated research agenda is needed to more fully understand the nature of a "pathological self." New avenues of research, such as the role of incongruent self-views, may improve our understanding of the self in CBT models of emotional disturbance.

Clinical application and future directions

Even though a dysfunctional self is clearly implicated in cognitive behavioral theories of anxiety and depression, self-representational theory and research have not had a significant impact on cognitive behavioral treatment. In this closing section, I speculate on how CBT could be improved by a greater appreciation of self-representational processes in a difficult case such as Derek. The cognitive behavioral therapist might start by determining the complexity of Derek's self-identity. Does he tend to identify with a few, highly valued negative self-attributes such as distrust of others, pessimism about his future, and the futility of effortful engagement in work, or is his self-identity more fragmented and diversified, with a more equalized valuation across various self-attributes? Cognitive intervention could be adjusted so it either focuses on scaling down the significance of certain self-attributes or bolstering the importance of under-valued attributes.

Another feature that the therapist might consider is the degree of congruence or interconnectedness of positive and negative self-attributes. It is likely that Derek has a few highly interconnected negative attributes. It may be that these connections could be loosened with learning experiences that provide a degree of incongruence between the negative attributes. For example, let's assume that Derek is highly pessimistic about his future and distrustful of the intentions of others. His belief might be "people enjoy seeing me fail and make a fool of myself." In this case, Derek could be asked to engage in some sort of team activity in which others were truly hoping he would succeed. A greater appreciation of the self could actually help the cognitive behavioral therapist develop homework assignments with greater accuracy in modifying specific elements of the dysfunctional self.

It is likely that very few therapists ever consider the role that incongruent aspects of the self might play in a person's emotional disturbance. Derek, for example, had a strong fear of being disappointed. Disappointment in one's self was distressing, so he always expected the worst of himself and others. A therapist who appreciates the importance of this incongruence could then introduce interventions that focus on tolerance of disappointment in self and others. However, it would be difficult to arrive at such a case formulation without an assessment of incongruent self-aspects.

There is little doubt that cognitive behavioral theories and treatment of the emotional disorders would benefit from a greater appreciation of self-representational processes. There are a number of promising research areas on the self that could enrich CBT theory and treatment. One issue that remains unresolved is the relative contribution of negative and positive self-structure in the emotional disorders. CBT researchers and clinicians tend to view clinical disorders as a preponderance of a negative self-representation, and yet numerous studies suggest that the greater problem might be ill-defined or deficit positive self-representation. Whether this represents a bias in our research or a valid account of the emotional disorders remains to be seen. Second, our research has tended to focus on a dysfunctional self as a causal factor in clinical disorders, and yet, it is highly likely that negative emotion itself has a profound influence on self structure. In CBT we have tended to neglect the influence of emotion on self-representation. Third, structural aspects of the self such as its complexity, level of cohesion or interconnectedness, differentiation, and the like no doubt interact with self-belief domains (interpersonal, achievement, vitality, etc.) and valence to determine the onset and course of emotional disturbance. More complex multidimensional modelling of the self and emotion could hold new insights into the etiology of anxiety and depression. There can be little doubt that a greater appreciation of the self in CBT research and treatment might be one of the most important imperatives for the next generation of cognitive behavioral therapists.

References

Aardema, F., Moulding, R., Radomsky, A. S., *et al.* (2013). Fear of self and obsessionality: Development and validation of the Fear of Self Questionnaire. *Journal of Obsessive–Compulsive and Related Disorders*, 2, 306–315.

Aardema, F., & O'Connor, K. (2007). The menace within: Obsessions and the self. *Journal of Cognitive Psychotherapy: An International Quarterly*, 21, 182–197.

American Psychiatric Association. (2013). *Diagnostic and Statistical Manual of Mental Disorders* (5th ed.). Washington, DC: American Psychiatric Association.

Beck, A. T. (1967). *Depression: Causes and Treatment*. Philadelphia: University of Pennsylvania Press.

Beck, A. T. (1976). *Cognitive Therapy and the Emotional Disorders*. New York, NY: New American Library.

Beck, A. T. (1987). Cognitive models of depression. *Journal of Cognitive Psychotherapy: An International Quarterly*, 1, 5–37.

Beck, A. T. (1996). Beyond belief: A theory of modes, personality, and psychopathology. In: P. M. Salkovsksi (Ed.), *Frontiers of Cognitive Therapy* (pp. 1–25). New York, NY: Guilford Press.

Beck, A. T. & Emery, G. (with Greenberg, R. L.)(1985). *Anxiety Disorders and Phobias: A Cognitive Perspective*. New York, NY: Basic Books.

Beck, A. T., Steer, R. A., Epstein, N., & Brown, G. (1990). Beck Self-Concept Test. *Psychological Assessment*, 2, 191–197.

Beck, A. T., Rush, A. J., Shaw, B. F., & Emery, G. (1979). *Cognitive Therapy of Depression*. New York, NY: Guilford Press.

Bhar, S. S., & Kyrios, M. (2007). An investigation of self-ambivalence in obsessive–compulsive disorder. *Behaviour Research and Therapy*, 45, 1845–1857.

Brown, G. P., & Beck, A. T. (2002). Dysfunctional attitudes, perfectionism, and models of vulnerability to depression. In G. L. Flett & P. L. Hewitt (Eds.), *Perfectionism: Theory, Research, and Treatment* (pp. 231–251). Washington, DC: American Psychological Association.

Brown, G. P. & Rafaeli, E. (2007). Components of self-complexity as buffers for depressed mood. *Journal of Cognitive Psychotherapy: An International Quarterly*, 21, 310–333.

Campbell, J. D., Assanand, S.,& Di Paula, A. (2003). The structure of the self-concept and its relation to psychological adjustment. *Journal of Personality*, 71, 115–140.

Clark, D. A. & Beck, A. T. (with Alford, B.)(1999). *Scientific Foundations of Cognitive Theory and Therapy of Depression*. New York, NY: Wiley.

Clark, D. A. & Hilchey, C. A. (2015). Depressive personality disorder. In: A. T. Beck, D. D. Davis, & A. Freeman (Eds.), *Cognitive Therapy of Personality Disorders* (3rd ed., pp. 223–243). New York, NY: Guilford Press.

Doron, G., & Kyrios, M. (2005). Obsessive compulsive disorder: A review of possible specific internal representations within a broader cognitive theory. *Clinical Psychology Review*, 25, 415–432.

Doron, G., Kyrios, M., & Moulding, R. (2007). Sensitive domains of self-concept in obsessive–compulsive disorder (OCD): Further evidence for a multidimensional model of OCD. *Journal of Anxiety Disorders*, 21, 433–444.

Doron, G., Moulding, R., Kyrios, M., & Nedeljkovic, M. (2008). Sensitivity of self-beliefs in obsessive-compulsive disorder. *Depression and Anxiety*, 25, 874–884.

Doron, G., Sar-El, D., & Mikulincer, M. (2012). Threats to moral self-perceptions trigger obsessive compulsive contamination-related behavioral tendencies. *Journal of Behavior Therapy & Experimental Psychiatry*, 43, 884–890.

Dozois, D. J. A. (2007). Stability of negative self-structures: A longitudinal comparison of depressed, remitted, and nonpsychiatric controls. *Journal of Clinical Psychology*, 63, 319–338.

Dozois, D. J. A., Bieling, P. J., Patelis-Siotis, I., *et al.* (2009). Changes in self-schema structure in cognitive therapy for major depressive disorder: A randomized clinical trial. *Journal of Consulting and Clinical Psychology*, 77, 1078–1088.

Dozois, D. J. A., & Dobson, K. S. (2001a). Information processing and cognitive organization in unipolar depression: Specificity and comorbidity issues. *Journal of Abnormal Psychology,* 110, 236–246.

Dozois, D. J. A., & Dobson, K. S. (2001b). A longitudinal investigation of information processing and cognitive organization in clinical depression: Stability of schematic interconnectedness. *Journal of Consulting and Clinical Psychology*, 69, 914–925.

Ellis, A. (1962). *Reason and Emotion in Psychotherapy.* Secaucus, NJ: The Citadel Press.

Ellis, A. (1977). The basic clinical theory of rational-emotive therapy. In A. Ellis & R. Grieger (Eds.), *Handbook of Rational-emotive Therapy* (pp. 3–34). New York, NY: Springer Publishing.

Guidano, V. F., & Liotti, G. (1983). *Cognitive Processes and Emotional Disorders.* New York, NY: Guilford Press.

Harter, S. (1999). *The Construction of the Self: A Developmental Perspective.* New York, NY: Guilford Press.

Higgins, E. T. (1987). Self-discrepancy: A theory relating self and affect. *Psychological Review*, 94, 319–340.

Ingram, R. E., & Price, J. M. (2010). Understanding psychopathology: The role of vulnerability. In R. E. Ingram & J. M. Price (Eds.), *Vulnerability to Psychopathology: Risk Across the Lifespan* (2nd ed., pp. 3–17). New York, NY: Guilford Press.

James, W. (1890). *Principles of Psychology.* Chicago, IL: Encyclopedia Britannica.

Kihlstrom, J. H., Beer, J. S., & Klein, S. B. (2003). Self and identity as memory. In M. R. Leary & J. P. Tangney (Eds.), *Handbook of Self and Identity* (pp. 68–90). New York, NY: Guilford Press.

Leary, M. R., & Tangney, J. P. (2003). The self as an organizing construct in the behavioral and social sciences. In M. R. Leary & J. P. Tangney (Eds.), *Handbook of Self and Identity* (pp. 3–14). New York, NY: Guilford Press.

Linville, P. W. (1985). Self-complexity and affective extremity: Don't put all your eggs in one cognitive basket. *Social Cognition*, 3, 94–120.

Linville, P. W. (1987). Self-complexity as a cognitive buffer against stress-related illness and depression. *Journal of Personality and Social Psychology*, 52, 663–676.

Mahoney, M. J. (1974). *Cognition and Behavior Modification.* Cambridge, MA: Ballinger Publishing Company.

Mahoney, M. J. (1995). Continuing evolution of the cognitive sciences and psychotherapies. In R. A. Neimeyer & M. J. Mahoney (Eds.), *Constructivism in Psychotherapy* (pp. 39–67). Washington, DC: American Psychological Association Publications.

Markus, H. (1977). Self-schemata and processing information about the self. *Journal of Personality and Social Psychology*, 35, 63–78.

Markus, H. (1990). Unresolved issues of self-representation. *Cognitive Therapy and Research*, 14, 241–253.

Melli, G., Aardema, F., & Moulding, R. (2015). Fear of self and unacceptable thoughts in obsessive–compulsive disorder. *Clinical Psychology and Psychotherapy*, doi: 10.1002/cpp.1950

Moulding, R., Aardema, F., & O'Connor, K. P. (2014). Repugnant obsessions: A review of the phenomenology, theoretical models, and treatment of sexual and aggressive obsessional themes in OCD. *Journal of Obsessive-Compulsive and Related Disorders*, 3, 161–168.

Nikodijevic, A., Moulding, R., Anglim, J., Aardema, F., & Nedeljkovic, M. (in press). Fear of self, doubt and obsessive compulsive symptoms. *Journal of Behavior Therapy and Experimental Psychiatry* (2015) http://dx.doi.org/10.1016/j.jbtep.2015.02.005

Rafaeli-Mor, E., & Steinberg, J. (2002). Self-complexity and well-being: A review and research synthesis. *Personality and Social Psychology Review*, 6, 31–58.

Seeds, P. M., & Dozois, D. J. A. (2010). Prospective evaluation of a cognitive vulnerability–stress model for depression: The interaction of schema self-structure and negative life events. *Journal of Clinical Psychology*, 66, 1307–1323.

Weissman, M. M., & Beck, A. T. (1978). *Development and validation of the Dysfunctional Attitudes Scale.* Paper presented at the annual meeting of the Association for the Advancement of Behavior Therapy, Chicago, IL.

World Health Organization. (2013). *International Classification of Diseases and Related Health Problems* (10th rev.). Geneva: World Health Organization.

Chapter

6

The self in acceptance and commitment therapy

Robert D. Zettle

Overview of ACT

Acceptance and commitment therapy (ACT) is regarded as part of the "third wave" of cognitive-behavioral therapy (CBT) that has emerged over the past quarter century (Hayes, 2004). It is a trans-diagnostic approach recognized by Division 12 of the American Psychological Association (Society of Clinical Psychology, n.d.) as having strong research support in the treatment of chronic pain and modest empirical support in addressing depression, mixed anxiety, obsessive–compulsive disorder, and psychosis. Rather than seeking to directly change problematic thoughts, emotions, and other private events, ACT and related approaches within the latest generation of CBT writ large incorporate mindfulness, acceptance, and decentering/defusion strategies to change the function of such psychological events and alter how clients relate to them (Hayes, Luoma, Bond, Masuda, & Lillis, 2006).

Unlike other third-wave approaches such as dialectical behavior therapy (Linehan, 1993), mindfulness-based cognitive therapy (MBCT; Segal, Williams, & Teasdale, 2002), and metacognitive therapy (Wells, 2009), ACT is unique in (a) being explicitly grounded within a modern pragmatic philosophy of behavioral science known as functional contextualism (Hayes, 1993), (b) being informed by relational frame theory as an associated account of human language and cognition (Hayes, Barnes-Holmes, & Roche, 2001), and (c) identifying increased psychological flexibility, or the ability to make behavioral adjustments in the service of one's values, as its superordinate goal. Some discussion of each of these defining features of ACT is necessary to understand its stance on the self.

Functional contextualism

As it pertains to psychology, functional contextualism can be seen as a refinement of many of the basic tenets first articulated within Skinner's (1974) philosophy of radical behaviorism (Vilardaga, Hayes, Levin, & Muto, 2009). These include the instigation of deliberate behavioral change as a pragmatic goal of psychology and viewing all human activity, including what psychologists say and do in studying it, as a function of the current situational and historical contexts within which behavior occurs. Beyond psychology, functional contextualism is more usefully viewed as a paradigmatic approach to a comprehensive behavioral science formed by integrating psychology with biology, sociology, anthropology, and any other related disciplines that can contribute to the goal of predicting and influencing human behavior with sufficient precision, scope, and depth. Interested readers are encouraged to consult Biglan and Hayes (1996) and Hayes, Barnes-Holmes, and Wilson (2012) for more detailed coverage of functional contextualism and contextual behavioral science, respectively, than can be provided here.

Of greatest relevance for the purpose of this chapter is recognition that functional contextualism holds "successful working" as its truth criterion. The words, terms, concepts, and other verbal constructions that proponents and practitioners of ACT use in speaking about the self are accordingly seen as mere tools. As with any tools, their value or "truth" is to be ultimately determined by whether they serve their intended practical purpose within ACT of increasing psychological flexibility and alleviating human suffering, and not by

The Self in Understanding and Treating Psychological Disorders, ed. Michael Kyrios, Richard Moulding, Guy Doron, Sunil S. Bhar, Maja Nedeljkovic, and Mario Mikulincer. Published by Cambridge University Press. © Cambridge University Press, 2016.

the degree to which the words or concepts map onto or correspond to some external reality (Pepper, 1942). In short, when the self is talked about in ACT, no assertion is being made about the ontological status of some psychological entity or agent. To the extent that certain "self-language" is used in speaking about and conducting ACT, it is because doing so in those particular ways has at least so far been useful.

Relational frame theory

The pragmatic and functional contextualistic perspective taken towards the verbal behavior of both clients and therapists within ACT has been explicated most thoroughly within relational frame theory (RFT; Hayes *et al.*, 2001). Many organisms show an ability to respond to the relationship among stimuli based on their physical properties (Reese, 1968; e.g., a pigeon can be trained to reliably peck the larger of two discs). However, in the absence of intellectual and developmental disabilities, only humans – from around the same age that language acquisition occurs – have demonstrated relational responding under arbitrary stimulus control as well as an ability to derive untrained relationships among stimuli/relata within a network (Barnes-Holmes *et al.*, 2001).

Deriving relationships among stimuli based on arbitrary rather than physical properties is viewed within RFT as generalized operant behavior that normally originates through informal discrete trial training involving vocal and verbal interactions between young children and their caretakers. For example, children may learn through conversations with adults that the relative value of coins may not be determined by differences in size; i.e., a smaller coin may buy more candy than a larger one. Once acquired, however, relational framing may be maintained not only by the prevention and solution of problems, but also through a self-sustaining coherence-producing process (Torneke, 2010). In much the same way that self-stimulatory behaviors may be maintained by the sensory consequences they produce (Lovaas, Newsome, & Hickman, 1987), constructing elaborate relational networks about our lives and who we are may be supported in part by their "making sense" (Wray, Dougher, Hamilton, & Guinther, 2012).

The developmental process of relational responding is perhaps illustrated most readily in the establishment of coordinational framing through naming. Multiple instances of adult reinforcement for correctly pointing to identified objects ("Where's the ball?") and naming them ("What is this?") by children establish generalized relational frames of coordination, equivalence, or identity between objects and words (i.e., "This is a that"). Unfortunately, as will be seen, similar relational frames surrounding the self (e.g., "I am a failure") can also be constructed with potentially profound psychological implications.

Defining properties of relational framing

From an RFT perspective, the emotional impact of such self-statements is best comprehended by considering the three defining properties of relational framing: (a) mutual entailment, (b) combinatorial entailment, and (c) transformation of stimulus functions.

Mutual entailment

The bidirectional nature of mutual entailment, or responding to one event in terms of the other and vice versa, is not limited to frames of coordination (e.g., if I'm told that Bill is older than Joe, Joe being younger than Bill can be derived), as illustrated by naming. There is a correspondence between words ("ball") and things ("spherical toys") such that they are equivalent to and can be derived from each other. Similarly, the statement "I am a failure" places "I" and "failure" in a relational frame of identity with each other such that "I" = "failure" and "failure" = "I."

Combinatorial entailment

The property of combinatorial entailment points to relationships that can be derived between relata that are each mutually entailed with a shared stimulus. This can be illustrated by comparative framing; for example, if I am a failure compared to Bill, and Bill is a failure compared to Joe, then I am also a failure relative to Joe.

Transformation of stimulus functions

Identifying oneself as a failure in either an absolute or comparative sense would ostensibly be devoid of any negative emotional impact were it not for the transformation of stimulus functions as the third defining feature of relational framing. The negative emotional connotations of the word "failure" can in effect become transferred and attached to who I take myself to be when I describe myself in that way. This dominance of certain derived stimulus functions over other derived and direct stimulus functions is what is referred to in ACT as fusion (Strosahl, Hayes, Wilson, & Gifford,

2004, p. 39). "I am a failure" and its psychological consequences exemplify fusion with a flawed conceptualized self. The self-statement has meaning and is responded to not as mere words, but as an essential and literally truthful declaration of who I am.

Deictic framing

There are multiple types of relational responding, with frames of coordination and comparison having been cited thus far. A type of framing that is particularly relevant in understanding ACT's approach to the self involves what are known as deictic relations. Verbal–social communities question and differentially reinforce accurate reporting by their members of experiences and behaviors that have occurred in the past, are ongoing now, and will be happening in the future. One's own behavior becomes established as a discriminative stimulus in this process (Skinner, 1945) and gives rise to a repertoire of self-awareness or the behavior of "seeing that I am seeing" (Skinner, 1988, p. 286). Such reporting, however, is only reinforced if it conforms to the deictic parameters of person ("I vs. you"), location ("here vs. there"), and time ("now vs. then"); these parameters also participate in frames of opposition or distinction with each other (e.g., there is no "here" without a "there" and no "I" without a "you"). Stated somewhat differently, young children who are asked, "What are you doing now?" are corrected if they erroneously report what some other child is currently doing across the room or what they were doing 10 minutes ago.

For the purpose of this chapter what is most critical to appreciate across multiple interchanges of this sort is that the one constant is the perspective or vantage point from which such self-reports are provided. From a behavior-analytic and RFT perspective, this particular dimension or sense of self – that which is referred to in ACT as "the observing self" (Hayes & Gregg, 2000) or self-as-context (Hayes, 1995) – is a byproduct of the verbal–social contingencies involved in shaping self-awareness, and it plays a key role in the development of perspective taking (McHugh & Stewart, 2012). To the degree to which such perspective taking has a transcendent quality to it, a sense of spirituality can also be seen as emerging from this same process (Hayes, 1984). Perhaps not surprisingly, then, and as will be discussed later, activating and strengthening this self-observational repertoire within ACT can have a transformational and calming impact.

Psychological flexibility

The overarching goal of ACT is to increase psychological flexibility or the ability to adjust one's behavior to be congruent with personal values (Hayes et al., 2012). Values, in turn, are defined as "freely chosen, verbally constructed consequences of ongoing dynamic, evolving patterns of activity, which establish predominant reinforcers for that activity that are intrinsic in engagement in the valued behavioral pattern itself" (Wilson & DuFrene, 2008, p. 64). It is useful to think of following one's values as an ongoing intrinsically reinforcing process that can be engaged in through a myriad of goal-directed approaches. For example, the value of being a loving parent could be realized by deliberate acts as large as saving for a child's college education or as small as reading a bedtime story or worrying about a child's future welfare. The purpose of ACT is to enhance the person's ability to live a meaningful and values-consistent life by removing barriers to psychological flexibility. Accordingly, to the extent that matters and issues pertaining to the self serve as such obstacles, they are strategically targeted within ACT. While almost all clients receive and benefit from some "self-work" in ACT, the degree of focus on this varies from client to client based on a case conceptualization of how three different senses of self contribute to psychological flexibility versus suffering.

Three senses of self

Although talk of three different senses or dimensions of self is common within ACT (Hayes et al., 2012, chapter 8), it should be reiterated that each can be viewed through a behavior-analytic lens (Lattal, 2012). From this perspective, "the self" in the aggregate within ACT can be conceptualized as an integrated set of behavioral repertoires (Wilson, Bordieri, & Whiteman, 2012) involving (a) a conceptualized self, (b) a knowing self, and (c) an observing self (Hayes & Gregg, 2000). As will become apparent, some of the experientially based techniques, exercises, and metaphors within ACT are designed to target only one of these dimensions, while others may simultaneously address two or even all three.

The conceptualized self

According to RFT and ACT, we continually construct various types of relational frames, including but by no means limited to those of coordination and comparison, about an almost limitless domain of objects and relata, including ourselves. These individual frames can, in turn, be related to each other, thereby creating coherent relational networks. For instance, we not only evaluate our worth against absolute standards and/or by socially comparing ourselves to others, but even more importantly construct narratives that logically explain and justify such formulations. What is referred to in ACT as the conceptualized self is essentially a storytelling repertoire about who we are and how and why we came to be that person (e.g., "I'll never amount to anything given the way others have mistreated me."). Unfortunately, psychological flexibility can be severely reduced when we closely identify with or "buy into" our life stories, particularly when they support a negatively evaluated conceptualized self. When we fuse with such narratives, our own self-awareness can become distorted. Being oblivious to and dismissive of any psychological experiences that would challenge the dysfunctional life story only helps maintain it. Moreover, acting in alternative, life-affirming ways (e.g., as if "I could amount to something") may not only be framed as impossibilities, but threaten the very sense of who we are (e.g., "I'm not the kind of person who could ever."). Sadly, clients may consequently rigidly prefer to "be right" about the life story they have constructed and that keeps them stuck rather than have their lives work for them.

ACT therapists have been advised to suggest that their clients in effect reinvent themselves everyday as a means of liberation from the arbitrary constraints imposed by the self-as-concept. Consistent with this, it is important to underscore that from an ACT perspective the concern is with psychological inflexibility that can arise from fusion with any life story, and not with the narrative per se. As evidenced by narcissism, attachment to a positive conceptualized self can be just as limiting as a negatively evaluated one. Thus, ACT does not primarily seek to tear down one relational network and replace it with another, but to assist clients in defusing from and deconstructing the narratives that have boxed them in and that have limited the ways in which they can lead a valued life. Clients may indeed incidentally end up telling a different story about their lives, but the old story can and often does reappear.

Weakening the conceptualized self

Behavior analysts typically have conceptualized therapeutic targets as either behavioral deficits or excesses.

From this vantage point, overidentification and fusion with the conceptualized self can be construed as a behavioral excess that has the effect of limiting psychological flexibility. ACT adopts a two-pronged strategy long-recognized by behavior analysts as effective in reducing behavioral excesses. One aspect of this overall strategy involves the use of defusion techniques and exercises to weaken behavioral control exerted by stories and other verbal constructions about the self. However, focusing exclusively on eliminating behavioral excesses, such as fusion with the conceptualized self, fails the "dead-man test" of Ogden Lindsley (Malott, Whaley, & Malott, 1991, p. 10). That is, it establishes not fusing with the life story as a singular client goal, which a dead man, as well as woman, could do even better. As will subsequently be seen, ACT accordingly combines defusion work surrounding the self-as-concept with efforts to also strengthen and reactivate repertoires of alternative and incompatible behavior involving the other two aspects of the self.

Efforts to loosen the grip of the conceptualized self can occur at multiple levels within ACT. At the simplest level are defusion exercises that target single self-relevant statements such as "I'm stupid." Nearly a hundred years ago, Titchener (1916, p. 425) argued that the literal meaning of words can at least be briefly suspended by rapidly repeating them aloud. ACT has adapted this procedure as a defusion exercise by having clients say aloud single self-critical labels over and over (e.g., "stupid, stupid, stupid..."). With enough repetitions, the key word loses its meaning (i.e., its derived stimulus function is no longer dominant) and only its direct stimulus function remains (i.e., the mere sound of the word). While the impact of this exercise may be rather fleeting, it – and other similar defusion techniques, such as expressing the negative self-statement in a cartoon voice or singing it as lyrics to a familiar tune (Strosahl et al., 2004, pp. 41–42) – can be repeated by clients as needed, to at least temporarily open up more space for psychological flexibility each time.

As discussed, fusion with a coherent and logically consistent narrative that justifies and explains the validity of negative self-statements (e.g., "why I am stupid") is more problematic, and also more of a challenge to weaken. ACT attempts to do so by asking clients to first articulate their life story before deconstructing and then rewriting it (Strosahl & Robinson, 2008; Zettle, 2007). Initially, clients are asked to write out their account of the key events in their lives that have led up to and substantially contributed to their presenting problems. Clients and therapists then collaborate by underlining factual descriptions within the documents (e.g., "My parents divorced when I was 8.") in order to separate them from their attributed consequences (e.g., "And as a result I've remained distrustful of those close to me."). Following this deconstruction, the client is asked to write another story using these same objective facts, but with a different array of consequences and overall ending (e.g., "My parents divorced when I was 8 which has caused me to value my marriage even more."). If necessary, this last step can be repeated several times with a variety of alternative endings. For instance, some of the endings may represent an improvement over the client's current status (e.g., having a better job), while others may represent a deterioration (e.g., having fewer friends). With a different ending, new facts may emerge that support it and be woven into the revised life story (Zettle, 2007, p. 104). However, as suggested earlier, the overall purpose is not to simply trade one fused narrative for another, but to experientially illustrate that an assortment of life scripts can be constructed, some of which afford more psychological flexibility than others. Clients can then be asked to reflect on which narrative they prefer – "If it were within your power to choose one of these storylines for yourself over the others, which one would be the most helpful to you in having the kind of life you'd want for yourself?"

Related research

A series of laboratory-based, analogue studies with non-clinical samples have consistently documented that rapidly saying negative self-labels aloud is more effective than performing an emotionally neutral distracting task or undertaking efforts to either suppress (e.g., "Don't think about X") or distract from (e.g., "Think of something other than X") the target words, in terms of reducing believability in and discomfort associated with the self-labels (Masuda, Hayes, Sackett, & Twohig, 2004; Masuda, Twohig, *et al.*, 2010). Related research suggests that a rationale alone for the defusion exercise in the absence of rapid word repetition is ineffective (Masuda, Feinstein, Wendell, & Sheehan, 2010) and that longer durations of saying the word (20–30 s) are required in order to impact believability than are required to impact emotional discomfort (3–10 s) (Masuda *et al.*, 2009). While these studies appear to display sufficient internal validity, the degree to which reduced believability ratings can be seen as a proxy for

defusion and the extent that their overall findings can be generalized to clinical populations are questions that require further research.

The need for such research is even more apparent in evaluating efforts to reduce fusion to storytelling within ACT. Williams (2007) compared a version of ACT that eliminated "discovering the self" phase work (Hayes, Strosahl, & Wilson, 1999, chapter 7) to a full protocol in treatment of PTSD in Australian veterans. Significant, but equivalent, benefits over six weeks of daily sessions were noted for the two conditions, with the full protocol group displaying greater continued improvement during three-month follow-up. Unfortunately, the study's sample size was limited ($N = 16$) and the self-focused work eliminated from the truncated version of ACT apparently was not limited to only defusion from the self-as-concept. As a consequence, further dismantling studies with additional clinical samples are recommended to isolate the unique contribution that targeting the conceptualized self may play within the overall success of ACT.

The knowing self

The knowing self consists of a repertoire of individual noticing, in a non-judgmental manner, the full panorama of ongoing psychological experiences. As suggested earlier, it constitutes a behavioral deficit in most clients, which ACT seeks to strengthen as an antidote to the pernicious effects of attachment to the conceptualized self. Because most clients are selectively attentive to the point of being hypervigilant to a limited range of psychological experiences, the immediate objective is to expand the scope of ongoing awareness and how clients respond to their experiences. For example, unwanted private events such as obsessive thoughts, negative emotions, and unpleasant memories are often avoided, or if encountered, quickly escaped from. As ACT sees it, such experiential avoidance contributes to psychological rigidity in several ways. First, although experiential control appears to be ineffective and even counterproductive in the long term (Hayes & Gregg, 2000), it may be sufficiently successful in the short-term to be maintained and strengthened through negative reinforcement. As time and energy invested in experiential avoidance are increased, less of each is available for valued living.

Excessive engagement in experiential control also both directly and indirectly contributes to a negative construction of the self, which in turn, as previously discussed, limits psychological flexibility. Clients, for example, may add "I'm the kind of person who can't control his/her emotions" to their life story and conceptualized self. Indirectly, selective focus on unwanted private events to be avoided precludes ongoing awareness of both neutral and positive psychological experiences (e.g., fleeting moments of feeling whole, competent, and that there is vitality to life), which if fully processed might counteract a negative self-concept.

Strengthening the knowing self

A wide array of techniques, exercises, and metaphors are available within ACT to facilitate client openness to whatever psychological experiences occur in the here and now (Strosahl et al., 2004), particularly those that may serve as barriers to value-congruent actions. The time and effort devoted to increasing contact with the present moment varies from client to client and can range from a structured schedule of mindfulness meditation similar to that developed by Jon Kabat-Zinn (Kabat-Zinn, Lipworth, & Burney, 1985) and adapted by MBCT (Segal et al., 2002), to the selective use of certain exercises, such as "soldiers in the parade" (Hayes et al., 1999, pp. 158–162), to repeatedly encouraging clients to "just notice" whatever private events are present.

The common objective of all such efforts is to strengthen the attentional flexibility of clients to observe ongoing unwanted thoughts, emotions, memories, and bodily sensations without attempting to push them away, while also increasing awareness of overlooked positive private events. For example, during the "soldiers in the parade" exercise clients are asked to close their eyes and visualize a parade in which each of their emerging thoughts appears on a sign carried by a marching soldier. All thoughts are to be observed in this manner including judgments about other thoughts (e.g., "That's a stupid thought"), with clients also asked to notice any fusion shifts in which they find themselves in the parade rather than merely watching it from a distance. While the "soldiers in the parade" exercise is focused primarily on increasing mindfulness of thinking, the mindfulness involved in "just noticing" spans the entire stream of present moment awareness and can be conducted with eyes closed or open. As its name suggests, the exercise encourages clients to simply make note of all ongoing experiences, which can include those that are both

internally (thinking about tomorrow's meeting) as well as externally generated (hearing an outside noise), while simultaneously neither pushing away those that are unwanted, nor clinging to those that are desired. As alluded to earlier, a repertoire of responding to one's own behavior, or what Skinner (1974) referred to as seeing that one sees, is thereby strengthened. This can be further facilitated by asking clients to "take inventory" (Zettle, 2007, p. 99) by explicitly reporting on what they "see" as they are "seeing" it; e.g., "I notice that I have the thought that …, I notice I'm feeling …," etc.

Related research

At least some indirect empirical support for the inclusion of formalized mindfulness meditation within ACT is provided by research documenting the beneficial impact of other therapeutic approaches, such as MBCT, that rely much more heavily on such practices (Hofmann, Sawyer, Witt, & Oh, 2010). More direct support for other techniques within ACT focused on the knowing self has been provided by a recent meta-analysis of laboratory-based studies. Levin and colleagues (2012) reported a medium effect size for specific exercises and metaphors within ACT designed to increase present moment awareness. However, most of the study samples were college students, thus creating concerns about generalization of the findings to clinical populations. As with the investigation of components targeting the conceptualized self, dismantling studies with clinical samples are recommend to more clearly ascertain how critical the efforts to increase ongoing awareness are to the impact of ACT.

The observing self

The repertoire of behavior that comprises the observing self or self-as-context can perhaps most simply be understood through its relationships to the knowing self and the conceptual self. If the knowing self can be viewed as "seeing that one sees," the observing self can be thought of as "seeing that this seeing" occurs from a consistent vantage point. Stated somewhat differently, I am aware that is I who sees whatever is seen and not someone else; what I see now, have seen in the past, and will see in the future, is through my eyes.

While the observing self can be viewed as closely dependent upon and an extension of present moment awareness, what it entails is most usefully seen as a counterweight to the conceptualized self. The "I" of the conceptualized self is constructed as a thing or entity (e.g., "I am this and that, etc."), while the "I" within the type of perspective taking that defines self-as-context is inherently transcendent (Hayes & Gregg, 2000). This sense of self is experienced as no-thing and as such, unlike self-as-concept, does not limit psychological flexibility by having to be defended when threatened by certain ongoing psychological experiences. Moreover, it is also the aspect of self that is addressed when clients are asked the following in ACT: "If nothing stood in your way, what would you want your life to be about?"

Strengthening the observing self

At the beginning of therapy, strong attachment to the conceptualized self typically overshadows the perspective-taking repertoire that clients acquired as children through the deictic processes discussed earlier. The objective in ACT, therefore, is not so much one of strengthening the observing self – constructed as a behavioral deficit – as it is of reactivating it. ACT does so in a number of ways (Strosahl *et al.*, 2004, p. 46), with only a few examples offered here. Some of these techniques simultaneously also target the other two dimensions of self, while others are more specifically focused on strengthening the observing self.

The "just noticing" exercise used to increase present moment awareness can be expanded to also address transcendent perspective-taking by asking clients to periodically "notice who is noticing." The purpose of what will be referred to here as the "I am" exercise is to activate the observing self, while also simultaneously weakening attachment to the conceptual self (Moran, 2013, pp. 123–130). Clients are provided with a sheet of paper with several blank lines under the heading of "I am ..." on which they are first asked to list specific personal identifiers (e.g., "I am ... a parent, a spouse, etc."). Clients are then asked one by one to cross off the line which they would be most willing to give up until all that remains is "I am." Two client reactions are fairly common. The first, reflective of fusion with the conceptualized self, is some protest and agonizing over eliminating each line of self-identifiers, followed by calming relief when reflecting on the observing self that is left.

The ACT experientially based technique that is perhaps most widely recognized as specifically designed to emphasize the continuity and transcendent quality of the observing self is appropriately known as the "observer exercise" (Hayes *et al.*, 1999, pp. 193–195). With their eyes closed, clients are guided through a review of both past and present moment experiences, while being asked to notice that the "you that you call you that is here now, was there then." Client reactions to the exercise can vary widely from intellectualizing about it to those that appear to be emotionally transforming (see Orsillo & Batten, 2005, p. 118).

Related research

Given the fairly ephemeral quality of the observing self, it should not be surprising that techniques to enhance it have not been investigated to the same degree as those targeting the other self dimensions within ACT. A recent laboratory-based study found that a version of the observer exercise that addressed pain-related experiences was more effective than a generic version of the exercise and an attention-placebo protocol in increasing tolerance to a cold pressor pain stimulus (Carrasquillo & Zettle, 2014). However, there was no difference when compared to a protocol that included pain tolerance techniques, such as relaxation, cognitive restructuring, and positive imagery; techniques typically emphasized with more traditional CBT approaches.

A pair of earlier and related studies suggests that other adjustments to the observer exercise informed by RFT may also increase its impact (Foody, Barnes-Holmes, Barnes-Holmes, & Luciano, 2013; Luciano *et al.*, 2011). Specifically, framing the deictic relationship between the self and private events within the observer exercise hierarchically (e.g., "Imagine yourself as being the captain of a boat and your thoughts and feelings as being the passengers.") was more effective in reducing self-reports of problematic behavior among adolescents (Luciano *et al.*, 2011) and distress in college students (Foody *et al.*, 2013) than placing the self and private events in a frame of distinction (e.g., "Just contemplate your thought as if you were contemplating a painting."). Whether similar findings would extend to the use of the observer exercise within ACT with clinical samples remains unclear.

Summary and conclusions

Clients in ACT are often counselled to hold thoughts about themselves and their life stories lightly. Similar advice can be extended to those who write and read about ACT. This chapter accordingly is but one of several contemporary narratives that could be told about how ACT regards the self and related matters. It is of necessity in some sense "my story" – other proponents, practitioners, and investigators of ACT might provide somewhat different accounts. Regardless of differences that might emerge across varied presentations and formulations of the current status of the self within ACT, all should be held lightly because of a common, shared feature. If scientific and clinical progress involving ACT is to continue, it is my sincere hope that all are wrong in some fundamental ways. However, as Kelly Wilson has frequently pointed out, we, unfortunately, don't know at this point in time exactly how or why they are wrong. ACT's perspective on the three selves, or dimensions of self, as discussed in this chapter, have so far seemed useful in contributing to the creation of a "science more adequate to the challenge of the human condition" (Hayes, Barnes-Holmes, & Wilson, 2012, p. 1). From the vantage point of functional contextualism, however, detecting and correcting errors of omission as well as commission in our current approach to the self within ACT is necessary to improve our ability to alleviate both subclinical and clinical forms of human suffering, and to promote well-being.

References

Barnes-Holmes, Y., Barnes-Holmes, D., Roche, B., *et al.* (2001). Psychological development. In S. C. Hayes, D. Barnes-Holmes, & B. Roche (Eds.), *Relational Frame Theory: A Post-Skinnerian Account of Human Language and Cognition* (pp. 157–180). New York, NY: Plenum.

Biglan, A., & Hayes, S. C. (1996). Should the behavioral sciences become more pragmatic? The case for functional contextualism in research on human behavior. *Applied and Preventive Psychology: Current Scientific Perspectives*, 5, 45–57.

Carrasquillo, N., & Zettle, R. D. (2014). Comparing a brief self-as-context exercise to control-based and attention placebo protocols for coping with induced pain. *The Psychological Record*, 64, 659–669.

Foody, M., Barnes-Holmes, Y., Barnes-Holmes, D., & Luciano, C. (2013). An empirical investigation of hierarchical versus distinction relations in a self-based ACT exercise. *International Journal of Psychology and Psychological Therapy*, 13, 373–388.

Hayes, S. C. (1984). Making sense of spirituality. *Behaviorism*, 12, 99–110.

Hayes, S. C. (1993). Analytic goals and varieties of scientific contextualism. In S. C. Hayes, L. J. Hayes, H. W. Reese, & T. R. Sarbin (Eds.), *Varieties of Scientific Contextualism* (pp. 11–27). Reno, NV: Context Press.

Hayes, S. C. (1995). Knowing selves. *The Behavior Therapist*, 18, 94–96.

Hayes, S. C. (2004). Acceptance and commitment therapy, relational frame theory, and the third wave of behavior therapy. *Behavior Therapy*, 35, 639–665.

Hayes, S. C., Barnes-Holmes, D., & Roche, B. (Eds.). (2001). *Relational Frame Theory: A Post-Skinnerian Account of Human Language and Cognition*. New York, NY: Plenum.

Hayes, S. C., Barnes-Holmes, D., & Wilson, K. G. (2012). Contextual behavioral science: Creating a science more adequate to the challenge of the human condition. *Journal of Contextual Behavioral Science*, 1, 1–16.

Hayes, S. C., & Gregg, J. (2000). Functional contextualism and the self. In C. Muran (Ed.), *Self-Relations in the Psychotherapy Process* (pp. 291–307). Washington, DC: American Psychological Association.

Hayes, S. C., Luoma, J. B., Bond, F. W., Masuda, A., & Lillis, J. (2006). Acceptance and commitment therapy: Model, processes and outcomes. *Behaviour Research and Therapy*, 44, 1–25.

Hayes, S. C., Strosahl, K. D., & Wilson, K. G. (1999). *Acceptance and Commitment Therapy: An Experiential Approach to Behavior Change*. New York, NY: Guilford.

Hayes, S. C., Strosahl, K. D., & Wilson, K. G. (2012). *Acceptance and Commitment Therapy: The Process and Practice of Mindful Change* (2nd ed.). New York, NY: Guilford.

Hofmann, S. G., Sawyer, A. T., Witt, A. A., & Oh, D. (2010). The effect of mindfulness-based therapy on anxiety and depression: A meta-analytic review. *Journal of Consulting and Clinical Psychology*, 78, 169–183.

Kabat-Zinn, J., Lipworth, L., & Burney, R. (1985). The clinical use of mindfulness meditation for the self-regulation of chronic pain. *Journal of Behavioral Medicine*, 8, 163–190.

Lattal, K. A. (2012). Self in behavior analysis. In L. McHugh & I. Stewart (Eds.), *The Self and Perspective Taking: Contributions and Applications from Modern Behavioral Science* (pp. 37–52). Oakland, CA: Context Press.

Levin, M. E., Hildebrandt, M. J., Lillis, J., & Hayes, S. C. (2012). The impact of treatment components suggested by the psychological flexibility model: A meta-analysis of laboratory-based component studies. *Behavior Therapy*, 43, 741–756.

Linehan, M. M. (1993). *Cognitive-Behavioral Treatment of Borderline Personality Disorder*. New York, NY: Guilford.

Lovaas, I., Newsome, C., & Hickman, C. (1987). Self-stimulatory behavior and perceptual reinforcement. *Journal of Applied Behavior Analysis*, 20, 45–68.

Luciano, C., Ruiz, F. J., Vizcaino Torres, R. M., *et al.* (2011). A relational frame analysis of defusion in acceptance and commitment therapy: A preliminary and quasi-experimental study with at-risk adolescents. *International Journal of Psychology and Psychological Therapy*, 11, 165–182.

Malott, R. W., Whaley, D. L., & Malott, M. E. (1991). *Elementary Principles of Behavior* (2nd ed.). Englewood Cliffs, NJ: Prentice-Hall.

Masuda, A., Feinstein, A. B., Wendell, J. W., & Sheehan, S. T. (2010). Cognitive defusion versus thought distraction: A clinical rationale, training, and experiential exercise in altering psychological impacts of negative self-referential thoughts. *Behavior Modification*, 34, 520–538.

Masuda, A., Hayes, S. C., Sackett, C. F., & Twohig, M. P. (2004). Cognitive defusion and self-relevant negative thoughts: Examining the impact of a ninety year old technique. *Behaviour Research and Therapy*, 42, 477–485.

Masuda, A., Hayes, S. C., Twohig, M. P., *et al.* (2009). A parametric study of cognitive defusion and the believability and discomfort of negative self-relevant thoughts. *Behavior Modification*, 33, 250–262.

Masuda, A., Twohig, M. P., Stormo, A. R., *et al.* (2010). The effects of cognitive defusion and thought distraction on emotional discomfort and believability of negative self-referential thoughts. *Journal of Behavior Therapy and Experimental Psychiatry*, 41, 11–17.

McHugh, L., & Stewart, I. (2012). *The Self and Perspective Taking: Contributions and Applications from Modern Behavioral Science*. Oakland, CA: Context Press.

Moran, D. J. (2013). *Building Safety Commitment*. Joliet, IL: Valued Living Books.

Orsillo, S. M., & Batten, S. J. (2005). Acceptance and commitment therapy in the treatment of posttraumatic stress disorder. *Behavior Modification*, 29, 95–129.

Pepper, S. C. (1942). *World Hypotheses: A Study in Evidence*. Berkeley: University of California Press.

Reese, H. W. (1968). *The Perception of Stimulus Relations: Discrimination Learning and Transposition*. New York, NY: Academic Press.

Segal, Z. V., Williams, J. M. G., & Teasdale, J. D. (2002). *Mindfulness-based Cognitive Therapy for Depression: A New Approach to Preventing Relapse*. New York, NY: Guilford.

Skinner, B. F. (1945). The operational analysis of psychological terms. *Psychological Review*, 52, 270–277.

Skinner, B. F. (1974). *About Behaviorism*. New York, NY: Knopf.

Skinner, B. F. (1988). Behaviorism at fifty. In A. C. Catania & S. Harnad (Eds.), *The Selection of Behavior* (pp. 278–292). New York, NY: Cambridge University Press. (Original work published 1964.)

Society of Clinical Psychology. (n.d.). Psychological treatments. Retrieved from http://www.psychologicaltreatments.org

Strosahl, K. D., Hayes, S. C., Wilson, K. G., & Gifford, E. V. (2004). An ACT primer: Core therapy processes, intervention strategies, and therapist competencies. In S. C. Hayes & K. D. Strosahl (Eds.), *A Practical Guide to Acceptance and Commitment Therapy* (pp. 31–58). New York, NY: Springer.

Strosahl, K. D., & Robinson, P. J. (2008). *The Mindfulness and Acceptance Workbook for Depression*. Oakland, CA: New Harbinger.

Titchener, E. B. (1916). *A Text-Book of Psychology*. New York, NY: MacMillan.

Torneke, N. (2010). *Learning RFT: An Introduction to Relational Frame Theory and its Clinical Application*. Oakland, CA: Context Press.

Vilardaga, R., Hayes, S. C., Levin, M., & Muto, T. (2009). Creating a strategy for progress: A contextual behavioral science approach. *The Behavior Analyst*, 32, 105–133.

Wells, A. (2009). *Metacognitive Therapy for Anxiety and Depression*. New York, NY: Guilford.

Williams, L. M. (2007). *Acceptance and commitment therapy: An example of a third-wave therapy for treatment of Australian Vietnam War veterans with posttraumatic stress disorder*. Unpublished doctoral dissertation. Charles Sturt University; Bathurst, New South Wales, Australia.

Wilson, K. G., Bordieri, M., & Whiteman, K. (2012). The self and mindfulness. In L. McHugh & I. Stewart (Eds.), *The Self and Perspective Taking: Contributions and Applications from Modern Behavioral Science* (pp. 181–197). Oakland, CA: Context Press.

Wilson, K. G., & DuFrene, T. (2008). *Mindfulness for Two: An Acceptance and Commitment Therapy Approach to Mindfulness in Psychotherapy*. Oakland, CA: New Harbinger.

Wray, A. M., Dougher, M. J., Hamilton, D. A., & Guinther, P. M. (2012). Examining the reinforcing properties of making sense: A preliminary investigation. *The Psychological Record*, 62, 599–622.

Zettle, R. D. (2007). *ACT for Depression: A Clinician's Guide to Using Acceptance and Commitment Therapy in Treating Depression*. Oakland, CA: New Harbinger.

Chapter

7

The self in schema therapy

Eshkol Rafaeli, Offer Maurer, Gal Lazarus, and Nathan C. Thoma

The self has garnered a great deal of interest since receiving its first prominent treatment in the writings of William James (1890). James distinguished between the "me" – the known, or experienced, object self, and the "I" – the experiencing, knowing subject self. Both were seen as playing central roles in thought, affect, and behavior. Modern treatments of the self, particularly social cognitive and neuroscience ones (e.g., Linville & Carlson, 1994; Zaki & Ochsner, 2011), have equated the "me" with the declarative knowledge we have about ourselves, and the "I" with the procedural knowledge that directs our actions, thoughts, and feelings.

For decades, the self (particularly the "me") was seen as unitary (Allport, 1955; Rogers, 1977; Wylie, 1974, 1979); for example, the vast literature on self-esteem was predicated on the idea that people have a unitary self and that a single dimension of esteem can apply to it. However, pioneering psychologists (James, 1890; Kelly, 1955) and sociologists (Mead, 1934) offered a multifaceted view of the self as something composed of various aspects, roles, and perspectives. Each of the multiple "me"s contains the information we have about ourselves as objects of knowledge – i.e., as we are in that particular aspect of ourselves (cf. Rafaeli & Hiller, 2010). Similarly, each of the multiple "I"s holds our subjective experience in one particular facet, part, or mode of our being.

Schema therapy (ST), the integrative model of psychotherapy described in this chapter, adopts this multifaceted view of the self as both a clinical challenge and a clinical opportunity in the understanding and treatment of psychopathology and distress. In the following sections, we review the development of the ST model, placing particular emphasis on the way ST has come to view and work with the multiplicity of selves – that is,

on the ST mode model. After reviewing the evidence base for the concepts and efficacy of ST, we devote the latter half of the chapter to the application of ST.

Schema therapy and the emergence of the mode model

ST was first proposed by Jeffrey Young (1990) as an expansion of cognitive behavioral therapy (and particularly of Beck's cognitive therapy) aimed at addressing a wide spectrum of long-standing emotional/relational difficulties. Such difficulties often fit the definition of one or more personality disorders, but may also be present in disorders marked by chronic mood problems, anxiety or obsessions, traumatic responses, or dissociation, formerly labeled "Axis-I" disorders.

As Young (1990) explains, a major impetus for the development of the ST model (originally titled a "schema-focused approach to cognitive therapy") was the realization that a sizable group of clients were not responding fully to traditional cognitive therapy. Quite consistently, these non-responders, as well as clients experiencing relapse following improvement, are those whose problems are more characterological. Young reasoned that effective work with such clients would require a shift in focus from surface-level cognitions or beliefs to deeper constructs – i.e., to the schemas (which gave this therapy its name).

Schemas (Greek for template, shape, or form) are enduring foundational mental structures which help us represent a complex world in ways that allow efficient, sometimes even automatic, action. The use of this term in psychology (in reference to basic cognitive processes) dates back to Bartlett (1932), but has its roots even earlier, in Kant's *Critique of Pure Reason* (1781).

The Self in Understanding and Treating Psychological Disorders, ed. Michael Kyrios, Richard Moulding, Guy Doron, Sunil S. Bhar, Maja Nedeljkovic, and Mario Mikulincer. Published by Cambridge University Press. © Cambridge University Press, 2016.

As a term tied to psychopathology, it first appeared in Beck's seminal work (e.g., 1976) on cognitive therapy for emotional disorders. Beck posited that symptoms ensue from the activation of one particular set of (negative) schemas – those related to the self, others, world, and future.

In ST, the notion of schemas goes beyond addressing cognitive features of the mind; schemas are thought to encompass emotions, bodily sensations, images, and memories: "hot," and not just "cold" cognition. Over the years, Young (1990) and his colleagues (Young, Klosko, & Weishaar, 2003) have worked on refining a taxonomy of early maladaptive schemas, which are thought to emerge when core emotional needs go unmet or are met inappropriately, usually by a child's caregivers.[1] These needs (e.g., for safety, security, validation, autonomy, spontaneity, and realistic limits) are seen as universal. In infancy and childhood, meeting these needs falls to the child's caregivers, and is considered necessary for a child to develop into psychological health as an adult. Young posited that enduring client problems often stem from present-day activation of the early maladaptive schemas. At times, problems directly involve the distress felt when the schemas are activated. Quite often, however, they result from the characteristic behaviors enacted as a response to the schema – which Young first referred to as "coping styles."

Starting in the mid 1990s, Young (e.g., McGinn & Young, 1996) began recognizing the necessity of revising ST to move beyond its predominant focus on universal needs, pervasive schemas, and characteristic coping styles. Needs, schemas, and coping styles are all trait-like, and therefore leave unexplained much of the phenomenology and symptomatology of the clients for whom ST was developed in the first place – individuals with borderline or narcissistic personality characteristics, who manifest quick and often intense fluctuation among various self-states or moods. This led to the development of the mode concept.

A mode refers to the predominant schemas, coping reactions, and emotional states that are active for an individual at a particular time. By definition, modes are transient states, and at any given moment, a person is thought to be predominantly in one mode. Most individuals inhabit various modes over time; the manner in which they shift from one mode to another – that is, the degree of separation or dissociation between the modes – differs and lies on a continuum. On the milder end, modes could be like moods (e.g., one may feel a bit listless in the morning, but gradually feel more animated and upbeat by the evening) – i.e., a sense of consistent selfhood, an overarching "I," is maintained. At the most extreme end, total separation and dissociation between modes takes the form of dissociative identity disorder, in which each mode may present as a different personality – i.e., distinct and seemingly unrelated "I"s.

The manner in which modes shift reflects the structure of the self, yet individuals may also vary in the content of the self – i.e., the specific identity of the modes they tend to inhabit. For example, persons suffering from borderline personality disorder (BPD) tend to experience abrupt transitions and a strong dissociation among a *specific* set of characteristic modes (e.g., detached protector, angry child, abandoned/abused child, punitive parent; Lobbestael, van Vreeswijk, and Arntz, 2008; Shafran *et al.*, 2015). People characterized by narcissism have a different set of characteristic modes (e.g., self-aggrandizer, detached self-soother, lonely/inferior child). Moreover, a key principle of ST is to remain very "experience-near" (Greenberg & Rice, 1996); thus, in describing a particular client's "mode-map" in exact terms, schema therapists would pay special attention to idiosyncratic deviations (of this particular person) from the prototypical set of modes (characteristic of others who may suffer from the same symptoms).

Modes as self-states

ST theorists (Rafaeli, Bernstein, & Young, 2011; Young *et al.*, 2003) have paid considerable attention to the developmental origins of schemas, and have argued that they come about when core emotional needs go unmet. Less attention has been given to the origins of modes, but given the centrality of the mode concept to the way ST is practiced today, such attention is very much needed. Luckily, developmental accounts of self-development can help here. Such accounts (e.g., Putnam, 1989; Siegel, 1999) tell a story that is about non-integration, rather than about fragmentation.

According to Putnam, Siegel, and other developmental theorists (e.g., Chefetz, 2015; van der Hart, Nijenhuis, & Steele, 2006), human infants come equipped with a basic set of loosely interconnected "behavioral states": psychological and physiological patterns that co-occur and that repeat themselves, often in highly predictable sequences, in a relatively stable and enduring manner. These states (or "states-of-mind"; Siegel, 1999) can be defined as the total pattern of activation – affect, arousal, motor activity, cognitive processing, access to knowledge and memory, and self-of-self – that occurs in the brain at a particular moment in time.

States-of-mind begin as ad hoc combinations of mental faculties organized in response to discrete challenges or situations in the infant's life. Yet situations tend to repeat themselves – and thus, to repeatedly activate the same states. Over time and repeated activation, basic states-of-mind cluster together into self sub-systems – ingrained and separate "self-states" (Siegel, 1999). These serve as the early prototypes of what ST refers to as modes.

Below, we review the four major mode, or self-state, categories discussed by ST: (a) child modes, (b) coping modes, (c) internalized parental modes, and (d) the healthy adult mode. We also note our current thinking regarding these modes' etiology and briefly explain how ST works with each category of modes.

A taxonomy of modes and their etiology

Child modes

When a child's needs are, on balance, appropriately met, the ensuing self-states tend to be flexible and adaptive. Through repeated experience of situations in which emotional needs are met (emotions are regulated, distress is soothed), the child (and later, the adult he or she will become) develops what in ST terms is referred to as a *Happy Child mode*. In this mode, the person experiences closeness, trust, and contentment, and becomes free to access inner sources of vitality, spontaneity, and positive motivation. These innate feelings of playfulness and freedom may not be very accessible to many adult (or even adolescent) clients whose childhood was not marked by the safety and encouragement which foster such curiosity and joy. Even (or rather, particularly) when that is the case, ST seeks to reconnect clients with their Happy Child mode by removing obstacles or creating opportunities to develop such feelings, even if no such opportunity existed in childhood.

When a child's experience is marked by repeated instances of unmet (or inadequately met) needs, a self-state referred to as the *Vulnerable Child (VC) mode* coalesces. The VC mode is present for everyone to some degree, but its specific nature differs from person to

person, depending primarily on the unique profile of met and unmet needs. For example, when childhood needs for safety and security were repeatedly met with frightening parental behaviors (e.g., anger or violence), fear and anxiety typically prevail in the VC mode. When needs for empathy and validation were left unmet, the VC mode typically involves a chronic sense of loneliness, of being unseen or easily misunderstood by others. When needs for praise and encouragement were met with frequent blame and criticism, the VC mode typically contains feelings of shame, a lack of self-worth, and an expectation of further blame and criticism.

Although the VC mode is rooted in childhood experiences, it can often be triggered in an adult's life by situations that bear even small degrees of similarity to the originating experience (e.g., anger, invalidation, or criticism – see Porges, 2011, for a detailed description of how such triggering may occur neurologically). When these occur, individuals essentially re-experience an earlier relational trauma (Howell, 2013), which activates concomitant distress (e.g., fear, loneliness, or shame, respectively). Typically, they are not aware that the distress is linked to earlier experiences; instead, when the VC mode becomes activated, people simply think and feel as they did as vulnerable or mistreated children, and expect others to treat them as they had been treated at that early age. In a sense, the activated VC mode bears the brunt of most maladaptive schemas (e.g., mistrust/abuse, emotion deprivation, or defectiveness/shame).[2]

A primary goal of ST is to heal the relational trauma of unmet needs. To do so, the VC mode needs to be activated and accessible so that it may receive the care it needs. At first, much of this care is offered by the therapists. Over time, as clients' healthy adult modes gain strength, they internalize this care and learn how to administer it to themselves or obtain it from others outside of therapy. This process by which therapists identify and partially gratify the unmet needs of the VC is the central therapeutic stance within ST and is referred to as *limited re-parenting*.

In addition to the Happy and Vulnerable child modes discussed above, early life experiences often give rise to two additional child modes. The first is the *Impulsive/Undisciplined Child (IUC) mode*, which often results from improper limit setting on the parents' part. It embodies those schemas characterized by externalizing behavior (e.g., entitlement and insufficient self-control schemas). The second is the *Angry Child (AC) mode*, which emerges in spontaneous angry, or even rageful, reactions to unmet needs. The function of the AC mode is a protective one, and it can be thought of as a nascent manifestation of a coping reaction. However, just like other coping reactions (and coping styles), it often fails to achieve its intended goal. When either the AC or the IUC modes is present, ST calls for empathic yet firm limit-setting. It also calls for empathic exploration so as to discover the unmet needs (which typically underlie the AC mode) or to distinguish whims and wishes from needs (if the IUC mode is present).

Coping modes

Like the Child Modes described above, *Maladaptive Coping Modes* also represent behavioral states that coalesce into modes due to repeated activation. However, whereas Child Modes (particularly the VC) represent the organic emotional reactions of the child, Coping Modes emerge from a child's rudimentary survival and adaptation psychological strategies, strategies enacted to withstand the (inevitably depriving) environment encountered by the child. In some cases, especially in environments that were extremely emotionally negligent or otherwise noxious, the strategies were put to use again and again, consolidating into an easily triggered coping mode. In other cases, the coping modes may have been less of a response to a depriving or abusive environment, and more of an internalization of it.

Maladaptive Coping Modes correspond to three coping styles (avoidance, overcompensation, or surrender), which parallel the basic general adaptation responses to threat: flight, fight, or freeze (Young *et al.*, 2003). For different people (and sometimes, even for the same person), these modes may take on varied forms: avoidance may involve dissociation, emotional detachment, behavioral inhibition, or withdrawal; overcompensation may involve grandiose self-aggrandisement or perfectionistic over-control; and surrender may involve compliance, victimhood, and/or dependence.

For ST to achieve its main goal (of healing the relational trauma and allowing the client to develop healthy ways of having needs met), it must contend with the coping modes – negotiate with them, bypass them, or weaken their hold, so that the VC mode becomes accessible. It may be easiest to understand this process by thinking of one particular (and prominent) coping mode – the avoidant mode referred to as the *Detached Protector*. In this mode, clients are disconnected from

emotions – painful ones, but also adaptive ones such as sadness over a loss, assertive anger over a violation, intimate warmth towards close others, or a sense of vitality and motivation. The detachment, distraction, and avoidance in this mode are maintained in various ways (e.g., self-isolation, emotional eating, excessive drinking or drug use). To achieve its goals of re-parenting the VC and healing the relational trauma, ST must bypass the Detached Protector – i.e., find a way to break through the protective shield of numbness, dissociation, and disconnection.

The Detached Protector is often the most prominent mode seen in individuals prone to dissociation and avoidance (e.g., ones with BPD). Other clinical groups are characterized by other coping modes. For example, *the Self-Aggrandizer*, a mode very prominent among those characterized by narcissistic personality disorder, is an overcompensating Coping Mode that attempts to shore up the fragile self-esteem, loneliness, and inferiority that make up the Vulnerable Child for such people. The *Bully/Attack Mode* is often seen in individuals with antisocial traits, and is a more extreme adult version of the Angry Child mode. The *Compliant Surrenderer*, a typical mode among individuals with dependent personality traits, is an example of a surrender Coping Mode.

Once coping modes coalesce, they tend to be deployed almost automatically whenever schemas are triggered, as a way of coping with the ensuing distress. Paradoxically, though, they actually lead to schema maintenance by blocking the opportunity for new corrective emotional learning. For this reason, coping modes are considered maladaptive by definition. Indeed, they are typically seen as a cause of many, if not most, present-day problems.

As noted earlier, ST seeks to weaken the hold of coping modes. At the same time, it must acknowledge that these modes involve behaviors that were, at some point, adaptive responses to harsh interpersonal environments. Thus, ST sees the reasons for the coping modes' historical emergence as valid; it also calls for empathy towards the way in which particular triggering situations activate the mode. Together, the ST approach to these modes balances validation and empathy (to the "why") with directive intervention (towards the "how"). This approach, termed *empathic confrontation*, empathizes with the reasons for the coping mode(s)' emergence, yet helps clients recognize the costs involved in the inflexible use of such modes, ultimately reducing their reliance on these modes.

Parental modes

A third, more pernicious class of modes, are the *Internalized Dysfunctional Parental Modes*. By internalization, a process which incorporates principles of implicit learning through modeling (e.g., Bandura, 2006), children learn to treat themselves the way early influential others had treated them – ways that are often quite dysfunctional. Notably, despite the term chosen to label these modes, the maltreatment may not necessarily be that of actual parental figures, but rather of harmful non-parental figures or of the broader social milieu. Still, good-enough parental support under adverse circumstances tends to mitigate their long-term negative impact dramatically, resulting in much weaker internal influence of malevolent self-states; at times, it is the absence of such support that is internalized.

Internalized Parental Modes represent distinct ways in which individuals may be their own worst enemies – a phenomenon recognized by many clinicians, with terms such as punitive super-egos (Freud, 1940), internalized bad objects (Klein, 1946), malevolent introjects (Chessick, 1996), perpetrator parts (van der Hart *et al.*, 2006), or internal critics (Greenberg & Watson, 2006). Young *et al.* (2003) recognize two prototypical forms of Internalized Parental Modes: a *Punitive Parent (PP)* and a *Demanding Parent (DP)*. In a PP mode, the client becomes aggressive, intolerant, impatient, and unforgiving towards himself (or others), usually due to the perceived inability to meet the mode's standards. When in a DP mode, he might feel as if he must fulfill rigid rules, norms, and values and must be extremely efficient in meeting all these. In either mode, he might become very critical of the self or of others, and, as a result of the VC mode's co-activation, may also feel guilty and ashamed of his shortcomings or mistakes, believing he should be severely punished for them (Arntz & Jacob, 2012). The goal in ST is to help the client recognize these modes, assertively stand up to their punitiveness or criticism, and learn to protect and shield the VC mode from their destructive effects.

Healthy Adult mode

Alongside painful child modes, maladaptive coping modes, and dysfunctional parental modes, most people also have self-states that are healthy and positive. One (the Happy Child mode) was discussed earlier. The other, referred to as the *Healthy Adult (HA) mode*, is the part of the self that is compassionate, capable, and well-functioning. When parents meet their child's basic needs in an attentive and suitable way, they serve as a model for healthy (rather than punitive, demanding, or neglectful) adults. Indeed, for many clients, the HA mode is modeled after these positive aspects of their caregivers. For others, who lacked such models, the task of constructing such a mode is more challenging, yet not impossible. In fact, a major aim of ST is to have the therapist's behaviors, and particularly their limited re-parenting efforts, serve as a model for the development or reinforcement of this mode. The HA mode, like an internalized therapist, has to respond flexibly to the various other modes. With time, it begins to nurture, protect, and validate the VC mode, set limits on the impulsivity of the IUC mode, validate the AC mode while containing its angry outbursts, negotiate with maladaptive coping modes so as to limit their presence, and mitigate the effects of dysfunctional parent modes.

Empirical evidence

ST, as an intervention model, has undergone a variety of empirical testing for several disorders, particularly personality disorders. In the first major test of ST, Giesen-Bloo *et al.* (2006) conducted a multicenter randomized controlled trial (RCT) of ST vs. transference-focused therapy (TFP), a psychodynamic therapy, in the treatment of 86 BPD patients, treated twice-weekly for three years. A significantly greater proportion of patients recovered or reliably improved in BPD symptoms at the end of treatment in the ST arm (45.5% recovered and 65.9% improved) than in the TFP arm (23.8% recovered and 42.9% improved). Given that patient retention is notoriously difficult in the treatment of personality disorders, it is important to note that dropout rates were considerably lower in ST (25%) than in TFP (50%). Among those who dropped out, ST patients had a median of 98 sessions (close to 1 year) while TFP patients had a median of 34 sessions (roughly 4 months).

Extending the generalizability of these findings, Nadort *et al.* (2009) conducted a feasibility study with 62 BPD patients in which the patients were randomly assigned to two conditions, with or without between-session phone contact with the therapist. There was no difference in outcome, indicating that it was the within-session work that contributed to outcome. Overall, the treatment was found to be feasible and effective when delivered in the community, with 42% of patients reaching recovery from BPD after 1.5 years of treatment.

In another multicenter RCT, Bamelis, Evers, Spinhoven, and Arntz (2014) extended the mode model to patients with various personality disorders (but not BPD). A total of 300 patients were randomized to either ST, psychodynamically oriented treatment-as-usual (TAU) in the community, or clarification-oriented psychotherapy (COP). At the end of two years of treatment, ST had significantly better outcomes than TAU and COP, with personality disorder recovery rates of 81.4%, 51.8%%, and 60.0%, respectively. Interestingly, a moderator effect showed that the second of two cohorts of schema therapists drove the positive findings. This second cohort was trained more extensively in implementation of ST techniques. Initial process ratings validate that these therapists did use more of the ST techniques than the earlier cohort. This provides initial evidence that it is methods of actively evoking modes (which facilitate working with different self-states within the therapy session) that serve as key active ingredients. Additionally, very promising results emerged for the use of ST in a group format with BPD patients (Farrell, Shaw, & Webber, 2009). A single-case series ($N = 12$) examining ST for chronic depression found that by the end of 60 sessions of treatment, 60% of patients responded well or remitted (Malogiannis *et al.*, 2014). Finally, some additional effectiveness studies have also yielded positive results (see Bamelis *et al.*, 2012, and Sempértegui, Karreman, Arntz, & Bekker, 2014, for reviews of evidence for efficacy of ST for BPD and other conditions). Overall, the evidence for the efficacy of ST can be considered promising but preliminary, as there have not yet been any direct replications of the RCTs reviewed above.

Although tests of ST as a complete intervention package provide indirect support for the utility of the theoretical model, more research is needed to further validate it as a model of pathology. Some research into the reliability and validity of modes has been conducted (see Lobbestael, 2012, and Sempértegui *et al.*, 2014, for reviews), mainly centering on the development of the Schema Mode Inventory (Lobbestael, van Vreeswijk, Spinhoven, Schouten, & Arntz, 2010), a measure of 14 clinically relevant schema modes. This measure taps into the main modes discussed in the present chapter, but also offers further differentiation of some modes (e.g., differentiating the Angry Child and the Enraged Child). Using this measure, modes have largely been found to relate to personality disorders in theoretically coherent ways (Lobbestael, 2012). For example, patients with BPD have been found to

be higher in the frequency of the Abandoned/Abused Child, the Punitive Parent, the Detached Protector, and the Angry Child than both healthy controls and Cluster C personality disorder patients. Experimental studies involving watching a traumatic film clip (Arntz, Klokman, & Sieswerda, 2005) as well as anger induction experiments (Lobbestael, Arntz, Cima, & Chakhssi, 2009) have begun to validate the theory that modes are state-like experiences that occur in response to triggers in the environment, and much more so for personality disorder patients. More work is needed to show that in addition to activated emotion, modes also involve characteristic ways of thinking and behaving. Finally, a priority for research into the mode model lies in the area of process-outcome research within intervention studies, to demonstrate that in-session mode states can be reliably recognized, and further, that working actively with modes transforms underlying schemas and leads to lasting mental health.

The application of schema therapy

Assessment and conceptualization phase

ST begins with an initial period of assessment, which typically requires at least 4–5 sessions but at times may be much longer (cf., Rafaeli *et al.*, 2011). Assessment may incorporate informal history taking, administration of questionnaires (such as the Young Schema Questionnaire), assignment of thought and mood monitoring to obtain examples from daily life, as well as the use of imagery techniques for assessment.

Following the assessment phase, a case conceptualization, developed collaboratively by therapist and client, is created to serve as a guide to the intervention phase. In this conceptualization, the problems and symptoms reported by the client or identified by the therapist are re-cast using the concepts of needs, schemas, coping responses, and modes. In many cases, the conceptualization is brought in, in draft form, by the therapist, and then edited collaboratively. At times, a visual representation of the client's modes is used alongside, or in place of, a more verbal conceptualization (see Rafaeli, Maurer, & Thoma, 2014, for an example).

The process of jointly conceptualizing the problems involves exploring the origins of the schemas and modes, as well as the ways in which they are tied to present-day problems. A good conceptualization "fits well": it refers to the schemas and modes using terms that are understandable, even familiar, to the client – ideally, ones actually provided by the client. Ultimately, the conceptualization aims to help both the client and the therapist differentiate, identify, and name the relevant modes that play a part in the client's experience. Several recent books and chapters (e.g., Arntz & Jacob, 2012; Rafaeli *et al.*, 2011) discuss the conceptualization process in detail.

A conceptualization emphasizing the role of modes has become central to ST in the last two decades. At first, the mode model was thought to be relevant mostly to clients characterized by strong fluctuations among various modes (e.g., those with BPD). However, recent developments (e.g., Bamelis, Renner, Heidkamp & Arntz, 2011; Lobbestael *et al.*, 2008) have shown mode-centered conceptualizations to be applicable across a wide range of disorders, including the formerly labeled Axis I disorders. Indeed, the formulation of an individually tailored mode model, which is based on relevant prototypical "maps" (see, for example, Arntz & Jacob, 2012) is the starting point of most ST interventions.

Intervention phase

Overview of the intervention strategy

The central project of ST is to help clients (adults or children) get their own needs met, even when these needs had not been met in the past. Doing so involves helping clients understand their core emotional needs and learn ways of getting those needs met in an adaptive manner. In turn, this requires altering long-standing cognitive, emotional, relational, and behavioral patterns – which are instantiated in the schemas and coping styles, but most importantly in the modes.

ST emphasizes the importance of deliberately inviting or activating all of a client's modes, including the maladaptive ones, in session. In doing so, schema therapists seek to give voice to all modes, to differentiate them, and then to respond differentially to each one. This differentiation is key to ST, as it prescribes very different responses to modes of various types. Vulnerable, Impulsive, Angry, and Happy Child modes are responded to with relevant forms of limited reparenting (appropriate nurturance and protection, limit-setting, encouragement for ventilation along with limit-setting, and playful joining, respectively). Maladaptive coping modes are responded to with empathic confrontation (empathy for the difficulty or distress which prompted the coping response, and

for the typical feeling that "there's no other choice," along with confrontation towards the maladaptive behavior itself). Internalized Dysfunctional Parental modes are confronted so that they become externalized and ego-dystonic. Finally, the Healthy Adult mode is responded to with recognition and mirroring, along with modelling of additional adaptive parental responses. The differential response to modes may be the therapist's purview at first, but over time, the therapist models this differential response and the client's Healthy Adult internalizes and practices it.

We find the analogy between ST and structural/systemic family therapy (e.g., Minuchin, Nichols, & Lee, 2007) useful here. In structural/systemic approaches, a family is viewed as a complex system, comprising multiple and mutually interacting individuals, with interventions typically aimed at altering the structure of this system. Similarly, in ST, the person is viewed as a complex system, comprising multiple and mutually interacting modes or self-states. ST aims to alter the way these parts work together: we hope to alter the overall configuration of modes, and the relative dominance or power of specific modes. However, unlike structural/systemic approaches, ST does not shy away from seeing particular units within the broader structure (i.e., modes within the self) as requiring specific and focused interventions.

To affect change, schema therapists draw on cognitive, emotion-focused, relational, and behavioral tools. The remainder of this chapter will review interventions which use these tools to address, specifically, coping, parental, and child modes.

Bypassing and overcoming coping modes

Coping modes emerge early in life to protect or shield the vulnerable child. With time, they become ingrained and inflexible. They often serve as the person's "greeting card" in new situations, almost ensuring that no real emotional contact will be possible. For example, a narcissistic client with a lonely/inferior child mode may find it almost inconceivable to allow this vulnerability to be seen by anyone, including his new therapist. Instead, he is likely to spend the majority of time, especially early in therapy, in compensatory modes (e.g., Self Aggrandizer, Bully-and-Attack). Of course, these modes interfere with most basic tasks of therapy – building rapport and trust, clarifying the client's needs or distress, and formulating an action plan. For these reasons, therapists often need to address these modes up front.

The approach advocated by ST in such moments is that of *empathic confrontation*. Empathic confrontation is first and foremost a relational stance. To carry it out well, therapists need to genuinely be empathic to the need or the distress which activated the coping mode. Usually, this empathy will also involve a respectful and curious attitude towards the coping mode itself. These, however, will be coupled with some confrontation regarding the inefficacy of the coping behavior itself. Confrontation may be cautious and friendly when it comes to avoidant behaviors, but will involve more direct and emphatic limit-setting when it comes to overcompensation behaviors.

Empathic confrontation may utilize cognitive or behavioral techniques (cf., Arntz & Jacob, 2012). For example, using cognitive techniques, the therapist might encourage the client to identify and label the coping mode, explore its origins, or draw up a list of pros and cons for maintaining it. Using behavioral techniques, the therapist might work on decreasing avoidant behaviors (e.g., by setting up an exposure hierarchy of avoided situations, or by assigning graded tasks related to assertive expression) or on curtailing overcompensatory ones (e.g., by rehearsing adequate interpersonal behaviors so as to train the client's social skills).

At times, emotion-focused techniques can deepen the effects of empathic confrontation. A key example of this involves a two-chair dialogue exploring the pros and cons of a coping behavior (see Kellogg, 2004, as well as Rafaeli *et al.*, 2014, for more details on chair-work in ST). A therapist may pull in a separate chair on which the client's coping mode would sit. In it, the client might be encouraged to voice his typical behavioral coping reaction (e.g., disengagement, surrender, escape, etc.) to some distressing situations. Dialogues between this mode and the child mode (and/or the therapist) can be very informative, especially among avoidant, compliant, or dependent clients. Ultimately, once the coping mode's voice is made clearer, the therapist may use empathic confrontation with it, so that it steps aside to allow the therapist to nurture the child mode, or to observe the key drama between the child and parent modes as it plays out.

Another emotion-focused technique, imagery for assessment, is often used early in therapy to bypass coping modes. When using imagery as an assessment tool, therapists invite the client to shut their eyes and visualize certain scenes, memories, or experiences in a vivid way. The client is asked to verbalize what they see, hear, and feel, and to do so as if they are present in the scene (thus, speaking in the first person and the present tense). The purpose is for the client to become absorbed in the scene – to "be" in it, rather than relate it from a distanced perspective (see Arntz, 2014, as well as Rafaeli *et al.*, 2014, for more details on imagery in ST).

Confronting parental modes

Dysfunctional parental modes are the echoed voices of toxic external figures: the father who denigrated his daughter; the mother who conveyed a sense of invalidation and conditional regard; the peer group that ostracized or bullied a newcomer. Tragically, the damage done by these figures at an early impressionable age is perpetuated by those parts, within the adult client, that learned or internalized the lessons too well. An important ST goal is to help clients recognize these pernicious voices of self-criticism and self-punishment as ego-alien in nature, and to help them limit these voices' influence – by changing, fighting, and (if possible) even banishing them.

A variety of tools can be deployed in ST for this purpose. Relationally, limited reparenting itself serves as an antidote to this mode, as it models the compassionate responses of a healthy nurturing parent. Schema therapists place themselves squarely on the side of compassion and self-acceptance – i.e., on the side of the (sometimes barely nascent) Healthy Adult. Together with the Healthy Adult, they attempt to dislodge internalized voices that purport to have a monopoly on "truth," "values," or "standards," but in fact use these to oppress, devalue, or torment the client (and particularly the client's Vulnerable Child).

Cognitively, the therapist may use psychoeducation to provide information about reasonable, non-punitive expectations and practices; help the client create a narrative linking the dysfunctional internalized mode to its external sources and origins; and develop schema flashcards or diaries (see Rafaeli *et al.*, 2010) to be better prepared when the dysfunctional mode is activated.

Many other cognitive (as well as behavioral) techniques which strengthen the Healthy Adult mode, encourage the Contented Child mode, or provide a safe space for the Vulnerable or Angry Child modes also exert a simultaneous effect on the dysfunctional internalized modes. One example would be the use of behavioral activation and scheduling methods to introduce pleasure (alongside mastery) behaviors into the client's day-to-day life. This common (yet very powerful) behavioral technique almost inevitably requires defeating the internalized voice that sees pleasure as decadent, undeserved, and unacceptable.

The strongest techniques for building the case *against* dysfunctional internalized modes – and the counterpart case *for* an alternative view of truth, values, and standards – are emotion-focused ones. Two-chair techniques opening up dialogues between the Vulnerable Child (and/or Healthy Adult) mode(s) on the one hand and the punitive/critical parent mode on the other are often very fruitful (and bear strong resemblance to work done in emotion-focused techniques (EFT) with critical voices; e.g., Greenberg & Rice, 1996). Moreover, a variation on imagery work in which the therapist helps rescript a difficult or painful experience with the internalized figure (see Arntz, 2014; Rafaeli *et al.*, 2014) is particularly useful here. Imagery tends to evoke strong emotions (for review, see Holmes & Matthews, 2010), thus enabling the repair of dysfunctional schemas or emotional schemes (cf., Lane, Ryan, Nadel, & Greenberg, 2014). It has been shown to enhance the re-interpretation of situations (Holmes, Mathews, Dalgleish, & Mackintosh, 2006), thus allowing the client to reattribute whatever happened (e.g., abuse or neglect) to external, rather than internal, causes, and reducing the attendant shame and guilt. Finally, it provides a unique opportunity for nurturance and care: the simultaneous evocation of emotion in both client and therapist allows clients to feel their pain in the presence of an empathic and caring other, sometimes for the first time; and it attunes therapists to the very vivid and specific experiences harbored by their clients. This shared experience has been recognized by many (e.g., Fosha, 2000) as ameliorative, and sets the stage for nurturance of the vulnerable child.

The specific use of imagery with rescripting, like the broader ST strategy regarding dysfunctional internalized modes, sometimes entails direct confrontation with this mode. Even when that is the case, the work is *never* focused only on the internalized perpetrator, and *always* requires care and attention to the vulnerable child involved; when confrontation is called for, we must stay cognizant of the experience – sometime terrifying, sometimes ambivalent – of the child who is witnessing it as it unfolds. At times, we will opt to use a more dialogical approach, viewing the internalized perpetrator as an internal representation of parents (or others) who just did not – and maybe *still* do not – know how to treat their children right, mainly

because of their own deficient upbringing. After realizing the therapist is not against them, these modes often come out, with some tentativeness, and seek counsel. Oftentimes they agree to change their ways after getting enough reassurance and guidance (Maurer, 2015).

Re-parenting the child modes and helping them get their needs met

Child modes hold the core emotional experiences of the person: the sadness, pain, or fear of the vulnerable child, the anger or rage of the angry child, the joy and curiosity of the contented child, and the reckless abandon of the impulsive child. Each of these emotional experiences reflects a need (including safety, nurturance, validation, mirroring, encouragement, and limit-setting). The cardinal task of schema therapy is to help clients recognize these needs and meet them in an adaptive manner.

The most important set of techniques in pursuing this task are relational ones. In particular, the therapists' care and validation (key parts of the limited re-parenting stance) are expressly directed at the client's vulnerability. In this stance, schema therapists offer direct (although limited) fulfillment of the needs of the vulnerable child for warmth, caring, validation, and of course safety. This fulfillment is genuine (with therapists encouraged to respond as they believe a good-enough parent would) and limited (with therapists clearly instructed to refrain from offering more than they would be able to sustain over time, and of course to remain within professional and ethical boundaries).

Re-parenting is a broad therapeutic stance which permeates all parts of the therapist's actions. At times, it comes out most vividly within the context of emotion-focused techniques – particularly when conducting imagery with rescripting. As we noted earlier, imagery with rescripting achieves several simultaneous effects. It strengthens the Healthy Adult, curtails the effects of Coping modes, and combats Internalized Parental modes. At the same time, it also carries an empowering message to the hurt Vulnerable Child. At times, therapists themselves ask for permission to enter the image; when this happens, they have the opportunity to provide direct re-parenting *within the imagery*.

Another EFT useful in addressing Child modes is the empty chair technique. In it, clients are encouraged to express their hurt or angry feelings towards an external person, while imagining this person to be present and sitting in another chair in the room. The therapist gently directs the client away from abstract or experience-distant statements (e.g., "she wouldn't have agreed to have this conversation") and re-focuses them on concrete, present-focused conversation (e.g., "Can you tell her what it's like for you to see that expression on her face right now?"). The main objective is to activate pent-up emotion in the client and not to engage in a logical or factual argument with the imagined other. The intent is to activate and express the basic emotions felt by the vulnerable or angry child (e.g., anger, fear, shame, and sadness) rather than the processed secondary emotions (e.g., hopelessness, anxiety, complaint, or blame) that emerge from coping modes.

Alongside relational and emotion-focused techniques, cognitive ones may also be useful in helping develop an understanding of the (universal and personal) origins of child modes. For example, the collaborative drafting of schema flashcards can help impart the psychoeducational message that vulnerabilities (and the unmet needs that underlie them) are themselves a healthy, if painful, response to triggering situations. Similarly, behavioral techniques can be quite useful in aiding child modes: rehearsing the expression of appropriate anger and assertiveness (angry child); developing methods for self-regulation and discipline (impulsive child); establishing self-reinforcement (contented child); and practicing the expression of needs (vulnerable child).

Empowering the healthy adult as a key to an integrated self

We are often asked whether the emphasis on differentiating modes and on responding to them differentially carries a risk of leading to a fragmented, non-unified self. The truth is quite the opposite. The distress which brings clients into therapy is a clear indication that their current self-organization is not working well for them. Child modes do not receive adequate care; coping modes typically try but fail to block the negative messages of the Internalized Parental modes.

To correct such disharmony, the guiding self-compassionate presence of a healthy adult is needed. Early on in therapy, this job may fall to the therapist. Using the various techniques discussed above, the therapist strives to clarify what the modes are, to give voice to adaptive and vulnerable modes, and to create adaptive boundaries between the modes. Over time, the therapist cultivates the client's own Healthy Adult mode, joins with it, and serves as a model for it.

It is this Healthy Adult mode which ultimately helps clients attain a better integration of the self.

Conclusion

In this chapter, we presented the theoretical model of ST, reviewed the evidence for its utility, and gave an overview of how it is applied. As should be clear by now, ST aims to facilitate an adaptive integration of self-states. In doing so, it is itself a deeply integrative approach. Its etiological/developmental ideas are drawn from attachment theory, object relations, self psychology, and relational psychoanalysis. Its pragmatism stems from Beck's cognitive therapy, from which it emerged. The experiential techniques that play a central role in it are rooted in gestalt and process-experiential approaches. Finally, the objectives of ST's mode work are both experiential and cognitive, and make extensive use of relational, cognitive, behavioral, and experiential tools.

Notes

1   Although the formation of schemas is driven to a large degree by unmet needs, other factors such as temperamental vulnerability and cultural norms play major roles as well.

2   The exception to this are those schemas tied to acting out – such as insufficient self-control, or entitlement – which are typically seen more vividly within the Impulsive Child mode.

References

Allport, G. W. (1955). *Becoming*. New Haven, CT: Yale University Press.

Arntz, A. (2014). Imagery rescripting for personality disorders. In N. Thoma & D. McKay (Eds.), *Engaging Emotion in Cognitive Behavioral Therapy: Experiential Techniques for Promoting Lasting Change*. New York, NY: Guilford.

Arntz, A., & Jacob, G. (2012). *Schema Therapy in Practice: An Introductory Guide to the Schema Mode Approach*. New York, NY: Wiley.

Arntz, A., Klokman, J., & Sieswerda, S. (2005). An experimental test of the schema mode model of borderline personality disorder. *Journal of Behavior Therapy and Experimental Psychiatry*, 36, 226–239.

Bamelis, L., Giesen-Bloo, J., Bernstein, D., & Arntz, A. (2012). Effectiveness studies of schema therapy. In M. Vreeswijk, J. Broersen, & M. Nadort (Eds.) *The Wiley-Blackwell Handbook of Schema Therapy: Theory, Research and Practice* (pp. 495–510). New York, NY: Wiley.

Bamelis, L. L. M., Evers, S. M. A. A., Spinhoven, P., & Arntz, A. (2014). Results of a multicentered randomized controlled trial on the clinical effectiveness of schema therapy for personality disorders. *American Journal of Psychiatry*, 171, 305–322.

Bamelis, L. L., Renner, F., Heidkamp, D., & Arntz, A. (2011). Extended schema mode conceptualizations for specific personality disorders: An empirical study. *Journal of Personality Disorders*, 25, 41–58.

Bandura, A. (Ed.). (2006). *Psychological Modeling: Conflicting Theories.* Piscataway, NJ: Transaction.

Bartlett, F. C. (1932). *Remembering: An Experimental and Social Study.* Cambridge: Cambridge University Press.

Beck, A.T. (1976). *Cognitive Therapy and the Emotional Disorders.* Oxford: International Universities Press.

Chefetz, R. (2015). *Intensive Psychotherapy for Persistent Dissociative Processes: The Fear of Feeling Real.* New York, NY: Norton.

Chessick, R.D. (1996). Archaic Sadism. *Journal of the American Academy of Psychoanalysis*, 24, 605–618.

Farrell, J. M., Shaw, I. A., & Webber, M. A. (2009). A schema-focused approach to group psychotherapy for outpatients with borderline personality disorder: A randomized controlled trial. *Journal of Behavior Therapy and Experimental Psychiatry*, 40, 317–328.

Fosha, D. (2000). *The Transforming Power of Affect: A Model for Accelerated Change.* New York, NY: Basic Books.

Freud, S. (1940). An outline of psycho-analysis. *International Journal of Psychoanalysis*, 21, 27–84.

Giesen-Bloo, J., Van Dyck, R., Spinhoven, P., *et al.* (2006). Outpatient psychotherapy for borderline personality disorder: A randomized trial of schema-focused therapy vs transference-focused psychotherapy. *Archives of General Psychiatry*, 63, 649–658.

Greenberg, L. S. & Rice, L. N. (1996). *Facilitating Emotional Change: The Moment-By-Moment Process.* New York, NY: Guilford.

Greenberg, L. S. & Watson J. C. (2006). *Emotion Focused Therapy for Depression.* Washington, DC: APA Press.

Holmes, E. A., & Mathews, A. (2010). Mental imagery in emotion and emotional disorders. *Clinical Psychology Review*, 30, 349–362.

Holmes, E. A., Mathews, A., Dalgleish, T., & Mackintosh, B. (2006). Positive interpretation training: Effects of mental imagery versus verbal training on positive mood. *Behavior Therapy*, 37, 237–247.

Howell, E. F. (2013). *The Dissociative Mind.* New York, NY: Routledge.

James, W. (1950). *The Principles of Psychology.* Cambridge, MA: Harvard University Press. (Original work published 1890.)

Kant, I. (1781/1929) *Critique of Pure Reason*, trans. N. Kemp Smith. Macmillan. (Original work published in 1781; Kemp Smith translation 1929.)

Kellogg, S. (2004). Dialogical encounters: Contemporary perspectives on 'chairwork' in psychotherapy. *Psychotherapy: Theory, Research, Practice, Training*, 41, 310–320.

Kelly, G. A. (1955). *The Psychology of Personal Constructs* (Vols. 1–2). New York, NY: Norton.

Klein, M. (1946). *Envy and Gratitude and Other Works 1946–1963.* London: Hogarth Press.

Lane, R. D., Ryan, L., Nadel, L., & Greenberg, L. (2015). Memory reconsolidation, emotional arousal and the process of change in psychotherapy: New insights from brain science. *Behavioral and Brain Sciences*, 38, 1–64.

Linville, P. W., & Carlston, D. E. (1994). Social cognition and the self. In P. G. Devine, D. L. Hamilton, & T. M. Olstrom (Eds.), *Social Cognition: Impact on Social Psychology* (pp. 143–193). San Diego, CA: Academic Press.

Lobbestael, J. (2012). Validation of the Schema Mode Inventory. In M. Vreeswijk, J. Broersen, & M. Nadort (Eds.) *The Wiley-Blackwell Handbook of Schema Therapy: Theory, Research, and Practice* (pp. 541–551). New York, NY: Wiley.

Lobbestael, J., Arntz, A., Cima, M., & Chakhssi, F. (2009). Effects of induced anger in patients with antisocial personality disorder. *Psychological Medicine*, 39, 557–568.

Lobbestael, J., Van Vreeswijk, M. F., & Arntz, A. (2008). An empirical test of schema mode conceptualizations in personality disorders. *Behaviour Research and Therapy*, 46, 854–860.

Lobbestael, J., van Vreeswijk, M., Spinhoven, P., Schouten, E., & Arntz, A. (2010). Reliability and validity of the short Schema Mode Inventory (SMI).*Behavioural and Cognitive Psychotherapy*, 38, 437.

Malogiannis, I. A., Arntz, A., Spyropoulou, A., *et al.* (2014). Schema therapy for patients with chronic depression: A single case series study. *Journal of Behavior Therapy and Experimental Psychiatry*, 45, 319–329.

Maurer, O. (2015). A failure with a capital F. In A. Rolef Ben Shahar & R. Shalit (Eds.), *Therapeutic Failures.* London: Karnac.

McGinn, L. K., & Young, J. E. (1996). Schema-focused therapy. In P. M. Salkovskis (Ed.), *Frontiers of Cognitive Therapy* (pp. 182–207) New York, NY: Guilford Press.

Mead, G. H. (1934). *Mind, Self and Society from the Perspective of a Social Behaviorist.* Chicago, IL: Chicago University Press.

Minuchin, S., Nichols, P. N., & Lee, W. (2007) *Assessing Families and Couples, From Symptom to System.* New York, NY: Pearson.

Nadort, M., Arntz, A., Smit, J. H., *et al.* (2009). Implementation of outpatient schema therapy for borderline personality disorder with versus without crisis support by the therapist outside office hours: A randomized trial. *Behaviour Research and Therapy*, 47, 961–973.

Porges, S. W. (2011). *The Polyvagal Theory: Neurophysiological Foundations of Emotions, Attachment, Communication, and Self-Regulation.* New York, NY: Norton.

Putnam, F. W. (1989). *Diagnosis and Treatment of Multiple Personality Disorder.* New York, NY: Guilford.

Rafaeli, E., Bernstein, D. P., & Young, J. (2011). *Schema Therapy: Distinctive Features.* New York, NY: Routledge.

Rafaeli, E., & Hiller, A. (2010). Self-complexity: A source of resilience? In J. Reich, A. Zautra, & J. Hall (Eds.), *Handbook of Adult Resilience* (pp. 171–192). New York, NY: Guilford Press.

Rafaeli, E., Maurer, O., & Thoma, N. (2014). Working with modes in schema therapy. In N. Thoma & D. McKay (Eds.), *Engaging Emotion in Cognitive Behavioral Therapy: Experiential Techniques for Promoting Lasting Change.* New York, NY: Guilford Press.

Rogers, T. B. (1977). Self-reference in memory: Recognition of personality items. *Journal of Research in Personality*, 1, 295–305.

Sempértegui, G. A., Karreman, A., Arntz, A., & Bekker, M. H. J. (2014). Schema therapy for borderline personality disorder: A comprehensive review of its empirical foundations, effectiveness and implementation possibilities. *Clinical Psychology Review*, 33, 426–447.

Shafran, R., Rafaeli, E., Gadassi, R., *et al.* (2015). Examining the schema-mode model in borderline and avoidant personality disorders using experience-sampling methods. Manuscript in preparation.

Siegel, D. J. (1999). *The Developing Mind: Toward a Neurobiology of Interpersonal Experience.* New York, NY: Guilford.

van der Hart, O., Nijenhuis E. R. S., & Steele, K. (2006). *The Haunted Self.* New York, NY: Norton.

Wylie, R. (1974). *The Self Concept* (Rev. ed., Vol. 1). Lincoln: University of Nebraska Press.

Wylie, R. (1979). *The Self-Concept* (Vol. 2). Lincoln: University of Nebraska Press.

Young, J. E. (1990). *Cognitive Therapy for Personality Disorders: A Schema-focused Approach.* Sarasota, FL: Professional Resource Exchange.

Young, J. E., Klosko, J. S., & Weishaar, M. E. (2003). *Schema Therapy: A Practitioner's Guide.* New York, NY: Guilford.

Zaki, J., & Ochsner, K. N. (2011). You, me, and my brain: Self and other representation in social cognitive neuroscience. In A. Todorov, S. T. Fiske, & D. Prentice (Eds.), *Social Neuroscience: Toward Understanding the Underpinnings of the Social Mind.* New York, NY: Oxford University Press.

Chapter

8

The self in depression

Patrick Luyten and Peter Fonagy

Introduction

There has been lively interest in the role of the self and self-experience in depression and mood disorders more generally. Vulnerability to depression has been related to various aspects of the self, including low, fragile, or vulnerable *self*-esteem (Kohut & Wolf, 1978; Mollon & Parry, 1984), problems with *self*-efficacy (Maddux & Meier, 1995), *self*-consistency (Joiner, Alfano, & Metalsky, 1993), *self*-derogation (Pyszczynski & Greenberg, 1987), *self*-criticism or *self*-critical perfectionism (Blatt, 2004), *self*-silencing (Jack, 1991), *self*-focused attention (Pyszczynski & Greenberg, 1987), and the development of a false *self* (Kohut & Wolf, 1978). Research on narcissism (a concept emerging from the psychoanalytic tradition that refers to the development of feelings of self-esteem and self-worth) is also relevant here, as theories rooted in this tradition have argued that vulnerability for depression is associated with disruptions in the development of narcissism, leading to a defensively grandiose but vulnerable or false *self* (Kernberg, 1975; Kohut & Wolf, 1978; Pincus, Cain, & Wright, 2014). Depression has also been linked to discrepancies between the ideal, wished for or "ought to be" and the actual or real *self* (Higgins, 1987). Similarly, ego psychological theories of depression, albeit using the more abstract notion of ego instead of the more experience-near concept of self, have focused on discrepancies between the ego and the superego or ego ideal (internalized "ought to be" or ideal self-aspects) in explaining vulnerability for depression (Bibring, 1953; Jacobson, 1971). Also, various authors have linked *self*-conscious emotions such as shame and guilt to depression (Kim, Thibodeau, &

Jorgensen, 2011). Finally, many theories have focused on impairments in representations or cognitive schemas of *self* in-relation-to-others as vulnerability factors for depression (Arieti & Bemporad, 1978; Beck, 1983; Blatt, 2004; Bowlby, 1973).

The list of theories linking aspects of the self to vulnerability to depression is long. This should not be surprising. Indeed, the phenomenology of depression suggests that depression is associated with an often serious disruption of the feeling of self and self-experience (see Figure 8.1). Depression is associated with a range of subjective experiences that seriously threaten the coherence of the self: feelings of sadness, guilt, shame, helplessness, hopelessness, and despair disrupt the continuity of the self and are felt as extremely painful and inescapable, to the point that the depressed individual may have the feeling that he/she can no longer bear the psychological pain associated with these subjective states.

We begin this chapter with an attempt at conceptual clarification based on contemporary developmental theory and neuroscience. Next, we discuss an integrative dialectic model of the development of the self that has its roots in the delineation of two qualitative types of self-experience in depression, which has led to a productive program of research on vulnerability for depression. We also discuss links between this approach and other theories about the self in depression. We then go on to discuss more recent approaches that focus on the self as a process, and on disruptions in this process that are associated with depression. For each of these approaches, we discuss implications for treatment. Finally, we also discuss neurobiological accounts of the self in relation to depression.

The Self in Understanding and Treating Psychological Disorders, ed. Michael Kyrios, Richard Moulding, Guy Doron, Sunil S. Bhar, Maja Nedeljkovic, and Mario Mikulincer. Published by Cambridge University Press. © Cambridge University Press, 2016.

Features of the self and theories about vulnerability for depression

- Low, fragile, or vulnerable self-esteem/vulnerable narcissism

- Development of a false self

- Problems with: self-efficacy, self-consistency, self-derogation, self-criticism, self-silencing, self-focused attention, self-consciousness

- Discrepancies between the ideal, wished for or "ought to be" self and the actual or real self; conflicts or discrepancies between ego and superego or ego ideal

- Impairments in representations or cognitive schemas of self and others

Figure 8.1 Self psychological approaches and the phenomenology of depression.

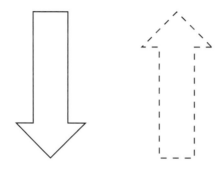

Phenomenology of depression

- Subjective experiences that seriously threaten the coherence of the self

- Feelings of sadness, guilt, shame, helplessness, hopelessness, and despair

- Felt as extremely painful and inescapable

What is the self?

Many theories referring to the role of the self in depression typically use metaphors (such as a "fragile self," or discrepancies between the ideal or wished for self and the actual self) to capture the psychological processes that may explain vulnerability for depression. These metaphors are tremendously helpful from a phenomenological perspective but also have led to the reification of these self-experiences, as if we truly "have" a false or fragile self, or that we "have" an ideal and an actual self. Although helpful clinically, they provide a metaphorical description of the phenomenological experience of depression, rather than a true explanation (see Figure 8.1). Most contemporary psychological approaches therefore assume that the self and the sense of self-coherence (i.e., the sense that one has continuity and consistency in thought and behavior) is an illusion (Bargh, 2011, 2014): it is the product of our capacity for social cognition or mentalizing, that is, our capacity to understand ourselves in terms of intentional mental states (i.e., our feelings, wishes, attitudes, and goals) that have some stability over time (Han, Northoff, & Joan, 2009; Northoff *et al.*, 2006).

In the remainder of this chapter, we focus on the differences between theories about the self in depression that are rooted in *mental representation* versus *mental process* approaches to the self. While the former typically focus on the *content* of representations

Table 8.1 Mental representation models of depression and the experience of self.

	Dimensions of self-experience in depression	
	Self-critical perfectionism/autonomy	Dependency/sociotropy
Self-experience	Self-experience is overly focused on achievement and autonomy	Self-experience is overly dependent on others
Phenomenology of depression	Themes of failure and/or defeat dominate: feelings of failure, self-hate, guilt, anhedonia, and loss of interest in others	Feelings of loss and deprivation dominate: helplessness, loneliness, and concerns about attractiveness and/or loveability
Developmental origins	Identification with high demands from attachment figures and/or the need for a defensive compensation for feelings of inferiority resulting from harsh parenting	Love and acceptance were strongly contingent upon the child's dependence on attachment figures
Typical interpersonal relationships	Critical, ambivalent: tend to evoke criticism and disapproval in others as a consequence of their high standards and critical attitudes	Clinging, claiming: elicit rejection and abandonment by others because of excessive demands for love and care
Therapeutic response	Respond primarily to interpretative aspects of the therapeutic process	Respond primarily to the interpersonal aspects of the therapeutic process
Mutative factor in treatment: emergence of the neglected and/or defended against self-experiences	Resolution of ruptures leads to recognition of underlying dependency needs	Resolution of ruptures leads to greater self-assertiveness and autonomy

of the self, the latter approaches view impairments in self-structures in depression as being the result of impairments in the *process* of social cognition or mentalizing (Fonagy, Moran, Edgcumbe, Kennedy, & Target, 1993; Luyten, Blatt, & Fonagy, 2013).

Mental representation models of the self in depression: depression and disruptions of the dialectic between the development of the self and relatedness

Both psychodynamic (Blatt, 2004; Luyten & Blatt, 2012) and cognitive-behavioral (Beck, 1983; Young, Klosko, & Weishaar, 2003) theorists have argued that distortions in the content of mental representations concerning the self (and others) confer vulnerability to depression (see Table 8.1). Beck (1983) described the concepts of *sociotropy* and *autonomy*, which refer to broad cognitive-affective schemas that organize the self and are presumed to confer vulnerability to depression, as well as to other types of psychopathology. These dimensions overlap both theoretically and empirically with psychodynamic formulations concerning *dependency* and *self-critical perfectionism*, respectively (Blatt, 2004; Luyten & Blatt, 2011,

2013). While sociotropy/dependency refers to a self-organization that is overly focused on others as a source of self-worth and self-esteem, autonomy/self-critical perfectionism refers to a sense of self that is overly focused on achievement and autonomy at the cost of developing a capacity for relatedness. These types of self-organization are considered to reflect a disruption of the normal dialectical interaction between two fundamental developmental lines. These are, first, an *anaclitic*, *relatedness* or *attachment* line, which normally leads to increasingly mature, complex, and mutually satisfying interpersonal relations; and second, an *introjective* or *self-definitional* line, which normally leads to the development of a stable, realistic, and essentially positive self and identity (Luyten & Blatt, 2013; Luyten *et al.*, 2011). Disruptions in this dialectic lead to an imbalance between these developmental lines, in which one is overemphasized or exaggerated while the other is neglected.

Empirical research suggests that autonomy/self-critical perfectionism involves one's identification with high demands from attachment figures and/or represents a defensive compensation for feelings of inferiority resulting from harsh parenting – in particular parental criticism and psychological control (Blatt & Luyten, 2009; Soenens, Vansteenkiste, & Luyten, 2010). Attempts to compensate for these feelings may lead to overcompensation, as is expressed in an exaggerated focus on achievement, often leading to mental and/or physical overexertion, and a so-called "false" self that is seen as strong, autonomous, and self-reliant, but in reality is fragile and vulnerable. These individuals have been described in the self psychology literature as experiencing a strong discrepancy between their "ought" or "ideal" self and their real self, or as characterized by strong conflicts between their ego ideal and/or superego and their ego, or as exhibiting high levels of self-criticism and self-derogation, depending on the specific theoretical approach. Excessive self-sacrificing tendencies may serve the purpose of seeking recognition and praise. Given this tendency for overexertion and self-sacrifice in combination with strong needs for autonomy and control, self-critical perfectionism is also implicated in fatigue- and pain-related exhaustion syndromes (see Chapter 19 in this book), as well as in eating disorders (Boone, Soenens, & Luyten, 2014; Egan, Wade, & Shafran, 2011).

Sociotropy/dependency refers to a self-organization that is overly focused on others as a source of self-esteem and self-worth, to the neglect of feelings of autonomy. This may range from individuals with a very fragile "self-structure" who thus are almost completely dependent on others for their self-esteem; this is, for instance, typically observed in individuals with borderline personality disorder. Indeed, studies suggest the existence of high levels of preoccupied and disorganized attachment in these individuals, which lead to idealization–denigration cycles in relationships and a lack of feelings of stability of the self – so-called *identity diffusion* (Fonagy & Luyten, 2016; Levy, Beeney, & Temes, 2011). In higher-functioning individuals (e.g., individuals with dependent or histrionic personality disorder), dependency needs are more modulated and are typically associated with a submissive yet passive–aggressive relational style. These individuals typically inhibit anger, as "anger threatens the very hand that feeds" (Blatt, 2004), which often is associated with "self-silencing" strategies (Jack & Dill, 1992), silencing their needs for autonomy and recognition because they fear abandonment and loneliness. Many of these individuals may also develop compulsive caregiving tendencies; that is, they care for others as they would like to be cared for themselves (Blatt, 2004). Developmentally, excessive dependency has been shown to be rooted in attachment figures' excessive emphasis on dependency, i.e., feelings of love, approval and recognition were excessively contingent upon the child's dependence, thwarting the development of the capacity for autonomy and self-efficacy.

Sociotropy/dependency and autonomy/self-critical perfectionism have also been shown to be associated with increased stress sensitivity and stress generation processes, particularly through their impact on close interpersonal relationships, which are expressed in dysfunctional interpersonal transactional styles (Luyten, Blatt, Van Houdenhove, & Corveleyn, 2006; Luyten *et al.*, 2011; Shahar & Priel, 2003). Highly dependent individuals tend to elicit rejection and abandonment by others because of excessive demands for love and care. They thus show hypervigilance for rejection and abandonment, leading to continuous doubts about the self, which hampers the development of feelings of autonomy, integrity and agency. Self-critical perfectionistic individuals tend to evoke criticism and disapproval in others as a consequence of their high standards and critical attitudes. Hence, others tend to confirm dependent individuals' fears of rejection and abandonment, and self-critical individuals' fears of disapproval, leading to interpersonal vicious cycles. Self-critical individuals therefore show hypervigilance for experiences of failure, typically leading to strong feelings of self-doubt and often even the conviction that, deep down inside, they are completely worthless. Needless to say, these feelings and fantasies seriously hinder the development of positive feelings of self-regard. These findings are in line with major models of depression linking the disorder to increased stress sensitivity and the active generation of stress (Hammen, 2005; Heim, Newport, Mletzko, Miller, & Nemeroff, 2008).

Despite these similarities in various theoretical formulations concerning these two types of self-organization in depression, there are also some interesting differences between theoretical orientations. For instance, there is a greater emphasis on the *function* of these types of self-construal within psychodynamic approaches. As an example, cognitive-affective schemas centered on sociotropy/dependency are not seen solely as reflecting an individual's high dependency needs resulting from a history of deprivation, but also as his/her best attempt, given his/her biological endowment and environmental context, to establish some sense of stability in the sense of self and others – however maladaptive the attempt may in fact be. This perspective has recently also been incorporated in schema therapy – for example, through the notion of experiential avoidance and the view that

Table 8.2 Mentalizing models of depression and the experience of self.

Non-mentalizing modes of experiencing the self (and others) in depression	
Psychic equivalence mode	• Inner (mental) reality is equated with outer reality ("mind–world isomorphism"); may lead to hyperembodiment • Intolerance of alternative perspectives; leads to "concrete" understanding: "things are what they are" ("depressive realism")
Teleological mode	• Extreme exterior focus: there is only goal-directed behavior and real physical causes • Observable change or action is experienced as the only true indicator of the intentions of the other
Extreme pretend mode	• The experience of self (thoughts and feelings) is decoupled from external reality • Leads to excessive rumination and in the extreme may manifest as "dissociation" of thought ("hypermentalizing" or "pseudomentalizing")
Painful experiences that threaten the coherence of the self-experience, leading to tendency to externalize these "alien-self" features	• The individual feels increasingly unable to bear the painfulness of subjective experiences • Suicidal thoughts and gestures and/or defensive externalization serve the purpose of getting rid of painful feelings and restoring the coherence of the self
Therapeutic response	• Validation of the patient's perspective • Suggest alternative perspectives (restoring mentalizing) • Link to current problems in relating to the self and others (restoring self-coherence of the self-experience)
Mutative factors in treatment	Restoring capacity for mentalizing leads to: • greater self-coherence and self-efficacy • greater capacity for relatedness • increased resilience in the face of adversity • restoring the capacity for social learning

schemas (and modes) may reflect compensatory strategies (Eurelings-Bontekoe, Luyten, Ijssennagger, van Vreeswijk, & Koelen, 2010; Young *et al.*, 2003).

Mentalizing and the self in depression: depression and disruptions in the capacity for reflecting about the self

More recent psychodynamic and cognitive-behavioral approaches have increasingly adopted a process approach to the disorganization of the self-experience and vulnerability for depression. Specifically, there is increasing interest in the role of impairments in metacognition – literally "thinking about thinking" – or mentalizing (also referred to as reflective functioning) in depression (Luyten, Fonagy, Lemma, & Target, 2012; Segal, Williams, & Teasdale, 2013; Watkins & Teasdale, 2004). These approaches center on the metacognitive processes that are involved in reflecting on the self and others (see Table 8.2). This approach is consistent with the so-called "third-wave" cognitive-behavioral approaches that focus on the roles of metacognitive

awareness and mindfulness in the treatment of depression.

These approaches complement views focusing on distorted cognitive-affective schemas in depression outlined earlier in this chapter. Specifically, they provide a better account of the disintegration of the feeling of *self* that is typical of many depressed patients and which is perhaps at the core of the depressive experience. These more phenomenological process-oriented approaches also provide more direct, and perhaps more effective, avenues for intervention with patients who are severely depressed: "lifting" these patients' depressed mood is often a prerequisite before they can engage with their therapist in any meaningful work relating to the content of their depressive experiences. This may be one of the reasons why mindfulness-based cognitive therapy has been shown to be effective in chronic depression (Kahl, Winter, & Schweiger, 2012; Mathew, Whitford, Kenny, & Denson, 2010). Similarly, the mentalizing approach originated in the treatment of patients with borderline personality disorder, who commonly experience intense, long-standing feelings of depression as well as serious disorganization of the self (Luyten & Fonagy, 2014).

Both mindfulness and mentalizing approaches to depression place emphasis on the influence of depressed mood on a person's metacognitive abilities. These approaches start from the point of view that, irrespective of the cause of a person's low mood and depression, he or she may well be completely unable to reflect on the self and others when depressed; when he or she does engage in reflective processes, they are very likely to be biased by his/her depressive thoughts. Hence, mindfulness and mentalizing approaches tend to avoid interventions that rely on insight and reflective capacities, particularly in the early stages of treatment, when patients are more likely to be severely depressed and to lack these capacities. Such interventions run the risk of the patient experiencing further pessimistic thoughts, for example, feeling helpless and hopeless, perceiving the therapist as lacking in empathy – or even as persecutory or accusatory – depending on the content of the patient's cognitive-affective schemas (that is, whether they tend toward sociotropy/dependency, or autonomy/self-critical perfectionism, as outlined earlier). A patient whose self-organization is strongly dependent may feel that the therapist fails to recognize his/her suffering or even blames the patient for his/her problems. In contrast, a patient who is more self-critical may feel that the therapist attempts to force interpretations on them and thwarts the patient's strivings for autonomy; these patients often drop out of treatment prematurely for this reason.

From the mentalizing perspective, three types of so-called *prementalizing modes* – modes of thinking that antedate full mentalizing – may be observed in individuals with depression (Lemma, Target, & Fonagy, 2011a; Luyten *et al.*, 2012). These modes of experiencing subjectivity seriously distort the patient's feeling of coherence of the self, which leads to increasing pressure to externalize unintegrated, unmentalized features of the self – a feature well known to anyone who has worked with seriously depressed patients.

In a *psychic equivalence mode*, inner and outer reality are equated, such that what the patient thinks or feels becomes hyper-real for them. For example, if a depressed patient *thinks* he is worthless, it means that he truly *is* worthless. Any attempt to correct these "dysfunctional thoughts" is itself meaningless – particularly when the patient is severely depressed – and only serves to reinforce psychic equivalence thinking. Psychic equivalence thinking can also lead the patient to equate psychological and physical pain, or emotional and physical exhaustion. The general concreteness of

these patients' experiences can mean that psychological pain literally feels like bodily pain, and depressive thoughts may feel as if they are actually pressing down on the self. This may go some way to explaining the high comorbidity between pain, fatigue, and depression (Luyten & Van Houdenhove, 2013). These individuals may also perceive negative remarks or criticism from others as a literal attack on the integrity of the self, which can lead to feelings of disintegration. This may result in *hyperembodiment* – a state in which all subjective experiences are experienced as too real; this often leads the individual into a "psychic retreat" because thoughts and feelings, in particular feelings of shame, are literally too painful for the patient to bear (Luyten, Fontaine, & Corveleyn, 2002). The so-called "depressive realism" that some depressed patients show also seems to be related to psychic equivalence thinking: while it may be "realistic" in some respects, reality simply is what it is, which leads to a sense of meaninglessness and apathy.

The *teleological mode* refers to a mode of functioning in which the patient recognizes a role for mental states as motivating the actions of the self and others, but this understanding is limited to goal-directed behaviors (hence the term "teleological") that can be directly attributed to observable (physical or biological) causes. In this mode, depressed patients may only feel loved or recognized when someone demonstrates love or recognition by observable, physical means, such as keeping them constant company. These patients may well engage in desperate strategies to get their attachment figures – including medical and mental health professionals – to show that they care for the patient. This is most notable in more dependent patients (e.g., by demanding that a loved one never leaves them alone, or by expecting their therapist always to be available for them). Another consequence of thinking in the teleological mode is that patients may deny that psychological factors play a role in their depressive illness, and steadfastly believe that there is a biological cause, as only biological factors can be recognized as real; this is often typical of more self-critical patients.

Depressed patients often seem to function in an extreme pretend mode, or *hypermentalizing* mode. This may appear on the surface to be genuine mentalizing, just as depressive realism may come across as appropriate realism. However, hypermentalizing can be distinguished from genuine mentalizing in a number of ways. Hypermentalizing accounts (a) are mostly overly analytical and lengthy; (b) are likely to be heavily focused on depressive themes and self-conscious emotions in particular (i.e., guilt, shame); (c) are often self-serving (e.g., they are constructed to encourage others to show empathy or compassion to the patient, or they may even be used to control or coerce others); and (d) may lack true affective grounding or, at the other extreme, may completely overwhelm the patient and others affectively. In addition, (e) the patient may show an inability to "switch perspectives" (e.g., from a focus on the self to others) when asked to; in contrast, genuine mentalizing is characterized by the ability to consider the mind of others at the same time as the self. Hypermentalizing is thus often accompanied by what is called *rumination* in cognitive-behavioral terms.

Depressed individuals' use of prementalizing modes typically gives rise to a pressure to externalize alien self-parts, that is, self-experiences that the individual cannot mentalize. As discussed previously, the capacity for mentalizing creates a feeling of coherence and stability of the self; thus, in an individual whose capacity to mentalize is impaired, this integrative process will be weak, and the incoherence in their self-representation is likely to become dominant. Torturous feelings of being "bad" or "worthless," for instance, will come to dominate the person's self-experience. They may deal with these experiences by externalizing them – that is, behaving toward others as though *the others* are responsible for the unmentalized self-experiences, and sometimes even generating the same experiences in others – that is, others then tend to engage in the same punitive or persecutory behaviors that the person internally inflicts upon themself (Fonagy & Target, 2000). Some patients instead engage in substance abuse, excessive eating or fasting, or other types of behavior that (in the teleological mode) temporarily relieve their tension and arousal (Fonagy & Target, 2000). Hence, the disintegration of the experience of coherence of the self because of the failure of mentalizing that is a result of depressed feelings appears to play an important role in explaining the association between depression and suicidal behaviors (Fonagy & Target, 1997, 2000; Luyten *et al.*, 2013).

Implications for intervention

All major therapies for depression focus on the experience of the self in depression. More traditional approaches, such as cognitive-behavioral therapy, psychodynamic psychotherapies, interpersonal therapy and emotion-focused therapy, focus on the *content* of self-experiences and self-organization that are presumed to confer vulnerability to depression. More recent approaches, as we have seen, also focus on the *process* of generation of a coherent self-experience and how this process is disrupted in depression. Increasingly, clinicians are integrating both perspectives; this approach is exemplified by dynamic interpersonal therapy (DIT) for depression, an integrative psychodynamic treatment that has recently been developed in the United Kingdom (Lemma *et al.*, 2011a; Lemma, Target, & Fonagy, 2011b). DIT has a content focus, the so-called *interpersonal affective focus*, which looks at the patient's typical recurring self-in-relation-to-others patterns. It also has a clear process focus, aimed at improving mentalizing capacities.

Changes in the capacity to reflect upon and make sense of one's own experiences may be the common factor that explains the effects of all evidence-based forms of psychosocial treatment; improvements in this capacity will help to restore the coherence of the self and facilitate the development of "broaden and build" cycles (Fredrickson, 2001) that allow a reorganization of the patient's self-experience. While different treatments may focus on the capacity to mentalize in different ways, they have a common outcome in process terms.

Traditional cognitive-behavioral approaches may promote mentalizing via drawing the patient's attention to his/her automatic thoughts and unhelpful attitudes, which may provide a new perspective on the self (Bjorgvinsson & Hart, 2006). Mindfulness-based approaches may foster mentalizing about inner mental states in particular, and on how inner mental states affect how the individual perceives and interprets the world around them, including their social relationships.

Interpersonal psychotherapy fosters mentalizing with regard to the self-in-relation-to-others, because of its focus on interpersonal relationships (Klerman, Weissman, Rounsaville, & Chevron, 1984). The use in traditional psychodynamic treatments of clarification, confrontation, and interpretation, and the examination of maladaptive representations of the self and others in the context of the therapeutic relationship (Leichsenring & Leibing, 2007), is also likely to foster mentalizing. Experiential therapies, which focus on the patient's affect states in the here-and-now within the context of an empathic and understanding therapeutic alliance, may, equally, foster mentalizing. For example, Greenberg, Watson, and Goldman's (1998) emotion-focused therapy for depression, which focuses on empathic understanding and experiential processing of core emotion-linked "depressogenic" schemas, is likely to promote mentalizing.

Neurobiology of the self in depression: the disruption of the self as an emergent structure

The focus on the self in theories of depression also provides links with the field of affective neuroscience. Congruent with the interpersonal, dialectic view of the self as a construct that results from the capacity of mentalizing, neurobiological studies suggest the existence of considerable overlap between the neural circuits involved in reflecting on the self and those that subserve the capacity to mentalize (Lieberman, 2007; Lombardo *et al.*, 2010).

Impairments in these neural circuits, including those in the medial prefrontal cortex, amygdala, hippocampus, and ventromedial parts of the basal ganglia (Drevets, Price, & Furey, 2008; Johnson, Nolen-Hoeksema, Mitchell, & Levin, 2009; Savitz & Drevets, 2009), have been found to be associated with depression (Fonagy & Luyten, 2009; Luyten & Fonagy, 2015). These dysfunctions have been linked to the failure of top-down regulation and/or impairments in bottom-up input as a consequence of the hypersensitivity of limbic structures, which may underlie the changes in autonomic regulation, emotion regulation, and neuroendocrine stress responses typically observed in individuals with depression (Drevets *et al.*, 2008; Johnson *et al.*, 2009; Savitz & Drevets, 2009). These findings suggest that depression is characterized by an inability to reappraise and suppress negative affect. To use our terminology, this represents a failure of controlled mentalizing, which leads to automatic, affect-dominated mentalizing becoming dominant. This model may partly explain the characteristic biased, non-reflective assumptions about the self (and others) as well as the emergence of prementalizing modes that are commonly shown by people with depression.

Although further studies are needed to provide more evidence regarding the neural substrates of depression, the findings to date are consistent with the view that depression is associated with a severe disruption of the experience of self, leading to an increasing focus on self-related thoughts and feelings.

Conclusions

Many theories in psychology and psychiatry have linked features of the self and disruptions in self-experience to depression. This chapter has outlined two general approaches. The first of these approaches focuses on content, distinguishing between two types of self-organization – one around issues of dependency, the other around self-criticism. The second approach sees the self as an emergent quality or process. The two approaches are complementary, and both are in line with current neurobiological understanding of the origins of the self. The self is inherently dialectical and its development is intrinsically linked to interactions with others. The sense and feeling of coherence of the self depend on the capacity for mentalizing. Disruptions in interactions with others, as well as in the capacity to mentalize, confer vulnerability for depression – and, unsurprisingly, both of these features are related. It is also important to consider the influence of depression on mentalizing and the feeling of self: disruptions in the self may thus be both a cause and a consequence of depression. These views open up interesting new perspectives for intervention and for considerations concerning the role of the self in depression and other types of psychopathology more generally.

References

Arieti, S., & Bemporad, J. (1978). *Psychotherapy of Severe and Mild Depression*. Northvale, NJ: Jason Aronson.

Bargh, J. A. (2011). Unconscious thought theory and its discontents: A critique of the critiques. *Social Cognition*, 29(6), 629–647. doi: 10.1521/soco.2011.29.6.629

Bargh, J. A. (2014). Our unconscious mind. *Scientific American*, 310(1), 30–37. doi: 10.1038/scientificamerican0114-30

Beck, A. T. (1983). Cognitive therapy of depression: New perspectives. In P. J. Clayton & J. E. Barrett (Eds.), *Treatment of Depression: Old Controversies and New Approaches* (pp. 265–290). New York, NY: Raven Press.

Bibring, E. (1953). The mechanism of depression. In P. Greenacre (Ed.), *Affective Disorders* (pp. 13–48). New York, NY: International Universities Press.

Bjorgvinsson, T., & Hart, J. (2006). Cognitive behavioural therapy promotes mentalizing. In J. G. Allen & P. Fonagy (Eds.), *Handbook of Mentalization-Based Treatment* (pp. 157–170). New York, NY: Wiley.

Blatt, S. J. (2004). *Experiences of Depression: Theoretical, Clinical and Research Perspectives*. Washington, DC: American Psychological Association.

Blatt, S. J., & Luyten, P. (2009). A structural–developmental psychodynamic approach to psychopathology: Two polarities of experience across the life span. *Development and Psychopathology*, 21(3), 793–814. doi: 10.1017/S0954579409000431

Boone, L., Soenens, B., & Luyten, P. (2014). When or why does perfectionism translate into eating disorder pathology? A longitudinal examination of the moderating and mediating role of body dissatisfaction. *Journal of Abnormal Psychology*, 123(2), 412–418. doi: 10.1037/a0036254

Bowlby, J. (1973). *Attachment and Loss: Separation.* New York, NY: Basic Books.

Drevets, W., Price, J., & Furey, M. (2008). Brain structural and functional abnormalities in mood disorders: Implications for neurocircuitry models of depression. *Brain Structure and Function*, 213(1), 93–118. doi: 10.1007/s00429-008-0189-x

Egan, S. J., Wade, T. D., & Shafran, R. (2011). Perfectionism as a transdiagnostic process: A clinical review. *Clinical Psychology Review*, 31(2), 203–212. doi: 10.1016/j.cpr.2010.04.009

Eurelings-Bontekoe, E. H. M., Luyten, P., Ijssennagger, M., van Vreeswijk, M., & Koelen, J. (2010). Relationship between personality organization and Young's cognitive model of personality pathology. *Personality and Individual Differences*, 49(3), 198–203. doi: 10.1016/j.paid.2010.03.034

Fonagy, P., & Luyten, P. (2009). A developmental, mentalization-based approach to the understanding and treatment of borderline personality disorder. *Development and Psychopathology*, 21(4), 1355–1381. doi: 10.1017/S0954579409990198

Fonagy, P., & Luyten, P. (2016). A multilevel perspective on the development of borderline personality disorder. In D. Cicchetti (Ed.), *Developmental and Psychopathology* (3rd ed.). New York, NY: Wiley.

Fonagy, P., Moran, G. S., Edgcumbe, R., Kennedy, H., & Target, M. (1993). The roles of mental representations and mental processes in therapeutic action. *Psychoanalytic Study of the Child*, 48, 9–48.

Fonagy, P., & Target, M. (1997). Attachment and reflective function: Their role in self-organization. *Development Psychopathology*, 9(4), 679–700.

Fonagy, P., & Target, M. (2000). Playing with reality: III. The persistence of dual psychic reality in borderline patients. *International Journal of Psychoanalysis*, 81(5), 853–874.

Fredrickson, B. L. (2001). The role of positive emotions in positive psychology. The broaden-and-build theory of positive emotions. *American Psychologist*, 56(3), 218–226. doi: 10.1037/0003-066X.56.3.218

Greenberg, L. S., Watson, J. C., & Goldman, R. (1998). Process-experiential therapy of depression. In L. S. Greenberg, J. C. Watson & G. Lietaer (Eds.), *Handbook of Experiential Psychotherapy* (pp. 227–248). New York, NY: The Guilford Press.

Hammen, C. (2005). Stress and depression. *Annual Review of Clinical Psychology*, 1(1), 293–319. doi: 10.1146/annurev.clinpsy.1.102803.143938

Han, S., Northoff, G., & Joan, Y. C. (2009). Understanding the self: A cultural neuroscience approach. *Progress in Brain Research*, 178, 203–212. doi: 10.1016/S0079-6123(09)17814-7

Heim, C., Newport, D. J., Mletzko, T., Miller, A. H., & Nemeroff, C. B. (2008). The link between childhood trauma and depression: Insights from HPA axis studies in humans. *Psychoneuroendocrinology*, 33(6), 693–710. doi: 10.1016/j.psyneuen.2008.03.008

Higgins, E. T. (1987). Self-discrepancy: A theory relating self and affect. *Psychological Review*, 94(3), 319–340.

Jack, D. C. (1991). *Silencing the Self: Women and Depression.* Cambridge, MA: Harvard University Press.

Jack, D. C., & Dill, D. (1992). The silencing the self scale: Schemas of intimacy associated with depression in women. *Psychology of Women Quarterly*, 16(1), 97–106. doi: 10.1111/j.1471-6402.1992.tb00242.x

Jacobson, E. (1971). *Depression: Comparative Studies of Normal, Neurotic and Psychotic Conditions.* New York, NY: International Universities Press.

Johnson, M. K., Nolen-Hoeksema, S., Mitchell, K. J., & Levin, Y. (2009). Medial cortex activity, self-reflection and depression. *Social Cognitive and Affective Neuroscience*, 4(4), 313–327. doi: 10.1093/scan/nsp022

Joiner, T. E., Alfano, M. S., & Metalsky, G. I. (1993). Caught in the crossfire: Depression, self-consistency, self-enhancement, and the response of others. *Journal of Social and Clinical Psychology*, 12(2), 113–134. doi: 10.1521/jscp.1993.12.2.113

Kahl, K. G., Winter, L., & Schweiger, U. (2012). The third wave of cognitive behavioural therapies: What is new and what is effective? *Current Opinion in Psychiatry*, 25(6), 522–528. doi: 10.1097/YCO.0b013e328358e531

Kernberg, O. F. (1975). *Borderline Conditions and Pathological Narcissism.* New York, NY: Jason Aronson.

Kim, S., Thibodeau, R., & Jorgensen, R. S. (2011). Shame, guilt, and depressive symptoms: A meta-analytic review. *Psychological Bulletin*, 137(1), 68–96. doi: 10.1037/a0021466

Klerman, G. L., Weissman, M. M., Rounsaville, B. J., & Chevron, E. S. (1984). *Interpersonal Psychotherapy of Depression.* New York, NY: Basic Books.

Kohut, H., & Wolf, E. S. (1978). The disorders of the self and their treatment: An outline. *International Journal of Psycho-Analysis*, 59, 413–426.

Leichsenring, F., & Leibing, E. (2007). Psychodynamic psychotherapy: A systematic review of techniques, indications and empirical evidence. *Psychology and Psychotherapy: Theory, Research and Practice*, 80(2), 217–228. doi: 10.1348/147608306X117394

Lemma, A., Target, M., & Fonagy, P. (2011a). *Brief Dynamic Interpersonal Therapy: A Clinician's Guide*. Oxford: Oxford University Press.

Lemma, A., Target, M., & Fonagy, P. (2011b). The development of a brief psychodynamic intervention (Dynamic Interpersonal Therapy) and its application to depression: A pilot study. *Psychiatry*, 74(1), 41–48. doi: 10.1521/psyc.2011.74.1.41

Levy, K. N., Beeney, J. E., & Temes, C. M. (2011). Attachment and its vicissitudes in borderline personality disorder. *Current Psychiatry Reports*, 13(1), 50–59. doi: 10.1007/s11920-010-0169-8

Lieberman, M. D. (2007). Social cognitive neuroscience: A review of core processes. *Annual Review of Psychology*, 58, 259–289. doi: 10.1146/annurev.psych.58.110405.085654

Lombardo, M. V., Chakrabarti, B., Bullmore, E. T., *et al.* (2010). Shared neural circuits for mentalizing about the self and others. *Journal of Cognitive Neuroscience*, 22(7), 1623–1635. doi: 10.1162/jocn.2009.21287

Luyten, P., & Blatt, S. J. (2011). Integrating theory-driven and empirically-derived models of personality development and psychopathology: A proposal for DSM-V. *Clinical Psychology Review*, 31(1), 52–68. doi: 10.1016/j.cpr.2010.09.003

Luyten, P., & Blatt, S. J. (2012). Psychodynamic treatment of depression. *Psychiatric Clinics of North America*, 35(1), 111–129. doi: 10.1016/j.psc.2012.01.001

Luyten, P., & Blatt, S. J. (2013). Interpersonal relatedness and self-definition in normal and disrupted personality development: Retrospect and prospect. *American Psychologist*, 68(3), 172–183. doi: 10.1037/a0032243

Luyten, P., Blatt, S. J., & Fonagy, P. (2013). Impairments in self structures in depression and suicide in psychodynamic and cognitive behavioral approaches: Implications for clinical practice and research. *International Journal of Cognitive Therapy*, 6(3), 265–279. doi: 10.1521/ijct.2013.6.3.265

Luyten, P., Blatt, S. J., Van Houdenhove, B., & Corveleyn, J. (2006). Depression research and treatment: Are we skating to where the puck is going to be? *Clinical Psychology Review*, 26(8), 985–999. doi: 10.1016/j.cpr.2005.12.003

Luyten, P., & Fonagy, P. (2014). Psychodynamic treatment for borderline personality disorder and mood disorders: A mentalizing perspective. In L. Choi-Kain & J. G. Gunderson (Eds.), *Borderline Personality Disorder and Mood: Controversies and Consensus* (pp. 223–251). New York, NY: Springer.

Luyten, P., & Fonagy, P. (2015). The neurobiology of mentalizing. *Personality Disorders: Theory, Research, and Treatment*, 6(4), 366–379. doi: 10.1037/per0000117

Luyten, P., Fonagy, P., Lemma, A., & Target, M. (2012). Depression. In A. Bateman & P. Fonagy (Eds.), *Handbook of Mentalizing in Mental Health Practice* (pp. 385–417). Washington, DC: American Psychiatric Association.

Luyten, P., Fontaine, J. R. J., & Corveleyn, J. (2002). Does the Test of Self-Conscious Affect (TOSCA) measure maladaptive aspects of guilt and adaptive aspects of shame? An empirical investigation. *Personality and Individual Differences*, 33(8), 1373–1387. doi:10.1016/S0191-8869(02)00197-6

Luyten, P., Kempke, S., Van Wambeke, P., *et al.* (2011). Self-critical perfectionism, stress generation, and stress sensitivity in patients with chronic fatigue syndrome: Relationship with severity of depression. *Psychiatry*, 74(1), 21–30. doi: 10.1521/psyc.2011.74.1.21

Luyten, P., & Van Houdenhove, B. (2013). Common and specific factors in the psychotherapeutic treatment of patients suffering from chronic fatigue and pain disorders. *Journal of Psychotherapy Integration*, 23(1), 14–27. doi: 10.1037/a0030269

Maddux, J. E., & Meier, L. J. (1995). Self-efficacy and depression. In J. E. Maddux (Ed.), *Self-Efficacy, Adaptation, and Adjustment* (pp. 143–169). New York, NY: Springer.

Mathew, K. L., Whitford, H. S., Kenny, M. A., & Denson, L. A. (2010). The long-term effects of mindfulness-based cognitive therapy as a relapse prevention treatment for major depressive disorder. *Behavioural and Cognitive Psychotherapy*, 38(5), 561–576. doi: 10.1017/S135246581000010X

Mollon, P., & Parry, G. (1984). The fragile self: Narcissistic disturbance and the protective function of depression. *British Journal of Medical Psychology*, 57(2), 137–145. doi: 10.1111/j.2044-8341.1984.tb01592.x

Northoff, G., Heinzel, A., de Greck, M., *et al.* (2006). Self-referential processing in our brain – A meta-analysis of imaging studies on the self. *Neuroimage*, 31(1), 440–457. doi: 10.1016/j.neuroimage.2005.12.002

Pincus, A. L., Cain, N. M., & Wright, A. G. (2014). Narcissistic grandiosity and narcissistic vulnerability in psychotherapy. *Personality Disorders*, 5(4), 439–443. doi: 10.1037/per0000031

Pyszczynski, T., & Greenberg, J. (1987). Self-regulatory perseveration and the depressive self-focusing style: A self-awareness theory of reactive depression. *Psychological Bulletin*, 102(1), 122–138. doi: 10.1037/0033-2909.102.1.122

Savitz, J., & Drevets, W. C. (2009). Bipolar and major depressive disorder: Neuroimaging the developmental-degenerative divide. *Neuroscience & Biobehavioral Reviews*, 33(5), 699–771. doi: 10.1016/j.neubiorev.2009.01.004

Segal, Z. V., Williams, J. M. G., & Teasdale, J. D. (2013). *Mindfulness-based Cognitive Therapy for Depression* (2nd ed.). New York, NY: The Guilford Press.

Shahar, G., & Priel, B. (2003). Active vulnerability, adolescent distress, and the mediating/suppressing role of life events. *Personality and Individual Differences*, 35(1), 199–218. doi: 10.1016/S0191-8869(02)00185-X

Soenens, B., Vansteenkiste, M., & Luyten, P. (2010). Towards a domain-specific approach to the study of parental psychological control: Distinguishing between dependency-oriented and achievement-oriented psychological control. *Journal of Personality*, 78(1), 217–256. doi: 10.1111/j.1467-6494.2009.00614.x

Watkins, E., & Teasdale, J. D. (2004). Adaptive and maladaptive self-focus in depression. *Journal of Affective Disorders*, 82(1), 1–8. doi: 10.1016/j.jad.2003.10.006

Young, P. J. E., Klosko, P. J. S., & Weishaar, M. E. (2003). *Schema Therapy: A Practitioner's Guide*. New York, NY: The Guilford Press.

The self in bipolar disorder

Nuwan D. Leitan

Chapter 9

Bipolar disorder (BD) is a serious disorder of mood associated with significant morbidity and mortality. Although originally understood through a psychological frame, the past few decades have seen the dominance of a biomedical paradigm in BD due to the importance of drug treatments and the condition's marked genetic loading. Consequently, psychological constructs like the "self" have not been systematically investigated to date in the context of BD, and there is no linking theory, much less consensus on how the term is best used. Nonetheless, the term appears frequently in various contexts, and the aim of this chapter is to explicate the divergent approaches to the concept of "self" as employed in the literature on BD. By systematically describing the various uses of the term "self" in BD, and reviewing empirical literature related to the term, it is hoped to clear the foundation for future theory, research and treatment in this potentially important domain.

Development of self in BD

The average age of onset for BD is between 18 and the early 20s, with more than 75% of individuals with the disorder developing clinical symptoms before the age of 18 (Merikangas *et al.*, 2007). Adolescence is associated with drastic changes in emotional, cognitive, and social identity and the formation of a sense of self has been identified as the key developmental task in this phase of life (Erikson, 1959). The onset of BD symptoms during adolescence has the potential to derail this important process, leading to disturbances in present and future sense of self and identity (Erikson, 1959; Marcia, 1966).

There has been limited research examining the development of self in BD; however, one qualitative study of young people with BD (aged 18–35) conducted by Inder *et al.* (2008) identified four core themes associated with the development of self and identity: confusion, contradiction, self-doubt, and self-acceptance. Confusion was underpinned by struggles in differentiating self from illness and the varying experiences of self caused by mood episodes. Contradiction was linked to polar experiences of self in depressive and manic states. Self-doubt arose from the lack of a stable sense of self, leading to excessive molding of the self to external factors. Finally, self-acceptance was seen as a way to consolidate and integrate aspects of the self in order to develop a more stable sense of self, but was sometimes seen as contingent on periods of mood stability. The research by Inder *et al.* presents preliminary evidence suggesting that BD symptoms in adolescents and young people present challenges to the development of a stable, coherent sense of self and identity, following similar difficulties found in other serious mental illnesses such as schizophrenia and borderline personality disorder (e.g., Sass, Pienkos, Nelson, & Medford, 2013). Associated research suggests that interpersonal and social rhythm therapy might be useful in stabilizing mood in this age group, thereby assisting in developing a more stable sense of self and identity in BD (Crowe *et al.*, 2009).

Conceptualizations of self in BD

Organization of self in BD

The oldest and most consistently researched approach to the self in BD is the notion of a "compartmentalized" or "modularized" self (Alatiq, Crane, Williams, & Goodwin, 2010b; Power, De Jong, & Lloyd, 2002;

The Self in Understanding and Treating Psychological Disorders, ed. Michael Kyrios, Richard Moulding, Guy Doron, Sunil S. Bhar, Maja Nedeljkovic, and Mario Mikulincer. Published by Cambridge University Press. © Cambridge University Press, 2016.

Taylor, Morley, & Barton, 2007). This idea is an extension of Showers' (1992) model of the "compartmentalized self" which was developed for application to the non-clinical self-concept and the "self" in unipolar depression. Showers' model considers the self-concept as represented in relational "self-aspects" (e.g., "me and boss," "me and parents," etc.). In people with a *compartmentalized* self-organization, each self-aspect is coded as *solely* positive or negative according to the individual's overall conceptualization of the relationship defined by the self-aspect. Contrastingly, in those with an *integrated* self-organization, each self-aspect is coded as a *mixture* of positive and negative self-beliefs, according to the individual's complex conceptualization of the relationship defined by the self-aspect. Showers proposes that in those with a compartmentalized self-organization, activation of one negative self-aspect triggers the activation of an overall negative self-concept because that self-aspect contains only negative self-beliefs (and vice versa for the activation of positive self-aspects). Notably, Showers also found that if positive self-aspects were perceived as important, compartmentalization was associated with high self-esteem and positive mood (or low depression), while if negative self-aspects were perceived as important, compartmentalization was associated with low self-esteem and negative mood (or high depression).

This "compartmentalized" or "modularized" model of self-organization is relevant to BD due to its potential to explain dramatic changes in mood, such as those observed in BD. The model suggests that in people with a compartmentalized self-organization, events which trigger a particular self-aspect that is positively valenced will activate an overwhelming sense of positive self-belief, potentially leading to hypomanic or manic behaviors. Conversely, in the same group of people, an adverse life event or environmental trigger activating a negatively valenced self-aspect will promote exclusively negative self-belief, potentially leading to dysphoric or depressive mood and behaviors. In comparison, for those with integrated self-organization, events which trigger a particular self-aspect will activate both positive and negative (balanced) self-belief because their self-aspects contain a mixture of positive and negative self-beliefs. In an initial study of the compartmentalized self in BD, Power *et al.* (2002) demonstrated that in BD patients in the euthymic phase, key self-aspects are compartmentalized as either completely positive or negative, leading to a modularized

self-concept, whereas in non-bipolar controls (diabetic sample) the same self-aspects were integrated.

Another model of self-organization which has been explored in relation to BD is "self-complexity" (Linville, 1985, 1987; see Bhar and Kyrios, Chapter 2 in this volume, for an introduction to self complexity). Linville (1985) suggested that low self-complexity could be a factor associated with dysregulated mood because activation of a self-aspect with a particular valence could trigger other self-aspects described by the same traits, leading to the perpetuation of an excessively negative or positive sense of self-belief. Contrastingly, if a particular self-aspect is activated in an individual with high self-complexity, activation is less likely to spread to other self-aspects because they are described using different traits. Alatiq *et al.* (2010b) and Taylor *et al.* (2007) explored self-compartmentalization and self-complexity in remitted BD patients compared to remitted unipolar depression patients and healthy controls. They found that self-compartmentalization was higher in BD and unipolar depression groups than healthy controls. Alatiq *et al.* (2010b) found no differences in self-complexity between groups while Taylor *et al.* (2007) found that remitted BD patients showed greater self-complexity than healthy controls when illness-related self-aspects (e.g., depression and mania-related) were included. Akin to Taylor *et al.*'s (2007) self complexity findings, Ashworth, Blackburn, and McPherson (1985) found that manic patients showed complex self-concepts relative to depressed patients.

Findings of high self-complexity in BD may have been due to the interaction between self-complexity and self-compartmentalization. If self-aspects are compartmentalized in BD, as found by both Alatiq *et al.* (2010b) and Taylor *et al.* (2007), then high complexity would allow activation to spread to more compartmentalized self-aspects, thus spiralling the activated state (either positive for mania or negative for depression) because those self-aspects do not contain mixed valence to moderate the activated state. This is consistent with the findings of Taylor *et al.* that high complexity was only found when highly compartmentalized illness-related concepts were included. Conversely, Linville's (1987) suggestion that high complexity could buffer against affective extremities would be supported if self-aspects were integrated, allowing activation to spread to more integrated self-aspects whose mixed valence would promote moderation of the initially activated state.

Hyperpositive self in BD

In exploring why large proportions of individuals with BD do not respond to cognitive therapy, Lam, Wright, and Sham (2005) proposed a "sense of hyperpositive self" as a potential factor. A hyperpositive self describes the proportion of individuals with BD who enjoy and aspire to be in a state of high arousal, positive mood, and behavioral hyperactivity and value traits such as being creative, entertaining, and outgoing. This group of patients may not always meet the criteria for mania or hypomania, but may be prone to dysregulation of goal-driven behavior and routine (Lam, Jones, Hayward, & Bright, 1999), which is in turn related to disruption of circadian rhythms and consequent triggering of mood episodes (Shen, Alloy, Abramson, & Sylvia, 2008). In a similar vein, it has been suggested that valuing internal states associated with mania and hypomania may be a factor in maintaining BD symptoms (Mansell, Morrison, Reid, Lowens, & Tai, 2007).

There is much evidence to suggest that vulnerability to mania and hypomania may be linked to traits associated with a hyperpositive sense of self such as goal-striving and goal-attainment (see Johnson, 2005) as well as creativity (see Murray & Johnson, 2010), and in turn these traits have been linked to a more severe course of BD (Johnson *et al.*, 2000). Two studies which explicitly examined sense of hyperpositive self in BD found that it was negatively correlated with depression and social performance, significantly predicted goal-attainment and preferred internal state of mania, and is associated with increased chance of relapse during cognitive therapy (Lam *et al.*, 2005; Lee, Lam, Mansell, & Farmer, 2010).

Self-discrepancy in BD

Discrepancies between specific dimensions of self have been linked to particular mood states. Actual:ideal self-discrepancies have been associated with depression (L. Scott & O'Hara, 1993; Strauman, 1989), while actual:ought self-discrepancy has been associated with anxiety (L. Scott & O'Hara, 1993; Strauman & Higgins, 1988). In an examination of self-discrepancy theory in BD, Bentall, Kinderman, and Manson (2005) found that depressed BD patients had higher levels of actual:ideal and actual:ought self-discrepancies compared to BD patients in other phases and healthy controls, while manic BD patients showed extremely low levels of actual:ideal self-discrepancy compared to healthy controls. The authors interpreted their latter

finding as consistent with the "manic defense" hypothesis (Neale, 1988), which contends that mania has the function of keeping depressive thoughts from entering consciousness and is triggered to block any stimuli that may promote depressive thinking. Aligning with this theory, the authors suggested that manic patients avoid distressing thoughts and negative affect about the self by overestimating success and underestimating weakness, thereby decreasing the discrepancy between selves.

Underpinned by evidence suggesting agitation is a common symptom of BD, Alatiq, Crane, Williams, and Goodwin (2010a) examined discrepancies between actual and feared "selves" in a student population. There were no group differences between BD and healthy controls. The authors suggest that this may drive motivation to avoid the feared self and consequently increase goal-directed behavior towards the ideal-self, thus potentially triggering elevated mood.

Self-related cognitive processing in BD

Self-referent processing in BD

Another broad stream of literature referring to the "self" in BD is associated with self-referent cognitive processing. This diverse group of studies is held together by the underlying idea that BD is associated with a dysfunction in in cognitive processing related to the self. Most of the empirical work conducted on self-referential processing in BD is an extension and replication of research conducted on unipolar depressed populations.

The primary theoretical basis for disturbed self-referent processing in unipolar depression is Beck's cognitive theory of depression (Beck, 1967), which posits that depressive symptoms occur as a result of negative schemas of self, world, and the future, which colours the processing of external and internal stimuli. There is little theoretical basis underpinning empirical work examining self-referent processing in BD, with the implicit assumption being the application of Beck's model to individuals in the depressive phase of BD and its mirror image, positing that manic symptoms occur as a result of overly positive schemas of self, world, and the future, applied to individuals in the manic phase of BD.

There has been a significant amount of empirical evidence suggesting a disturbance to self-referent processing in BD. These studies consistently demonstrate that in comparison to healthy controls, BD participants endorse and recall more negative than positive self-referent adjectives and attribute more negative than positive events to self, and this is often mediated by depressive symptomatology (e.g., Lyon, Bentall, & Startup, 1999; Molz Adams, Shapero, Pendergast, Alloy, & Abramson, 2014). Further, a pilot study of offspring of parents with BD found that there were no differences between high-risk children and low-risk children in the endorsement of positive and negative self-referent adjectives; however, high-risk children better recalled negative self-referent adjectives than low-risk children, providing preliminarily evidence that recall of self-referent material may be a vulnerability factor for BD (Gotlib, Traill, Montoya, Joormann, & Chang, 2005).

Aberrant self-referent processing in BD could also be understood as "damaged (or defensive)" self-esteem. Damaged self-esteem refers to high explicit self-reported self-esteem and negative implicit attitudes toward the self (also implied by the "manic defense hypothesis"). A number of studies have found such discrepancies in explicit and implicit self-associations (Jabben et al., 2014; Lyon et al., 1999). Damaged self-esteem has been linked to narcissistic behavior (Bosson, Swann Jr, & Pennebaker, 2000), high goal standards (Zeigler-Hill, 2006) and depressive attributional style (Creemers, Scholte, Engels, Prinstein, & Wiers, 2012).

Self-esteem in BD

Unlike other sections in this chapter, there has been a plethora of empirical evidence linking self-esteem to various domains of BD, thus here I will focus on empirical findings. There is significant evidence to suggest that BD is associated with low self-esteem during both euthymic and depressive phases and high self-esteem during manic/hypomanic episodes (Pavlickova et al., 2013, etc.). One study found that levels of self-esteem in BD patients were normal but more unstable in comparison to unipolar depressive patients and healthy controls (Knowles et al., 2007), a pattern which has also been found in children of parents with BD (Jones, Tai, Evershed, Knowles, & Bentall, 2006). Low self-esteem in BD has been linked to increased suicidality risk and worse prognosis (e.g., Halfon, Labelle, Cohen, Guilé, & Breton, 2013). Interestingly, studies which have examined vulnerability factors for BD have found that self-esteem does not predict vulnerability to BD (e.g.,

Pavlickova, Turnbull, & Bentall, 2014). Taken together, this evidence suggests that individuals' perception of their self-worth or self-value may be a perpetuating factor or symptom associated with the onset of BD rather than a vulnerability factor preceding onset.

Self-stigma in BD

Self-stigma refers to the process of internalizing negative external perceptions of mental illness leading to negative feelings about the self and behaving in ways consistent with the stigmatizing beliefs of the public (e.g., not pursuing a job because of discrimination) or anticipation of negative social reactions to mental illness (Ritsher, Otilingam, & Grajales, 2003). BD is an illness which is particularly prone to stigmatization (e.g., Mileva, Vázquez, & Milev, 2012), and recent literature has shown high levels of self-stigma in people with BD (see Ellison, Mason, & Scior, 2013).

Self-stigma in BD has been associated with poor psychosocial functioning (Vazquez et al., 2011), including low perceived social support (Cerit, Filizer, Tural, & Tufan, 2012), impaired social functioning (Perlick et al., 2001), low self-esteem, and high social anxiety (Hayward, Wong, Bright, & Lam, 2002). Evidence for the relationship between self-stigma and BD has been mixed with some studies finding associations with increased depressive (Cerit et al., 2012; Vazquez et al., 2011) and manic symptomatology (Vazquez et al., 2011), while others have found no association with depressive (Hayward et al., 2002) or manic symptomology (Cerit et al., 2012; Hayward et al., 2002).

Embodied self in BD

Some of the more contemporary conceptualizations of "self" in BD emphasize the phenomenological dimension of the concept. A developing phenomenological literature suggests that disturbances of the "lived/embodied/minimal" self, defined in greater detail below, may be intimately involved in psychopathology (Cermolacce, Naudin, & Parnas, 2007; Fuchs & Schlimme, 2009). This conceptualization of self is not purely cognitive but embodied, embedded and dependent on successful interactions in the world. Correspondingly, these phenomenological conceptualizations of self are either explicitly or implicitly associated with embodiment theory (Cermolacce et al., 2007).

Fuchs and Schlimme (2009) describe embodiment as the embedding of cognitive processes in the brain and the origin of these processes in an organism's sensory–motor experience in relation to its environment. Thus, for phenomenologists, the self is intertwined with the conscious stream of subjective experiences with a world which *affords* certain actions and prevents others according to ones' sensorimotor capabilities (Cermolacce *et al.*, 2007). BD may be associated with diminished subjective experience in the world due to the body standing in the way of environmental interaction instead of providing access to the world; correspondingly, the awareness of self becomes disturbed.

For example, Fuchs (2005) describes melancholic depression as a *corporealization* of the body as it loses fluidity, becomes heavier and more rigid and eventually the loss of bodily mediation of emotional experience leads to a sense of detachment from emotions and a diminished sense of self, sometimes to a point to which the sense of existence in the world may be denied. This description of disturbed self in melancholic depression is relevant for BD because depressive episodes in BD have a more severe, melancholic flavor than those in unipolar depression (Mitchell *et al.*, 2001).

Conversely, mania and hypomania in BD may be associated with a diminished subjective experience in the world due to the body and behavior becoming separated from an individual's sense of self; correspondingly, the self becomes distorted. Qualitative and quantitative empirical research has suggested that manic and hypomanic phases of BD are associated with a lack of self-control and a feeling of being "out of control" (Crowe *et al.*, 2012; Russell & Moss, 2013). These feelings are reflected in a sense of fast motion perception and thinking, feeling overwhelmed, loss of autonomy, and overall a lack of self-control of behavior (Crowe *et al.*, 2012; Russell & Moss, 2013). Thus, the body and its behaviors phenomenally become separated from consciousness, and immersed in the world without a sense of self. Such issues have led to a call for interventions which encourage and foster self-control (e.g., Jones & Burrell-Hodgson, 2008).

The only study to date examining the embodied self in BD was conducted by Haug *et al.* (2014), who examined disturbances of self-awareness or "sense of self," defined as being immersed in the world, continuous, and coherent, in individuals with schizophrenia and psychotic BD. The authors found high levels of disturbed sense of self, which was associated with poorer social functioning in both individuals with schizophrenia and psychotic BD.

The self in current and emerging psychological treatments for BD

CBT is a well-recognized evidence-based intervention for BD. In one variant of CBT for BD, the integrative cognitive model of Mansell *et al.* (2007), self plays an integral role in the explanation of mood swings. Mansell and colleagues propose that mood swings are maintained by interpreting changes in energy and mood as providing information about the self. This information may be positive ("my increased speed of thought shows how intelligent I am"), or negative ("my increased sensitivity to colors means I am going mad"). Self-involving thoughts are therefore central to this particular model.

It is informative to compare this involvement of "the self" in CBT with the metaphysically different "self" in so-called third-wave mindfulness-based therapies for BD (Perich, Manicavasagar, Mitchell, & Ball, 2014). Mindfulness-based approaches contrast with CBT by encouraging a change in relationship to thoughts rather than a change in content of thoughts. The self in these third-wave approaches is not a *cognizer*, but a *witness of experiences* (including thoughts, sensations, perceptions, emotions, etc.). The metaphysical assumptions of mindfulness approaches grow out of eastern religion, and encourage a radically different view of the self. A recent online mindfulness-based intervention for BD developed by Murray *et al.* (2015) encapsulated this conceptualization of self in their treatment model (also refer to Chapter 6 by Robert Zettle in this book for more on this conceptualization of self in BD).

Although traditional psychological therapies are widely used as adjuncts to pharmacotherapy in the treatment of BD, studies have found that psychological treatments have limited efficacy (Parikh *et al.*, 2012; J. Scott *et al.*, 2006). Thus, it may be important to consider alternative and/or adjunctive therapies, in particular for self-stigma and phenomenological self-related issues, which are not commonly targeted by the traditional psychosocial therapies described above.

Recently, it has been suggested that peer support may be an effective way of helping manage self-stigma in mental illness (e.g., Corrigan, Kosyluk, & Rüsch, 2013). Additionally, it has been found that peer support may also have beneficial impact on self-esteem (Watson, Corrigan, Larson, & Sells, 2007). Although peer support interventions have been encouraged by both individuals with BD (Todd, Jones, & Lobban, 2013) and experts (Lewis, 2005), and found to be efficacious (Morriss *et al.*, 2011; Proudfoot, Jayawant, *et al.*, 2012), only one study has examined their impact on self-stigma in BD, finding them only as effective as an online psychoeducational program without peer support (Proudfoot, Parker, *et al.*, 2012). Despite this finding, peer support interventions should be further researched on the basis of positive findings for other severe mental illnesses (Corrigan, Sokol, & Rüsch, 2013; Thomas *et al.*, in preparation).

Another area which has not been a focus of traditional psychosocial interventions for BD is the embodied, phenomenological dimension of the illness (Leitan & Murray, 2014). There is a longstanding continental literature which is emerging in mainstream psychology which suggests that working with the body's interaction with the world, as well as the mind, may be beneficial in the treatment of severe mental illness (Röhricht, 2009). There are a number of therapies under the umbrella of "body psychotherapies" which are held together by their common aim to release and re-shape somatic memories in order to release associated psychological constraints (Totton, 2003). One of the core tenets of the majority of body psychotherapies is their focus on improving self-awareness and integrating the body in self-awareness (Röhricht, 2009). Although body psychotherapies have not been widely applied to BD, research has suggested that they are efficacious in treating schizophrenia, including qualitative accounts of improved self-confidence, self-awareness, self-reflection, and bodily self-perception (Röhricht, Papadopoulos, Holden, Clarke, & Priebe, 2011; Röhricht, Papadopoulos, Suzuki, & Priebe, 2009). These findings encourage research into the use of body psychotherapies to treat the maladaptive phenomenological dimension of BD.

Conclusion

The term "self" has been used in a multiplicity of divergent ways in the BD literature. This chapter has endeavored to summarize how BD might impact on the development of self, how the self has been conceptualized in BD, how BD influences cognitive processing related to the self and the role of the body and experience in the relationship between self and BD. The chapter concluded by presenting initial thoughts about how the self fits into current and emerging treatments for BD.

This exercise demonstrates the lack of an underlying theory linking the concept of self in BD and the consequent immaturity of thinking about the self in the treatment of BD. By bringing together a divergent literature, this chapter highlights the potential importance of the self for BD theory and practice. It is hoped that this will form the foundation for future theorizing to begin to develop a more coherent conceptualization of self in BD, which may have potentially important consequences for BD treatment.

References

Alatiq, Y., Crane, C., Williams, J. M. G., & Goodwin, G. M. (2010a). Self-discrepancy in students with bipolar disorder II or NOS. *Journal of Behavior Therapy and Experimental Psychiatry*, 41, 135–139.

Alatiq, Y., Crane, C., Williams, J. M. G., & Goodwin, G. M. (2010b). Self-organization in bipolar disorder: Replication of compartmentalization and self-complexity. *Cognitive Therapy and Research*, 34, 479–486.

Ashworth, C. M., Blackburn, I. M., & McPherson, F. M. (1985). The performance of depressed and manic patients on some repertory grid measures: A longitudinal study. *British Journal of Medical Psychology*, 58 (Pt 4), 337–342.

Beck, A. T. (1967). *Depression: Clinical, Experimental, and Theoretical Aspects*. New York, NY: Harper & Rowe.

Bentall, R. P., Kinderman, P., & Manson, K. (2005). Self-discrepancies in bipolar disorder: Comparison of manic, depressed, remitted and normal participants. *British Journal of Clinical Psychology*, 44, 457–473.

Bosson, J. K., Swann Jr, W. B., & Pennebaker, J. W. (2000). Stalking the perfect measure of implicit self-esteem: The blind men and the elephant revisited? *Journal of Personality and Social Psychology*, 79, 631–643. doi: 10.1037/0022-3514.79.4.631

Cerit, C., Filizer, A., Tural, Ü., & Tufan, A. E. (2012). Stigma: A core factor on predicting functionality in bipolar disorder. *Comprehensive Psychiatry*, 53, 484–489.

Cermolacce, M., Naudin, J., & Parnas, J. (2007). The "minimal self" in psychopathology: Re-examining the self-disorders in the schizophrenia spectrum. *Consciousness and Cognition*, 16, 703–714. doi: http://dx.doi.org/10.1016/j.concog.2007.05.013

Corrigan, P. W., Kosyluk, K. A., & Rüsch, N. (2013). Reducing self-stigma by coming out proud. *American Journal of Public Health*, 103, 794–800.

Corrigan, P. W., Sokol, K. A., & Rüsch, N. (2013). The impact of self-stigma and mutual help programs on the quality of life of people with serious mental illnesses. *Community Mental Health Journal*, 49, 1–6.

Creemers, D. H. M., Scholte, R. H. J., Engels, R. C. M. E., Prinstein, M. J., & Wiers, R. W. (2012). Implicit and explicit self-esteem as concurrent predictors of suicidal ideation, depressive symptoms, and loneliness. *Journal of Behavior Therapy and Experimental Psychiatry*, 43, 638–646. doi: http://dx.doi.org/10.1016/j.jbtep.2011.09.006

Crowe, M., Inder, M., Carlyle, D., *et al.* (2012). Feeling out of control: A qualitative analysis of the impact of bipolar disorder. *Journal of Psychiatric and Mental Health Nursing*, 19, 294–302.

Crowe, M., Inder, M., Joyce, P., *et al.* (2009). A developmental approach to the treatment of bipolar disorder: IPSRT with an adolescent. *Journal of Clinical Nursing*, 18, 141–149. doi: 10.1111/j.1365-2702.2008.02571.x

Ellison, N., Mason, O., & Scior, K. (2013). Bipolar disorder and stigma: A systematic review of the literature. *Journal of Affective Disorders*, 151, 805–820.

Erikson, E. H. (1959). Identity and the life cycle: Selected papers. *Psychological Issues*, 1.

Fuchs, T. (2005). Corporealized and disembodied minds. A phenomenological view of the body in melancholia and schizophrenia. *Philosophy, Psychiatry and Psychology*, 12, 95–107.

Fuchs, T., & Schlimme, J. E. (2009). Embodiment and psychopathology: A phenomenological perspective. *Current Opinion in Psychiatry*, 22, 570–575.

Gotlib, I. H., Traill, S. K., Montoya, R. L., Joormann, J., & Chang, K. (2005). Attention and memory biases in the offspring of parents with bipolar disorder: Indications from a pilot study. *Journal of Child Psychology and Psychiatry and Allied Disciplines*, 46, 84–93.

Halfon, N., Labelle, R., Cohen, D., Guilé, J. M., & Breton, J. J. (2013). Juvenile bipolar disorder and suicidality: A review of the last 10 years of literature. *European Child and Adolescent Psychiatry*, 22, 139–151.

Haug, E., Oie, M., Andreassen, O. A., *et al.* (2014). Anomalous self-experiences contribute independently to social dysfunction in the early phases of schizophrenia and psychotic bipolar disorder. *Comprehensive Psychiatry*, 55, 475–482.

Hayward, P., Wong, G., Bright, J. A., & Lam, D. (2002). Stigma and self-esteem in manic depression: An exploratory study. *Journal of Affective Disorders*, 69, 61–67. doi: http://dx.doi.org/10.1016/S0165-0327(00)00380-3

Inder, M. L., Crowe, M. T., Moor, S., *et al.* (2008). "I actually don't know who I am": The impact of bipolar disorder on the development of self. *Psychiatry*, 71, 123–133.

Jabben, N., de Jong, P. J., Kupka, R. W., *et al.* (2014). Implicit and explicit self-associations in bipolar disorder: A comparison with healthy controls and unipolar depressive disorder. *Psychiatry Research*, 215, 329–334.

Johnson, S. L. (2005). Mania and dysregulation in goal pursuit: A review. *Clinical Psychology Review*, 25, 241–262.

Johnson, S. L., Sandrow, D., Meyer, B., *et al.* (2000). Increases in manic symptoms after life events involving goal attainment. *Journal of Abnormal Psychology*, 109, 721–727.

Jones, S. H., & Burrell-Hodgson, G. (2008). Cognitive-behavioural treatment of first diagnosis bipolar disorder. *Clinical Psychology and Psychotherapy*, 15, 367–377.

Jones, S. H., Tai, S., Evershed, K., Knowles, R., & Bentall, R. (2006). Early detection of bipolar disorder: A pilot familial high-risk study of parents with bipolar disorder and their adolescent children. *Bipolar Disorders*, 8, 362–372.

Knowles, R., Tai, S., Jones, S. H., *et al.* (2007). Stability of self-esteem in bipolar disorder: Comparisons among remitted bipolar patients, remitted unipolar patients and healthy controls. *Bipolar Disorders*, 9, 490–495.

Lam, D., Jones, S., Hayward, P., & Bright, J. (1999). *Cognitive Therapy for Bipolar Disorder: A Therapist's Guide to the Concept, Methods and Practice*. Chichester: John Wiley and Son Ltd.

Lam, D., Wright, K., & Sham, P. (2005). Sense of hyper-positive self and response to cognitive therapy in bipolar disorder. *Psychological Medicine*, 35, 69–77.

Lee, R., Lam, D., Mansell, W., & Farmer, A. (2010). Sense of hyper-positive self, goal-attainment beliefs and coping strategies in bipolar I disorder. *Psychological Medicine*, 40, 967–975. doi: S0033291709991206 [pii] 10.1017/S0033291709991206

Leitan, N. D., & Murray, G. (2014). The mind–body relationship in psychotherapy: Grounded cognition as an explanatory framework. *Frontiers in Psychology*, 5, 472.

Lewis, L. (2005). Patient perspective on the diagnosis, treatment, and management of bipolar disorder. *Bipolar Disorders (Supplement)*, 7, 33–37.

Linville, P. W. (1985). Self-complexity and affective extremity: Don't put all of your eggs in one cognitive basket. *Social Cognition*, 3, 94–120. doi: 10.1521/soco.1985.3.1.94

Linville, P. W. (1987). Self-complexity as a cognitive buffer against stress-related illness and depression. *Journal of Personality and Social Psychology*, 52, 663–676.

Lyon, H. M., Bentall, R. P., & Startup, M. (1999). Social cognition and the manic defense: Attributions, selective attention, and self-schema in bipolar affective disorder. *Journal of Abnormal Psychology*, 108, 273–282.

Mansell, W., Morrison, A. P., Reid, G., Lowens, I., & Tai, S. (2007). The interpretation of, and responses to, changes in internal states: An integrative cognitive model of mood swings and bipolar disorders. *Behavioural and Cognitive Psychotherapy*, 35, 515–539.

Marcia, J. E. (1966). Development and validation of ego-identity status. *Journal of Personality and Social Psychology*, 3, 551–558.

Merikangas, K. R., Akiskal, H. S., Angst, J., *et al.* (2007). Lifetime and 12-month prevalence of bipolar spectrum disorder in the National Comorbidity Survey replication. *Archives of General Psychiatry*, 64, 543–552. doi: 64/5/543 [pii] 10.1001/archpsyc.64.5.543

Mileva, V. R., Vázquez, G. H., & Milev, R. (2012). Effects, experiences, and impact of stigma on patients with bipolar disorder. *Neuropsychiatric Disease and Treatment*, 9, 31–40.

Mitchell, P. B., Wilhelm, K., Parker, G., *et al.* (2001). The clinical features of bipolar depression: A comparison with matched major depressive disorder patients. *Journal of Clinical Psychiatry*, 62, 212–216.

Molz Adams, A., Shapero, B. G., Pendergast, L. H., Alloy, L. B., & Abramson, L. Y. (2014). Self-referent information processing in individuals with bipolar spectrum disorders. *Journal of Affective Disorders*, 152–154, 483–490.

Morriss, R. K., Lobban, F., Jones, S., *et al.* (2011). Pragmatic randomised controlled trial of group psychoeducation versus group support in the maintenance of bipolar disorder. *BMC Psychiatry*, 11, 114.

Murray, G., & Johnson, S. L. (2010). The clinical significance of creativity in bipolar disorder. *Clinical Psychology Review*, 30, 721–732.

Murray, G., Leitan, N. D., Berk, M., *et al.* (2015). Online mindfulness-based intervention for late-stage bipolar disorder: Pilot evidence for feasibility and effectiveness. *Journal of Affective Disorders*, 178, 46–51. doi: 10.1016/j.jad.2015.02.024

Neale, J. M. (1988). *Defensive Functions of Manic Episodes. Delusional Beliefs*. New York, NY: John Wiley & Sons.

Parikh, S. V., Zaretsky, A., Beaulieu, S., *et al.* (2012). A randomized controlled trial of psychoeducation or cognitive-behavioral therapy in bipolar disorder: A Canadian Network for Mood and Anxiety Treatments (CANMAT) study. *Journal of Clinical Psychiatry*, 73, 803–810.

Pavlickova, H., Turnbull, O., & Bentall, R. P. (2014). Cognitive vulnerability to bipolar disorder in offspring of parents with bipolar disorder. *British Journal of Clinical Psychology*, 54, 386–401.

Pavlickova, H., Varese, F., Turnbull, O., *et al.* (2013). Symptom-specific self-referential cognitive processes in bipolar disorder: A longitudinal analysis. *Psychological Medicine*, 43, 1895–1907.

Perich, T., Manicavasagar, V., Mitchell, P. B., & Ball, J. R. (2014). Mindfulness-based approaches in the treatment of bipolar disorder: Potential mechanisms and effects. *Mindfulness*, 5, 186–191. doi: 10.1007/s12671-012-0166-6

Perlick, D. A., Rosenheck, R. A., Clarkin, J. F., *et al.* (2001). Stigma as a barrier to recovery: Adverse effects of perceived stigma on social adaptation of persons diagnosed with bipolar affective disorder. *Psychiatric Services*, 52, 1627–1632.

Power, M. J., De Jong, F., & Lloyd, A. (2002). The organization of the self-concept in bipolar disorders: An empirical study and replication. *Cognitive Therapy and Research*, 26, 553–561.

Proudfoot, J., Jayawant, A., Whitton, A., *et al.* (2012). Mechanisms underpinning effective peer support: A qualitative analysis of interactions between expert peers and patients newly-diagnosed with bipolar disorder. *BMC Psychiatry*, 12, 196.

Proudfoot, J., Parker, G., Manicavasagar, V., *et al.* (2012). Effects of adjunctive peer support on perceptions of illness control and understanding in an online psychoeducation program for bipolar disorder: A randomised controlled trial. *Journal of Affective Disorders*, 142, 98–105.

Ritsher, J. B., Otilingam, P. G., & Grajales, M. (2003). Internalized stigma of mental illness: psychometric properties of a new measure. *Psychiatry Research*, 121, 31–49.

Röhricht, F. (2009). Body oriented psychotherapy. The state of the art in empirical research and evidence-based practice: A clinical perspective. *Body, Movement and Dance in Psychotherapy*, 4, 135–156.

Röhricht, F., Papadopoulos, N., Holden, S., Clarke, T., & Priebe, S. (2011). Therapeutic processes and clinical outcomes of body psychotherapy in chronic schizophrenia – An open clinical trial. *Arts in Psychotherapy*, 38, 196–203.

Röhricht, F., Papadopoulos, N., Suzuki, I., & Priebe, S. (2009). Ego-pathology, body experience, and body psychotherapy in chronic schizophrenia. *Psychology and Psychotherapy: Theory, Research and Practice*, 82, 19–30.

Russell, L., & Moss, D. (2013). A meta-study of qualitative research into the experience of 'symptoms' and 'having a diagnosis' for people who have been given a diagnosis of bipolar disorder. *Europe's Journal of Psychology*, 9, 643–663.

Sass, L. A., Pienkos, E., Nelson, B., & Medford, N. (2013). Anomalous self-experience in depersonalization and schizophrenia: A comparative investigation. *Consciousness and Cognition*, 22, 430–441.

Scott, J., Paykel, E., Morriss, R., *et al.* (2006). Cognitive-behavioural therapy for severe and recurrent bipolar disorders: Randomised controlled trial. *British Journal of Psychiatry*, 188, 313–320.

Scott, L., & O'Hara, M. W. (1993). Self-discrepancies in clinically anxious and depressed university students. *Journal of Abnormal Psychology*, 102, 282–287.

Shen, G. H., Alloy, L. B., Abramson, L. Y., & Sylvia, L. G. (2008). Social rhythm regularity and the onset of affective episodes in bipolar spectrum individuals. *Bipolar Disorders*, 10, 520–529. doi: 10.1111/j.1399-5618.2008.00583.x

Showers, C. (1992). Compartmentalization of positive and negative self-knowledge: Keeping bad apples out of the bunch. *Journal of Personality and Social Psychology*, 62, 1036–1049.

Strauman, T. J. (1989). Self-discrepancies in clinical depression and social phobia: Cognitive structures that underlie emotional disorders? *Journal of Abnormal Psychology*, 98, 14–22.

Strauman, T. J., & Higgins, E. T. (1988). Self-discrepancies as predictors of vulnerability to distinct syndromes of chronic emotional distress. *Journal of Personality*, 56, 685–707.

Taylor, J. L., Morley, S., & Barton, S. B. (2007). Self-organization in bipolar disorder: Compartmentalization and self-complexity. *Cognitive Therapy and Research*, 31, 83–96.

Thomas, N., Nunan, C., Leitan, N. D., *et al.* (in preparation). The effect of an 8-week peer-facilitated course on personal recovery.

Todd, N. J., Jones, S. H., & Lobban, F. A. (2013). What do service users with bipolar disorder want from a web-based self-management intervention? A qualitative focus group study. *Clinical Psychology and Psychotherapy*, 20, 531–543.

Totton, N. (2003). *Body Psychotherapy: An Introduction.* Maidenhead: Open University Press.

Vazquez, G. H., Kapczinski, F., Magalhaes, P. V., *et al.* (2011). Stigma and functioning in patients with bipolar disorder. *Journal of Affective Disorders*, 130, 323–327. doi: 10.1016/j.jad.2010.10.012

Watson, A. C., Corrigan, P., Larson, J. E., & Sells, M. (2007). Self-stigma in people with mental illness. *Schizophrenia Bulletin*, 33, 1312–1318. doi: 10.1093/schbul/sbl076

Zeigler-Hill, V. (2006). Discrepancies between implicit and explicit self-esteem: Implications for narcissism and self-esteem instability. *Journal of Personality*, 74, 119–144. doi: 10.1111/j.1467-6494.2005.00371.x

Chapter

10

The self in social anxiety

Bree Gregory, Lorna Peters, and Ronald M. Rapee

Cognitive-behavioral models of social anxiety (e.g., Clark & Wells, 1995; Rapee & Heimberg, 1997) emphasize the role of self-related concepts in maintaining the disorder. Although not exhaustive, these self concepts can include negative self-beliefs, biased self-judgments, negative self-perceptions, self-focused attention, and negative mental imagery of the perceived self. The following chapter examines how these constructs of the self are integrated into models of social anxiety, and how they inform treatment practices for social anxiety disorder (SAD; also known as social phobia).

Social anxiety disorder

SAD is a debilitating disorder characterized by an intense fear of social or performance situations where there is a possibility the individual will be scrutinized by others (American Psychiatric Association, 2013). Such situations span from ones featuring the near-ubiquitous fear of public speaking to those requiring conversing with authority figures, initiating and maintaining conversations, making requests of others, being assertive, or performing everyday activities (e.g., eating, writing, drinking) within view of other people. For socially anxious individuals, the underlying fear in these situations is that they will say or do something that will elicit negative judgment and/or that their actions will be perceived as embarrassing or humiliating by others. Accordingly, individuals with SAD limit the potential scrutiny from others by engaging in avoidance behaviors where possible, or they endure the social situation with significant distress.

Recognized as a prevalent, complex, and disabling disorder that, if left untreated, runs a chronic course

(Stein & Stein, 2008; Wong, Gordon, & Heimberg, 2014), SAD has received increasing attention since its recognition as a mental disorder in the third edition of the *Diagnostic and Statistical Manual of Mental Disorders* (DSM-3; American Psychiatric Association, 1980). Individuals with SAD have impairments extending beyond social concerns, including impairments in employment, academic performance, and general mental health (e.g., Ruscio *et al.*, 2008). These difficulties are often compounded by a high degree of comorbidity with other mental disorders, with psychiatric comorbidity associated with an increase in anxiety symptom severity, impairment level, and a decrease in overall quality of life (for a review see Szafranski, Talkovsky, Farris, & Norton, 2014). The high personal, social, and economic cost of SAD (Stein & Stein, 2008) has led to the development of a number of cognitive models aimed at improving understanding and treatment of the disorder.

The self in cognitive models of SAD

In defining the construct of the self, the present chapter focuses on the contributions made by researchers in the social-cognitive psychology domain, where the majority of self-based research has been conducted and utilized by practitioners. Here, the self is viewed as an organized knowledge structure (comprised of schemas) that includes information about beliefs, past experiences, and self-related evaluations that guide the way in which a person samples and processes information and experiences (for a review see Ellemers, Spears, & Doosje, 2002). The following pages will briefly describe how self-related constructs are considered in cognitive models of SAD. We will first examine models

The Self in Understanding and Treating Psychological Disorders, ed. Michael Kyrios, Richard Moulding, Guy Doron, Sunil S. Bhar, Maja Nedeljkovic, and Mario Mikulincer. Published by Cambridge University Press. © Cambridge University Press, 2016.

that have been at the forefront of clinical research and treatment practices since their conception, including influential models by Beck and Emery (1985), Clark and Wells (1995), and Rapee and Heimberg (1997). We then turn our focus to examine more recent cognitive models of SAD (e.g., Hofmann, 2007), some of which have placed the concept of self at the center of the disorder (e.g., Moscovitch, 2009; Stopa, 2009).

Beck and Emery's (1985) cognitive model of anxiety

Beck and Emery propose that anxiety disorders are maintained by a cognitive–affective–physiological interaction that is fueled by self-knowledge stored in long-term memory. This knowledge stems from past experiences and forms a cognitive set of assumptions (schemas) composed of rigid and inflexible beliefs about the self, others, and the world. Beck and Emery's cognitive model therefore takes a schema-based information-processing perspective. They suggest that individuals with anxiety have hyperactivated negative schemas, leading to preferential processing of threat-consistent information, and schemas that are hyposensitive to cues signaling safety, leading to underestimations of personal coping recourses and of the level of safety in the environment.

For individuals with SAD, social situations involving perceived social scrutiny activate these dysfunctional schemas (Beck & Emery, 1985). At the deepest level of the cognitive system are unconscious, unconditional beliefs about the self (e.g., "I am boring") and negative views of others (e.g., "people are judgmental"). At the surface level are more conscious conditional rules (e.g., "if I make a mistake, others will laugh at me"). Information consistent with these self-beliefs (e.g., "people think I am a failure") becomes selected preferentially and information inconsistent with these beliefs (e.g., positive social interaction) is ignored or discarded. Such selective processing of negative self and social information increases the sense of vulnerability, heightening anxiety and confirming and perpetuating negative views of the self.

Clark and Wells' (1995) cognitive model of SAD

According to Clark and Wells, heightened self-focused attention, negative observer-perspective images of the perceived self, and negative self-evaluation all contribute to maintaining the dysfunctional patterns of social anxiety. Derived from self-presentation models (see Schlenker & Leary, 1982), a core feature of the model is that socially anxious individuals hold a strong desire to convey a favorable impression of themselves to others in social situations, but believe that they may not have the ability to do so. These negative performance expectations trigger a processing mode termed "processing of the self as a social object" (Clark, 2001, p. 401). When engaged in this processing mode, socially anxious individuals shift their attention from the environment to detailed monitoring of themselves (called self-focused attention). Self-focused attention increases awareness of feared anxiety responses and perpetuates the belief that other people perceive the individual in the same negative manner in which the individual sees themselves.

This negative impression of the "observable self" (p. 71) is often described by individuals with social anxiety as a "compelling *feeling*" (p. 71); however, Clark and Wells (1995) suggest that this negative representation of the self can also include negative imagery. Negative self-images are conceptualized as distorted mental pictures representing an individual's feared outcome (e.g., being embarrassed in social situations). These images tend to be idiosyncratic, are viewed from the observer perspective, and can hijack attentional resources. Focusing on this self-image in social situations increases the perception that others are noticing anxiety symptoms consistent with the image. In this way, self-focused attention directed toward somatic symptoms, thoughts, and/or images is said to increase anxiety in social situations as well as to bias processing of information.

Consistent with Beck and Emery's (1985) model, the tendency of socially anxious individuals to interpret situations in a threatening manner is also linked to dysfunctional beliefs by Clark and Wells (1995). The authors distinguish between three categories of beliefs: beliefs in excessively high standards (e.g., "I must get everyone's approval"), conditional beliefs about social evaluation (e.g., "If someone does not approve of me it must be my fault"), and unconditional beliefs about the self (e.g., "I am uninteresting"). The model also suggests that the use of safety behaviors and engagement in post-event rumination following a social event not only exacerbate anxiety, but increase self-focused attention and prevent disconfirmation of these negative self-beliefs.

Rapee and Heimberg's (1997) cognitive model of SAD

Similar to Clark and Wells (1995), Rapee and Heimberg (1997) suggest that when social situations are encountered, individuals with SAD focus on an internal mental representation of the self as seen by the audience. This mental representation is described as a distorted image that may be based on past negative social experiences that are consistent with negative core beliefs and self-schemas (as described by Beck & Emery, 1985; the importance of imagery is further emphasized in the updated model by Heimberg, Brozovich, & Rapee, 2010). Along the lines of self-presentation theory (Schlenker & Leary, 1982), a core feature of the model is the comparison of this mental representation of self with the perceived expectation of the audience. According to the model, individuals with SAD have a strong desire to be accepted by others. They also believe that others hold high expectations for their social performance, but at the same time assume that they will be unable to live up to these standards. As a result, individuals with SAD expect greater negative evaluation from others (the updated model also emphasizes the role of positive evaluation, see Heimberg *et al.*, 2010), which in turn produces heightened anxiety.

Whereas Clark and Wells' (1995) model suggests that self-focused attention is the central attentional process maintaining anxiety, Rapee and Heimberg (1997) assert that socially anxious individuals attend to both this internal mental representation of the self *and* to external threat cues (e.g., behaviors indicating negative evaluation from audience members). Rapee and Heimberg argue that this attentional monitoring is not done in isolation; rather, there exists an interactive relationship between monitoring the mental representation of self and the monitoring of attention toward social threat in the environment. For example, biased detection of audience behaviors (e.g., yawning) results in greater focus on internal self-representations (e.g., cognitions regarding how boring one is). Focusing on internal self-representations also leads to an increase in internal anxiety sensations, as well as an increase in the detection of negative audience behaviors (those that are in line with negative self-appraisals). Accordingly, both monitoring of mental representations of the self and external cues in the environment can heighten anxiety, hinder social performance, and preclude the perception of information inconsistent with social fears.

Hofmann's (2007) cognitive model of SAD

Consistent with previous conceptualizations of SAD, Hofmann (2007) suggests that individuals with social anxiety experience apprehension in social situations because they perceive the social standards (i.e., expectations and social goals) of performance to be excessively high and doubt their ability to meet those standards. In this way, the model incorporates theory described in self-presentation models of the disorder (as in Clark & Wells, 1995; Rapee & Heimberg, 1997). According to Leary and Kowalski (1995), the goal for most socially anxious individuals in a social situation is to make a desired impression on others. However, Hoffman argues that socially anxious individuals have a deficiency in their ability to define attainable social goals. Moreover, they experience difficulty in selecting achievable behavioral strategies to reach these goals. These processes lead to increases in social apprehension and self-focused attention. This attention is directed at both internal and external threat cues (as in the Rapee and Heimberg model); however, the model emphasizes the role of heightened self-focused attention in SAD (consistent with the model of Clark and Wells).

In discussing the role of negative self-perception as a maintaining factor in the disorder, Hofmann (2007) explicitly incorporates research relating to self-discrepancy theory (Higgins, 1987), making a conceptual departure from previous cognitive-behavioral models (Beck & Emery, 1985; Clark & Wells, 1995; Rapee & Heimberg, 1997). Self-discrepancy theory postulates that people compare themselves to internalized standards, or domains of the self. Three basic domains of the self exist: the actual self (i.e., perceived attributes that either themselves or others believe they possess), the ideal self (i.e., perceived attributes that either themselves or others hope, or wish they possessed), and the ought self (i.e., perceived attributes that themselves or others believe it is their duty or responsibility to possess). The model emphasizes that discrepancies among socially anxious individuals' self-domains may underlie their fear that they will be unable to convey a desired impression to others in social situations.

Moscovitch's (2009) cognitive model of SAD

Moscovitch argues that previous cognitive-behavioral models of SAD (Clark & Wells, 1995; Rapee & Heimberg, 1997; Hofmann, 2007) are unsatisfactory because they confuse feared stimuli (i.e., the focus of anxiety) with feared consequences (i.e., feared outcomes when stimuli are present; Moscovitch, 2009, p. 2). Instead, he contends that practitioners involved in assessing and treating socially anxious individuals should re-focus their attention from targeting patients' generic feared social situations (e.g., fear of evaluation) to targeting the core feared stimuli in SAD; namely, specific self-attributes that individuals with social anxiety perceive to be flawed or deficient. This view is built on the consensus that a negative, distorted self-view is central to SAD (e.g., Clark & Wells, 1995; Rapee & Heimberg, 1997).

Moscovitch (2009) proposes a typology of self-fears that include concerns about social skills and behaviors (e.g., "I will do something stupid"), showing signs of anxiety (e.g., "I will sweat"), physical appearance (e.g., "I am ugly") and character (e.g., "I am boring"). During the development of the Negative Self-Portrayal Scale (used to assess perceived deficiencies in self-attributes; Moscovitch & Huyder, 2011), these four deficiencies were reduced to three subscales, concerns about: social competence, physical appearance, and showing signs of anxiety. As the core fear or threat in SAD, the model suggests that it is the activation of these self-attributes in anticipation of or during social situations that leads to emotional distress and maladaptive behavioral responses, including the use of safety behaviors designed to conceal perceived flaws in self-attributes and to prevent feared consequences. Thus, whereas Clark and Wells (1995) assert that people with social anxiety fear they will behave in a socially inept fashion, Moscovitch (2009) emphasizes broader feared self-dimensions.

Stopa's (2009) model of SAD

Stopa argues that despite consensus that self-related constructs are an important maintaining factor in SAD (Clark & Wells, 1995; Hofmann, 2007; Rapee & Heimberg, 1997), previous conceptualizations of the disorder take a limited view of the self into consideration. These models often recognize only one or two aspects of the self and do not capture the construct's full complexity. Stopa (2009) acknowledges that this oversimplification may be due to the models' aims to provide theoretical frameworks from which treatment may be derived. However, in doing so, she states that we may be ignoring important information regarding aspects of the self and self-processes that may

significantly contribute to the continuation of social anxiety.

Stopa (2009) proposes that the self can be organized into three broad aspects: content, structure, and process. Content refers to information about the self and the way this information is represented. For example, knowledge about oneself can exist in the form of verbal statements (e.g., "I am boring") or be represented visually as images. Structure describes the way information about the self is organized, which can determine what aspects of self-knowledge are accessed at any given time. For example, individuals may have a more compartmentalized sense of self (i.e., little to no overlap between different self-attributes across self-aspects) or an integrated self-organization (i.e., duplication of different self-attributes across self-aspects; see Showers, 1992). Process refers to how attention is allocated to self-relevant information and the strategies that are used to evaluate and monitor information about the self.

To date, Stopa (2009) argues that cognitive-behavioral models have primarily focused on the content of the self-concept (e.g., the way that self-images, self-schemas, and negative thoughts and beliefs about the self contribute to SAD) and on one aspect of self-related processes, attentional biases. In contrast, relatively few researchers have incorporated the aspect of self-structure into models of SAD; yet knowing how self-knowledge and information is stored and organized could lead to more targeted and effective interventions.

The self: evidence for self-constructs and treatment

It is clear that a number of self-related constructs feature prominently across the cognitive-behavioral models of SAD. Among these, several have been the focus of a large body of research and discussion, including negative self-imagery, the role of maladaptive self-beliefs, and self-focused attention. The following section of the chapter will therefore review the evidence for these particular self-constructs in maintaining social anxiety. The emphasis placed on these self-related constructs is also reflected in evidence-based treatments for the disorder. The most thoroughly studied and established therapeutic approach to SAD is cognitive-behavior therapy (CBT; see Butler, Chapman, Forman, & Beck, 2006). CBT for SAD is a time-limited, present-oriented, non-pharmacological approach that aims to teach clients the cognitive and behavioral competencies needed to function adaptively on an interpersonal level. The following pages will also detail how these self-constructs have featured in contemporary CBT protocols for SAD.

Self-imagery and imagery rescripting

Several cognitive-behavioral models of SAD posit that negative self-images play a role in the maintenance of the disorder (Clark & Wells, 1995; Hofmann, 2007; Rapee & Heimberg, 1997). Research has found that individuals with social anxiety report experiencing negative self-images in social situations (for a review see Ng, Abbott, & Hunt, 2014). These self-images are often recurrent as they tend to occur in different social situations and are linked in meaning and content to prior unpleasant social events (Hackmann, Clark, & McManus, 2000). Research has also demonstrated the deleterious effects of negative-self imagery. For example, negative self-images tend to increase the perceived visibility of anxiety symptoms, poor performance appraisal (Hirsch, Mathews, Clark, Williams, & Morrison, 2003; Stopa & Jenkins, 2007), negative thoughts, and self-focused attention (Makkar & Grisham, 2011). This relationship between self-focused attention and negative self-images is consistent with the models' emphases on the role of heightened self-focused attention (Clark & Wells, 1995; Hofmann, 2007), and preferential allocation of attention (Rapee & Heimberg, 1997) in social anxiety. Focusing on these distorted self-images has also been found to increase post-event rumination following a speech task (Makkar & Grisham, 2011), as predicted by Hofmann (2007), and increase the use of safety behaviors (Hirsch, Meynen, & Clark, 2004), as predicted by Clark and Wells (1995). Focusing on these negative self-images has also been found to decrease explicit self-esteem (Hulme, Hirsch, & Stopa, 2012).

A number of contemporary CBT treatment programs for SAD (e.g., Clark et al., 2003; Rapee, Gaston, & Abbott, 2009) have been developed that include techniques (e.g., video feedback, behavioral experiments, and surveying other people's observations) to modify distorted self-images. To correct negative self-images using video feedback, clients are asked to (1) visualize how they think they will appear prior to watching the video, (2) specifically operationalize what their negative behaviors will look like (e.g., how red the blushing will be), and (3) watch the video from an observer point-of-view, ignoring the negative thinking and feelings that may bias the perception of performance (e.g., Harvey, Clark, Ehlers, & Rapee, 2000). In this way, video feedback offers clients the opportunity to discover that they do not appear as they think they do, consequently learning that their self-impressions are inaccurate (e.g., Rapee & Hayman, 1996). Studies documenting the effectiveness of video feedback as a tool to modify distorted self-images during CBT have found that videotaped feedback decreases social anxiety ratings, perceived social cost ratings, and increases positive appraisals of performance (e.g., Laposa & Rector, 2014; see also Rapee et al., 2009). Having video feedback across CBT sessions also tends to increase performance ratings and to decrease self-focused attention for the following feedback session (Laposa & Rector, 2014).

Despite support for the efficacy of video feedback in modifying distorted images and social anxiety, these techniques are primarily present-focused and do not directly modify the early memories and experiences that tend to be linked to self-images. While this may not be an issue for some clients (e.g., those who have an image unrelated to a past event), for clients who experience negative imagery that is linked to a past traumatic event, Wild and Clark (2011) suggest that use of only present-focused techniques may produce modest treatment responding. The authors argue that for these clients, new advances in CBT treatment techniques, such as "imagery rescripting" (i.e., a pre-existing negative self-image is identified, challenged, and then transformed into a more benign mental image or a new positive mental image, see Wild & Clark, 2011), may prove more efficacious.

Investigators have begun to examine the efficacy of using imagery rescripting as an intervention to correct distorted self-images and to improve social anxiety symptoms (e.g., Wild, Hackmann, & Clark, 2008). CBT for SAD including imagery rescripting has been found to be superior to in vivo exposure with applied relaxation (Clark et al., 2006). Other smaller trials have found that imagery rescripting is associated with reductions in fear of negative evaluation, negative core beliefs, and social anxiety (e.g., Frets, Kevenaar, & Heiden, 2014; Lee & Kwon, 2013; Nilsson, Lundh, & Viborg, 2012; Wild, Hackmann, & Clark, 2007, 2008). However, these studies examine the efficacy of imagery rescripting as a standalone procedure, rather than within the context of CBT. To overcome this issue, McEvoy and Saulsman (2014) developed the imagery-enhanced cognitive group behavioral therapy protocol (IE-CGBT). IE-CGBT includes techniques such as video feedback and imagery rescripting, and utilizes imagery-based techniques in all components of the CBT program (i.e., cognitive restructuring, behavioral experiments, and attention training). In comparing IE-CGBT to a control treatment without the self-imagery enhancements, McEvoy, Erceg-Hurn, Saulsman, and Thibodeau (2015) found that more clients completed treatment in the IE-CGBT condition (91% vs. 65%). Furthermore, while effect sizes were large for both treatment protocols, they were significantly higher for IE-CGBT. A higher proportion of the IE-CGBT clients also achieved clinically significant change according to the reliable change index. These findings suggest that modifying distorted self-images through IE-CGBT may be an efficacious treatment protocol for SAD. However, these findings are preliminary and more research is needed to replicate and extend these results.

Maladaptive self-beliefs and treatment

Maladaptive beliefs about the self that are negatively biased and inaccurate are thought to play a key role in maintaining SAD (Clark & Wells, 1995; Hofmann, 2007; Rapee & Heimberg, 1997). Indeed, all current cognitive conceptualizations of the disorder are based on the premise that individuals with social anxiety have maladaptive cognitive schema that activate negative beliefs (Turner, Johnson, Beidel, Heiser, & Lydiard, 2003). Despite this theoretical consensus, relatively few studies have investigated the role of maladaptive beliefs in SAD in a consistent manner. This may be a result of different terminology being used to formally test the construct. For example, the term self-perception includes positive and negative statements about the self and about an individual's beliefs and expectations for the self (Baldwin, 1994). Research has also used the terms self-presentations (e.g., Anderson, Goldin, Kurita, & Gross, 2008), self-views (Goldin *et al.*, 2013), and maladaptive beliefs interchangeably. Studies have also typically assessed transient thought-like constructs (e.g., self-appraisals, thoughts, and attributions), rather than the enduring core beliefs theorized by cognitive models (e.g., Abbott & Rapee, 2006; Hofmann, Moscovitch, Kim, & Taylor, 2004; Moscovitch *et al.*, 2013; Schulz, Alpers, & Hofmann, 2008).

A recently proposed measure, the Self-Beliefs Related to Social Anxiety Scale (SBSA; Wong & Moulds, 2009), offers some insight into the role of maladaptive self-beliefs and social anxiety. A benefit of using the SBSA is that it maps directly onto the three maladaptive beliefs proposed by Clark and Wells (1995): high standard beliefs, conditional beliefs, and unconditional beliefs about the self. Research has shown that stronger high-standard beliefs predict less behavioral avoidance, stronger unconditional beliefs predict more behavioral avoidance, and stronger conditional beliefs predict more cognitive avoidance (Wong & Moulds, 2011). The authors also found that higher levels of ruminative processing predicted stronger conditional and unconditional beliefs about the self, but not high standard beliefs (Wong & Moulds, 2012). Both of these studies used undergraduate samples, so more research is needed to examine whether these findings translate to clinical populations.

Consistent with the model presented by Beck and Emery (1985), several studies have examined the relationship between early maladaptive schemas and social anxiety (e.g., Calvete, Orue, & Hankin, 2015; Gonzalez-Diez, Calvete, Riskind, & Orue, 2015), as these map onto the content of maladaptive self-beliefs. For example, Pinto-Gouveia, Castilho, Galhardo, and Cunha (2006) found that socially anxious individuals score higher on themes of disconnection/rejection using the Young Schema Questionnaire (Young & Brown, 1990) than do individuals with panic and obsessive–compulsive disorder. This finding may indicate that individuals with social anxiety have expectations that their need for stable, trustworthy, nurturing, and empathetic relationships will not be met. They may also believe they are defective or inferior in some way.

Studies have begun to examine whether treatment changes the nature of maladaptive self-beliefs and social anxiety. A key component of CBT is training patients to restructure maladaptive beliefs. This is most often achieved via the systematic collection and rational disputation of evidence for and against the identified core belief (e.g., identified via the downward arrow techniques). Behavioral experiments allow the client to engage in activities that will undermine their maladaptive belief(s). Cognitive restructuring then allows the individual to derive more rational and accurate beliefs about their self. Clients also discuss the consequences of their negative self-beliefs across life domains and develop action plans (see Rapee *et al.*, 2009). Studies have found that following CBT, socially anxious individuals endorse significantly fewer negative self-beliefs, and have reductions in social anxiety (e.g., Boden *et al.*, 2012; Koerner, Antony, Young, & McCabe, 2013; Rapee *et al.*, 2009). More research is needed to examine self-beliefs and social anxiety, particularly within the context of treatment. Including measures within treatment would allow for more information about when and how self-beliefs change during treatment.

Self-focused attention and treatment

Several cognitive-behavioral models of SAD (Clark & Wells, 1995; Hofmann, 2007; Rapee & Heimberg, 1997) suggest that self-focused attention contributes to the etiology, maintenance, and exacerbation of social anxiety. Studies have supported this proposition (for a review see Bögels & Mansell, 2004). Inducing self-focused attention (either through mirrors, video cameras, or a live audience) has been linked to impairments in social performance, higher frequency of self-critical thoughts, and increases in social anxiety (e.g., Bögels & Lamers, 2002; Zhou, Hudson, & Rapee, 2007; however, see Jakymin & Harris, 2012). Self-focused attention has also been associated with heightened self-examination, enhanced negative affect in the form of self-criticism and self-dissatisfaction, and poorer social self-efficacy (e.g., Kashdan & Roberts, 2004).

A number of interventions have been designed to modify attentional processing in SAD. Attention training, or task concentration training (TCT), aims to reduce social anxiety by changing an individual's attentional focus (Mulkens, Bögels, de Jong, & Louwers, 2001). In TCT, clients are taught to focus on the task at hand (e.g., the content of the conversation), with the ultimate aim being to reduce self-focused attention. The intervention has three phases: (1) gaining insight into attentional processes and the effects of self-focused attention on the self, (2) directing attention outward on non-threatening stimuli, and (3) directing attention outward on threatening stimuli. Studies have found that TCT helps reduce fears of blushing and of showing bodily symptoms, and reduces social anxiety (e.g., Bögels, 2006; Mulkens *et al.*, 2001).

Studies also suggest that maladaptive attention processes can be changed through attention bias modification procedures (e.g., Amir, Weber, Beard, Bomyea, & Taylor, 2008; Amir *et al.*, 2009; Schmidt, Richey, Buckner, & Timpano, 2009). While these procedures may not modify self-related concepts directly, modifying attention so that an individual has less bias toward negative external sources (e.g., social threat behaviors from an audience) may subsequently shift the mental representation of self (as hypothesized by Rapee & Heimberg, 1997). Attention modification comprises of a dot-probe detection task where threatening or natural emotional expressions are cued at different locations on a computer screen. In brief, the computerized procedure facilitates the disengagement from threatening stimuli by repeatedly redirecting participants' attention from social threat cues to induce selective processing of neutral, or non-threatening, cues (Amir *et al.*, 2008). Despite the support for the use of attention training in modifying the focus of attention and reducing social anxiety, more recent studies have struggled to replicate these effects (e.g., Boettcher, Berger, & Renneberg, 2012; Julian, Beard, Schmidt, Powers, & Smits, 2012). More research is therefore needed to examine the potential of attention modification programs as successful social anxiety interventions. Additionally, few studies have examined the effect of attention modification programs in influencing internal representations of self, as proposed in the Rapee and Heimberg (1997) model.

Conclusion

Our review of the self in cognitive-behavioral models of SAD suggests that self-constructs have an important role to play in maintaining social anxiety. This is particularly evident in the constructs of self-images, self-beliefs, and self-focused attention. Empirical research examining these constructs both within and outside the context of treatment appears to support many of the models' propositions relating to these self-constructs. However, there is still much to learn about how the self is positioned within models of SAD, and particularly how SAD treatment affects the self and social anxiety.

A large proportion of the evidence examining treatment effects for CBT interventions employs a pre–post methodology. While this is informative, more research is needed to examine within-treatment changes in self-constructs. Such information will help improve understanding of how, when, and why treatment influences self-related constructs and social anxiety. More research is also needed examining the recently developed interventions targeting self-constructs, such as imagery rescripting. Preliminary evidence suggests that the addition of these interventions to currently used treatment practices (e.g., CBT) may improve the efficacy of changing these constructs and social anxiety. Finally, more research is needed to examine the role of self-structure and social anxiety.

References

Abbott, M. J., & Rapee, R. M. (2006). Post-event rumination and negative self-appraisal in social phobia before and after treatment. *Journal of Abnormal Psychology*, 113, 136–144. doi: 10.1037/0021-843X.113.1.136

American Psychiatric Association. (1980). *Diagnostic and Statistical Manual of Mental Disorders* (3rd ed.). Washington, DC: American Psychiatric Association.

American Psychiatric Association. (2013). *Diagnostic and Statistical Manual of Mental Disorders* (5th ed.). Washington, DC: American Psychiatric Association.

Amir, N., Beard, C., Taylor, C. T., *et al.* (2009). Attention training in individuals with generalized social phobia: A randomized controlled trial. *Journal of Consulting and Clinical Psychology*, 77, 961–973. doi: 10.1037/a0016685

Amir, N., Weber, G., Beard, C., Bomyea, J., & Taylor, C. T. (2008). The effect of a single-session attention modification program on response to a public-speaking challenge in socially anxious individuals. *Journal of Abnormal Psychology*, 117, 860–868. doi: 10.1037/a0013445

Anderson, B., Goldin, P. R., Kurita, K., & Gross, J. J. (2008). Self-representation in social anxiety disorder: Linguistic analysis of autobiographical narratives. *Behaviour Research and Therapy*, 46, 1119–1125. doi: 10.1016/j.brat.2008.07.001

Baldwin, M. W. (1994). Primed relational schemas as a source of self-evaluation reactions. *Journal of Social and Clinical Psychology*, 13, 380–403. doi: 10.1521/jscp.1994.13.4.380

Beck, A. T., & Emery, G. (1985). *Anxiety Disorders and Phobias: A Cognitive Perspective*. New York, NY: Basic Books.

Boden, M. T., John, O. P., Goldin, P. R., *et al.* (2012). The role of maladaptive beliefs in cognitive-behavioral therapy: Evidence from social anxiety disorder. *Behaviour Research and Therapy*, 50, 287–291. doi: 10.1016/j.brat.2012.02.007

Boettcher, J., Berger, T., & Renneberg, B. (2012). Internet-based attention training for social anxiety: A randomized controlled trial. *Cognitive Therapy and Research*, 36, 522–536. doi: 10.1007/s10608-011-9374-y

Bögels, S. M. (2006). Task concentration training versus applied relaxation, in combination with cognitive therapy, for social phobia patients with fear of blushing, trembling, and sweating. *Behaviour Research and Therapy*, 44, 1199–1210. doi: 10.1016/j.brat.2005.08.010

Bögels, S. M., & Lamers, C. T. J. (2002). The causal role of self-awareness in blushing-anxious, socially anxious and social phobics individuals. *Behaviour Research and Therapy*, 40, 1367–1384. doi: 10.1016/S0005-7967(01)00096-1

Bögels, S. M., & Mansell, W. (2004). Attention processes in the maintenance and treatment of social phobia: Hypervigilance, avoidance, and self-focused attention. *Clinical Psychology Review*, 24, 827–856. doi: 10.1016/j.cpr.2004.06.005

Butler, A. C., Chapman, J. E., Forman, E. M., & Beck, A. T. (2006). The empirical status of cognitive-behavioral therapy: A review of meta-analyses. *Clinical Psychology Review*, 26, 17–31. doi: 10.1016/j.cpr.2005.07.003

Calvete, E., Orue, I., & Hankin, B. L. (2015). A longitudinal test of the vulnerability–stress model with early maladaptive schemas for depression and social anxiety symptoms in adolescents. *Journal of Psychopathology and Behavioral Assessment*, 37, 85–99. doi: 10.1007/s10862-014-9438-x

Clark, D. M. (2001). A cognitive perspective on social phobia. In W. R. Crozier & L. E. Alden (Eds.), *International Handbook of Social Anxiety* (pp. 405–430). Chichester: Wiley.

Clark, D. M., Ehlers, A., Hackmann, A., *et al.* (2006). Cognitive therapy versus exposure and applied relaxation in social phobia: A randomised control trial. *Journal of Consulting and Clinical Psychology*, 74, 568–578. doi: 10.1037/0022-006X.74.3.568

Clark, D. M., Ehlers, A., McManus, F., *et al.* (2003). Cognitive therapy vs. fluoxetine in generalized social phobia: A randomized controlled trial. *Journal of Consulting and Clinical Psychology*, 71, 1058–1067. doi: 10.1037/0022-006X.71.6.1058

Clark, D. M., & Wells, A. (1995). A cognitive model of social phobia. In R. G. Heimberg, M. R. Liebowitz, D. A. Hope, & F. R. Schneier (Eds.), *Social Phobia: Diagnosis, Assessment, and Treatment* (pp. 69–93). New York, NY: The Guilford Press.

Ellemers, N., Spears, R., & Doosje, B. (2002). Self and social identity. *Annual Review of Psychology*, 53, 262–286. doi: 10.1146/annurev.psych.53.100901.135228

Frets, P. G., Kevenaar, C., & Heiden, C. (2014). Imagery rescripting as a stand alone treatment for patients with social phobia: A case series. *Journal of Behavior Therapy and Experimental Psychiatry*, 45, 160–169. doi: 10.1016/j.jbtep.2013.09.006

Goldin, P. R., Jazaieri, H., Ziv, M., *et al.* (2013). Changes in positive self-views mediate the effect of cognitive-behavioral therapy for social anxiety disorder. *Clinical Psychological Science*, 2, 187–201. doi: 10.1177/2167702613476867

Gonzalez-Diez, Z., Calvete, E., Riskind, J. H., & Orue, I. (2015). Test of a hypothesized model of relationships between cognitive style and social anxiety: A 12-month prospective study. *Journal of Anxiety Disorders*, 30, 59–65. doi: 10.1016/j.janxdis.2014.12.014

Hackmann, A., Clark, D. M., & McManus, F. (2000). Recurrent images and early memories in social anxiety disorder. *Behaviour Research and Therapy*, 38, 601–610. doi: 10.1016/S0005-7967(99)00161-8

Harvey, A. G., Clark, D. M., Ehlers, A., & Rapee, R. M. (2000). Social anxiety and self-impression: Cognitive preparation enhances the beneficial effects of video feedback following a stressful social task. *Behaviour Research and Therapy*, 38, 1183–1192. doi: 10.1016/S0005-7967(99)00148-5

Heimberg, R. G., Brozovich, F. A., & Rapee, R. M. (2010). A cognitive-behavioral model of social anxiety disorder: Update and extension. In: S. G. Hofmann, & P. M. DiBartolo (2nd Eds.), *Social Anxiety: Clinical, Developmental, and Social Perspectives* (pp. 395–422). New York, NY: Academic Press.

Higgins, T. E. (1987). Self-discrepancy: A theory relating self and affect. *Psychological Review*, 94, 319–340. doi: 10.1037/0033-295X.94.3.319

Hirsch, C., Mathews, A., Clark, D. M., Williams, R., & Morrison, J. (2003). Negative self-imagery blocks inferences. *Behaviour Research and Therapy*, 41, 1383–1396. doi: 10.1016/S0005-7967(03)00057-3

Hirsch, C., Meynen, T., & Clark, D. (2004). Negative self-imagery in social anxiety contaminates social interactions. *Memory*, 12, 496–506. doi: 10.1080/09658210444000106

Hofmann, S. G. (2007). Cognitive factors that maintain social anxiety disorder: A comprehensive model and its treatment implications. *Cognitive Behaviour Therapy*, 26, 195–209. doi: 10.1080/16506070701421313

Hofmann, S. G., Moscovitch, D. A., Kim, H., & Taylor, A. (2004). Changes in self-perception during treatment of social phobia. *Journal of Consulting and Clinical Psychology*, 72, 588–596. doi: 10.1037/0022-006X.72.4.588

Hulme, N., Hirsch, C., & Stopa, L. (2012). Images of the self and self-esteem: Do positive self-images improve self-esteem in social anxiety? *Cognitive Behaviour Therapy*, 41, 163–173. doi: 10.1080/16506073.2012.664557

Jakymin, A. K., & Harris, L. M. (2012). Self-focused attention and social anxiety. *Australian Journal of Psychology*, 64, 61–67. doi: 10.1111/j.1742-9536.2011.00027.x

Julian, K., Beard, C., Schmidt, N. B., Powers, M. B., & Smits, J. A. J. (2012). Attention training to reduce attention bias and social anxiety stressor reactivity: An attempt to replicate and extend previous findings. *Behaviour Research and Therapy*, 50, 350–358. doi:1 0.1016/j.brat.2012.02.015

Kashdan, T. B., & Roberts, J. E. (2004). Social anxiety's impact on affect, curiosity, and social self-efficacy during a high self-focus threat situation. *Cognitive Therapy and Research*, 28, 199–141. doi: 10.1023/B:COTR.0000016934.20981.68

Koerner, N., Antony, M. M., Young, L., McCabe, R. E. (2013). Changes in beliefs about the social competence of self and others following group cognitive-behavioral treatment. *Cognitive Therapy and Research*, 37, 256–265. doi: 10.1007/s10608-012-9472-5

Laposa, J. M., & Rector, N. A. (2014). Effects of videotaped feedback in group cognitive behavioral therapy for social anxiety disorder. *International Journal of Cognitive Therapy*, 7, 360–372. doi: 10.1521/ijct.2014.7.4.360

Leary, M. R., & Kowalski, R. M. (1995). The self presentation model of social phobia. In R. G. Heimberg, M. R. Liebowitz, D. A. Hope, & F. R. Schneier (Eds.), *Social Phobia: Diagnosis, Assessment, and Treatment* (pp. 94–112). New York, NY: Guilford Press.

Lee, S. R., & Kwon, J. (2013). The efficacy of imagery rescripting (IR) for social anxiety disorder: A randomized controlled trial. *Journal of Behavioural Therapy and Experimental Psychiatry*, 44, 351–360. doi: 10.1016/j.jbtep.2013.03.001

Makkar, S. R., & Grisham, J. R. (2011). Social anxiety and the effects of negative self-imagery on emotion, cognitive, and post-event processing. *Behaviour Research and Therapy*, 49, 654–664. doi: 10.1016/j.brat.2011.07.004

McEvoy, P. M., & Saulsman, L. M. (2014). Imagery-enhanced cognitive behavioural group therapy for social anxiety disorder: A pilot study. *Behaviour Research and Therapy*, 55, 1–6. doi: 10.1016/j.brat.2014.01.006

McEvoy, P. M., Erceg-Hurn, D. M., Saulsman, L. M., & Thibodeau, M. A. (2015). Imagery enhancements increase the effectiveness of cognitive behavioural group therapy for social anxiety disorder: A benchmarking study. *Behaviour Research and Therapy*, 65, 42–51. doi: 10.1016/j.brat.2014.12.011

Moscovitch, D. A. (2009). What is the core fear in social phobia? A new model to facilitate individualized case conceptualisation and treatment. *Cognitive and Behavioral Practice*, 16, 123–134. doi: 10.1016/j.cbpra.2008.04.002

Moscovitch, D. A., & Huyder, C. (2011). The negative self-portrayal scale: Development, validation, and application to social anxiety. *Behavior Therapy*, 42, 183–196. doi: 10.1016/j.beth.2010.04.007

Moscovitch, D. A., Rowa, K., Paulitzki, J. R., *et al.* (2013). Self-portrayal concerns and their relation to safety behaviors and negative affect in social anxiety disorder. *Behaviour Research and Therapy*, 51, 476–486. doi: 10.1016/j.brat.2013.05.002

Mulkens, S., Bögels, S. M., de Jong, P. J., & Louwers, J. (2001). Fear of blushing: Effects of task concentration training versus exposure in vivo on fear and physiology. *Journal of Anxiety Disorders*, 15, 413–432. doi: 10.1016/S0887-6185(01)00073-1

Ng, A. S., Abbott, M. J., & Hunt, C. (2014). The effect of self-imagery on symptoms and processes in social anxiety: A systematic review. *Clinical Psychology Review*, 34, 620–633. doi: 10.1016/j.cpr.2014.09.003

Nilsson, J., Lundh, L., & Viborg, G. (2012). Imagery rescripting of early memories in social anxiety disorder: An experimental study. *Behaviour Research and Therapy*, 50, 387–392. doi: 10.1016/j.brat.2012.03.004

Pinto-Gouveia, J., Castilho, P., Galhardo, A., & Cunha, M. (2006). Early maladaptive schemas and social phobia. *Cognitive Therapy and Research*, 30, 571–584. doi: 10.1007/s10608-006-9027-8

Rapee, R. M., Gaston, J. E., & Abbott, M. J. (2009). Testing the efficacy of theoretically derived improvements in the treatment of social phobia. *Journal of Consulting and Clinical Psychology*, 77, 317–327. doi: 10.1037/a0014800

Rapee, R. M., & Hayman, K. (1996). The effects of video feedback on the self-evaluation of performance in socially anxious subjects. *Behaviour Research and Therapy*, 34, 315–322. doi: 10.1016/0005-7967(96)00003-4

Rapee, R. M., & Heimberg, R. G. (1997). A cognitive-behavioral model of anxiety in social phobia. *Behaviour Research and Therapy*, 35, 741–756. doi: 10.1016/S0005-7967(97)00022-3

Ruscio, A. M., Brown, T. A., Chiu, W. T., *et al.* (2008). Social fears and social phobia in the United States: Results from the national comorbidity survey replication. *Psychological Medicine*, 38, 15–28. doi: 10.1017/S0033291707001699

Schlenker, B. R., & Leary, M. R. (1982). Social anxiety and self-presentation: A conceptualization and model. *Psychological Bulletin*, 92, 641–669. doi: 10.1037/0033-2909.92.3.641

Schmidt, N. B., Richey, J. A., Buckner, J. D., & Timpano, K. R. (2009). Attention training for generalized social anxiety disorder. *Journal of Abnormal Psychology*, 118, 5–14. doi: 10.1037/a0013643

Schulz, S. M., Alpers, G. W., & Hofmann, S. G. (2008). Negative self-focused cognitions mediate the effect of trait social anxiety on social anxiety. *Behaviour Research and Therapy*, 46, 438–449. doi: 10.1016/j.brat.2008.01.008

Showers, C. (1992). Compartmentalization of positive and negative self-knowledge: Keeping bad apples out of the bunch. *Journal of Personality and Social Psychology*, 62, 1036–1049. doi: 10.1037/0022-3514.62.6.1036

Stein, M. B., & Stein, D. J. (2008). Social anxiety disorder. *The Lancet*, 371, 1115–1125. doi: 10.1016/S0140-6736(08)60488-2

Stopa, L. (2009). Why is the self important in understanding and treating social phobia? *Cognitive Behaviour Therapy*, 38, 48–54. doi: 10.1080/16506070902980737

Stopa, L., & Jenkins, A. (2007). Images of the self in social anxiety: Effects on the retrieval of autobiographical memories. *Journal of Behavior Therapy and Experimental Psychiatry*, 38, 459–473. doi: 10.1016/j.jbtep.2007.08.006

Szafranski, D. D., Talkovsky, A. M., Farris, S. G., & Norton, P. J. (2014). Comorbidity: Social anxiety disorder and psychiatric comorbidity are not shy to co-occur. In J. W. Weeks (Ed.), *The Wiley-Blackwell Handbook of Social Anxiety Disorder* (pp. 201–222). Chichester: John Wiley & Sons. doi: 10.1002/9781118653920.ch10

Turner, S. M., Johnson, M. R., Beidel, D. C., Heiser, N. A., & Lydiard, R. B. (2003). The social thoughts and beliefs scale: A new inventory for assessing cognitions in social phobia. *Psychological Assessment*, 15, 384–391. doi: 10.1037/1040-3590.15.3.384

Wild, J., & Clark, D. M. (2011). Imagery rescripting of early traumatic experience in social phobia. *Cognitive and Behavioral Practice*, 18, 433–443. doi: 10.1016/j.cbpra.2011.03.002

Wild, J., Hackmann, A., & Clark, D. M. (2007). When the present visits the past: Updating traumatic memories in social anxiety disorder. *Journal of Behavior Therapy and Experimental Psychiatry*, 38, 386–401. doi: 10.1016/j.jbtep.2007.07.003

Wild, J., Hackmann, A., & Clark, D. M. (2008). Rescripting early memories linked to negative images in social anxiety disorder: A pilot study. *Behavior Therapy*, 39, 47–56. doi: 10.1016/j.beth.2007.04.003

Wong, J., Gordon, E. A., & Heimberg, R. G. (2014). Cognitive-behavioral models of social anxiety disorder. In J. W. Weeks (Ed.), *The Wiley-Blackwell Handbook of Social Anxiety Disorder* (pp. 3–23). John Wiley & Sons, Ltd, Chichester, UK. doi: 10.1002/9781118653920.ch1

Wong, Q. J. J., & Moulds, M. L. (2009). Impact of rumination versus distraction on anxiety and maladaptive self-beliefs in socially anxious individuals. *Behaviour*

Research and Therapy, 47, 861–867. doi: 10.1016/j. brat.2009.06.014

Wong, Q. J. J., & Moulds, M. L. (2011). The relationship between the maladaptive self-beliefs characteristic of social anxiety and avoidance. *Journal of Behavior Therapy and Experimental Psychiatry*, 42, 171–178. doi: 10.1016/j.jbtep.2010.11.004

Wong, Q. J. J., & Moulds, M. L. (2012). Does rumination predict the strength of maladaptive self-beliefs characteristic of social anxiety over time? *Cognitive*

Therapy and Research, 36, 94–102. doi: 10.1007/s10608-010-9316-0

Young, J. E., & Brown, G. (1990). *Young Schema Questionnaire*. New York, NY: Cognitive Therapy Center of New York.

Zhou, J. B., Hudson, J. L., & Rapee, R. M. (2007). The effect of attentional focus on social anxiety. *Behaviour Research and Therapy*, 45, 2326–2333. doi: 10.1016/j. brat.2007.03.014

Chapter

11

The self in posttraumatic stress disorder

Mardi J. Horowitz and Monica A. Sicilia

Posttraumatic stress disorder (PTSD; American Psychiatric Association, 2013) is likely to impair a sense of identity in anyone, for a time. However, PTSD is more likely to develop if a person has pre-existing vulnerabilities in coherence of self-organization. If aspects of the personality have not been integrated in a way that allows for a cohesive and continuous but flexible experience of self, or more accurately selves, processing and incorporating the traumatic experience and its repercussions will present heightened challenges (Horowitz, 2011, 2014). While significant distress and functional impairment generally accompanies self-organizations that are characterized by dissociation, dissociation of certain aspects of self may occur across a range of functioning and with varied degrees of distress (Bromberg, 1998; Horowitz, 2011, 2014). Regardless of level of self-organization, sense of self and identity may be impacted in a multitude of ways in the wake of trauma. This chapter will discuss how this can occur. Person schema theory (Horowitz, 2011, 2014) will serve as a foundation for understanding the impact of trauma on self, general phases of self-experiences after trauma, and the ways in which trauma can, when personality growth occurs, lead to greater self-cohesion.

Person schema theory

Person schema theory (Horowitz, 2011, 2014) describes how parts of the self – images, bodily sensations, beliefs, values, defined roles, ways of being, identity concepts – come together to form organizing schemas that create a more or less cohesive and continuous sense of self or "me" and allow that self to navigate in the world. Levels of the model are nested in increasingly complex

configurations of self-structures. Each level of organization involves conscious and unconscious elements. For example, at the most basic level of the model, parts of self, sensory experiences that pertain to the self may be encoded implicitly, making them inaccessible to a conscious elaboration of one's experience but still allowing them to inform a sense of self and guide behavior. Self schemas link parts of self by collating different types of information formed in different types of memory (Horowitz, 1991, 1998; Kihlstrom, 1987; Piaget, 1962). The associational links of the self schema create a map containing cognitive-affective information based on past experience that forms the basis for generalizations about the self and self in relation to others (Baldwin, 1992; Bowlby 1969; Horowitz, 1991; Ryle, 1997; Stern, 1985; Young, Klosko, & Weishaar, 2003).

When internal or external stimuli activate a particular self schema, conscious and communicative expressions of self, or self-representations, arise and contribute to a conscious sense of identity. Conscious and unconscious components of self schemas inform self states, which reflect temporary, subjective experiences of self. Supra-ordinate self schemas connect individual self schemas but may or may not be connected themselves. Thus, while supra-ordinate self schemas represent higher, more complex levels of connectivity between any given grouping of self schemas, they may exhibit dissociation from another configuration of self schemas. Self-coherence refers to the individual's ability to associate or segregate self schemas; it reflects the overall functioning of the self-organization described here.

It is important to note at this point that, according to person schema theory (Horowitz, 2011, 2014), all aspects of self develop and function within the

The Self in Understanding and Treating Psychological Disorders, ed. Michael Kyrios, Richard Moulding, Guy Doron, Sunil S. Bhar, Maja Nedeljkovic, and Mario Mikulincer. Published by Cambridge University Press. © Cambridge University Press, 2016.

context of relational matrices. Role relationship models (RRMs; Horowtiz, 2014) highlight this feature of the theory. RRMs, like internal working models (IWMs; Bowlby, 1969), are schemas that organize expectations for future interactions based on past experiences.[1] They incorporate information, including thoughts, feelings, and bodily sensations, about self and other within the relational context. When current interpersonal experience or the expectation of such primes an RRM, a configuration of relational expectations, self states, and self-representations becomes active. This can lead to recurrent patterns in relationships that engender distress and reify RRMs that do not accurately reflect important aspects of current realities. In this way, relationship patterns and the self schemas that are associated with them are learned in the past but may be maintained in the present (Horowitz, 2011, 2014; Levenson, 1995, 2003; Schacht, Binder, & Strupp, 1984; Wachtel, 1993). They may also be challenged in the present, opening the possibility of linking past, present, and future self schemas. Therapeutic interventions that facilitate trauma mastery aim to do just this within the context of a new relational experience.

Case example: a transient regression in sense of self and roles of attachment

The following vignette highlights how disturbances in a conscious sense of identity following trauma, such as diminished self-esteem, lapses in self-confidence, or depersonalization, reflect unconscious shifts in self-concepts that can be ameliorated as an aspect of trauma mastery (Aldwin, Sutton, & Lachman, 1996; Horowitz, 2011; Park, Cohen, & Murch, 1996).

While traveling on business in another country, Harold and his wife escaped a hotel fire, but experienced minor smoke inhalation injuries. Harold and his wife agreed that she would return home at once while Harold completed essential business appointments. Five days later, he began to feel tense and anxious, and had a sense of depersonalization. Harold became too talkative and attention-seeking from women he met with during his daily business dealings. One night he awakened from a nightmare and remembered himself screaming "Mommy, mommy!" He canceled meetings, immediately flew home, and sought professional consultation. On evaluation, he reported intrusive memories of the fire and of unbidden images of his wife leaving him at the airport. He was embarrassed in retrospect by his memories of seeking excessive closeness in his engagement with female colleagues. He feared travel and avoided planning future business appointments out of the city even though his financial future depended on it. He had states of tension, panic, and hyperventilation.

In the first phase of therapy attention focused on increasing his sense of safety and on the story of how the fire and its sequel led to an activation of latent self-concepts in which he needed attention and reinforcement of his goals and sense of values from a woman. The second phase of therapy focused on integrating this usually dormant role relationship model, of a dependent boy requiring maternal attention for guidance, and feeling abandoned without it, with his role relationship model as a competent person who interacted as an equal with a woman to whom he felt close. In other words, a helpful interpretation of his syndrome included the concept that his altered behavioral pattern after the fire occurred with activation of a usually dormant role, that of a dependent self looking for a secure attachment figure, rather than his usually active self-concept as an autonomous adult. In the third phase of a brief therapy attention focused on when he shifted between his competent versus incompetent self states, and how these were affected by emotional events in his relationship with his wife. Harold could recognize both self states as parts of his identity. He could also reflect on when each was activated and the conflict he experienced between them, which led to his embarrassment and shame. This work increased his sense of personal stability and enabled him to engage even more mutually with his wife than before the hotel fire.

The impact of trauma on the self

Transient regressions to earlier schemas of self are among the possible effects of trauma. Increased use of defensive dissociation, denial, and avoidance may also occur in an attempt to preserve pre-trauma schemas of self and other. These states may give way to or alternate with a sense of a fractured or disintegrating self marked by depersonalization, derealization, intrusive phenomena, or symptoms of hyperarousal (e.g., Herman, 1992; Horowitz, 2011). The interpersonal sequelae of trauma also contribute to the impact that trauma can have on the self. A person may be stigmatized or disrupted in relationships because of the inciting events. This can strip away external sources of validation by

Table 11.1 Levels of integration of self–other schematization.

Level	Description
Harmonious	Internal desires, needs, frustrations, impulses, choices, and values are appraised as "of the self." Realistic pros and cons are examined to reach choices of rational action and restraint. Grounded in self, one views others as separate people with their own intentions, expectations, and emotional reactions. Perspectives on relationships approximate social realities. Past and present views of self and relationships are integrated, allowing a sense of constancy and modification of ambivalence. State transitions are smooth, appropriate, and adroit. Warm and caring relationships are maintained over time in spite of episodic frustrations. Emotional governance prevents out of control states.
Mildly conflicted	While good-enough relationships are formed in his or her closest work and intimate affiliations, the person displays states that contain varied intentions, manifesting as conflicting approach and distancing tendencies. On examination, these alternations are based on fluctuating attitudes about self in the relationship. Most commonly, fears of rejection may limit warm and caring attachments to others, or fears of subordination limit high levels of cooperation. The person appraises self with a variety of critical judgments: some too harsh, some too lax. State transitions occur between positive and negative moods, but the shifts in state are remembered and not explosive surprises or emergence of alternative selves.
Vulnerable	A sense of self-regard deteriorates under stress, criticism, and increased pressures to perform. To protect from feelings of inferiority or enfeeblement, grandiose supports of self-esteem may be utilized. Concern for the well-being of others may be considered less important than using others as tools for self-enhancement. Surprising shifts from vigor and boldness to states of apathy, boredom, or unpleasant restlessness may occur. Because of insufficient self-organization, the person may shift between being loving; suddenly, overly demanding; and suddenly appeasing. Emotional governance is reduced. Undermodulated rage may erupt at others who are perceived as insulting and are blamed for otherwise shameful deflations in the individual's own self-esteem.
Disturbed	Life seems organized by using various self states and some of them seem like a break with reality. Errors in self–other attribution occur. Undesirable self attributes and emotions are projected from self to other. The actions of self may be confused in memory in terms of who did or felt what, and shifts in self state may be accompanied by apparent forgetting of what happened in the alternative state of mind. Memories frequently combine fantasies with once-real elements. State transitions can be explosive. Dissociative identity experiences recur under stress and forgetting and then remembering may occur in segregated states of mind and views of self.
Fragmented	A massive chaos of selfhood can occur and, as a counter to cope with the high distress, the person frequently feels aroused to high defensiveness and accusation of others, as if under attack. As a needed repair of damage to self, the individual may regard self as merged with another person. Or, the person may withdraw in a hibernated, frozen, self-protecting coping effort that, to others, appears bizarre and self-damaging. Parts of the bodily self may be infused with the "badness" and disowned from self-images. This sense of chaos is very painful and can give rise to poorly regulated emotional impulses, including potentially suicidal or homicidal urges, intensified because the strange behaviors lead to social stigmatization.

others and habitual environments, leading towards identity disturbances. As a result of trauma, persons may experience themselves as unattractive and contact with others may be avoided to protect against an expected rejection. In these ways, trauma can strain relationships and create conflict between new realities and old internalized RRMs. These disturbances in sense of self, self in relation to others, and identity may interact with and exacerbate posttraumatic symptoms such as intrusive memories, phobic avoidances, anxiety, and depression. They may also contribute to emotional under-regulation of angry or guilty moods and substance abuse.

As the examples above illustrate, trauma impacts the survivor's entire world through its impact on self-organization. Self-organization mediates experience. Relative coherence of self-organization enables greater flexibility in dealing with new and unexpected cognitive-affective experience. Put another way, coherence of self-organization enables more realistic appraisal of self and others and more effective decision-making. Levels of integration of self–other schematization reflect coherence of self-organization and the abilities it supports. These levels are summarized in Table 11.1 (reproduced from table 6.1, p. 51, of Horowitz, 2014), where they range from the most coherent level, *harmonious*, to the most disorganized level, *fragmented*.[2]

When someone experiences a trauma, the severity of the trauma interacts with the individual's level of personality integration resulting in a variety of responses to the traumatic stressor (Horowitz, 2014; see also Agabi & Wilson, 2005, for a review of the prevalence of the Person × Situation model of resilience and vulnerability to posttraumatic stress in trauma research). Recent research on the relationship between pathological narcissism, which might describe vulnerable levels of self–other schematization, and posttraumatic stress syndromes supports this theory. Using a multidimensional measure of narcissism, Bachar, Hadar, and Shalev (2005) found that narcissistic traits predicted PTSD status in Israeli civilians both one and four months after they were exposed to war trauma. Similarly, Besser, Zeigler-Hill, Pincus, and Neria (2013) reported positive associations between pathological narcissistic traits and symptoms of PTSD in Israeli civilians following exposure to war trauma. The findings of these studies suggest that the level of personality functioning reflected in pathological narcissism interacts with stress and can lead to syndrome development.

Reflective functioning and dissociation

Notably, the capacity to reflect on self increases as one moves from fragmented towards harmonious levels of functioning. Studies that have shown a correlation between maltreatment in childhood and deficits in reflective functioning and identity formation (Beegly & Cicchetti. 1994; Schneider-Rosen & Cicchetti, 1984, 1991, cited in Fonagy, Gergely, Jurist, & Target, 2001) highlight the way trauma can impact personality integration. Fonagy *et al.* (2004) also point out that deficits in mentalization, the ability and willingness to reflect on one's own and others' mental states,[3] can contribute to survivors' vulnerability to further abuse. The authors postulate that because those who show deficits in understanding mental states, such as abused children, seek physical proximity not stress-inducing mental proximity, they may move closer to their abusers (or abusive/neglecting others) while lacking the mentalizing skills that might help them accurately appraise danger and protect themselves. At the same time, deficits in mentalization and the comprehension of internal states that it facilitates can lead to externalization and projection of aggression, including the expectation of neglect/abandonment. Within this iteration of the model, re-enactments of traumatic experiences remain an attempt by an individual with impaired self-regulation and characteristic dissociative defenses

to achieve regulation by turning a passive experience of trauma into an active experience of greater mastery and control.

The perspective presented here presupposes a multiplicity or a "committee of selves" (Horowitz, 2014, p. 23), which function optimally when the ability to access each other exists and is intact. This is not to say, however, that dissociation among self states is fundamentally maladaptive. To the contrary, dissociation is often needed to titrate overwhelming experience (Horowitz, 2014). It is also, as Bromberg (1998) has pointed out, essential as a means of heightening focus and preventing the stagnation of an overly determined self structure; dis-integration leads to growth when reorganization occurs as part of a re-integrating process (Horowitz, 2011, 2014). In these capacities, which arguably involve the capacity for mentalization, dissociation can enhance the self. However, following trauma, dissociation can also become a rigid defensive response to the threat of retraumatization and result in the siloing of self states, identity disturbances, and stress response syndromes (Bromberg, 1998; Horowitz, 2014). Rigid defenses developed in response to trauma affect the neurobiological systems that control perception, arousal, memory, emotion, and behavior; the effects on the self can be pervasive and lasting.

Neurobiological underpinnings of the impact of trauma on self

In his review of the research on the impact of trauma on neurobiological development, van der Kolk (2003) notes that because neurological systems mature and become functional at different times over the course of development, the impact of trauma differs by age. For example, the amygdala, which registers danger and triggers fear, is one of the first brain structures to begin functioning. However, the hippocampus, responsible for spatial and temporal localization of danger, develops over the course of the first five years of life and the prefrontal regions that enable a more sophisticated evaluation of danger and organization of response mature through early adulthood. Because early trauma affects hippocampal development, some scholars speculate that early trauma is more likely than later trauma to create a neurobiological system that is highly susceptible to misinterpreting stimuli as dangerous and less able to respond with effective self-protective behaviours (Nadel, 1992, cited in van der Kolk, 2003).

Chronic trauma can extend and compact the impact of early trauma on neurobiology. Van der Kolk (2003) suggests that:

> … prolonged alarm reactions alter limbic, midbrain, and brain stem functions through "use-dependent" modifications. Chronic exposure to fearful stimuli affects the development of the hippocampus, the left cerebral cortex, and the cerebellar vermis and alters the capacity to integrate sensory input (Teicher, Anderson, & Polcari, 2002). This changes the degree to which cortical and cerebellar structures can help the growing child modulate the limbic, midbrain, and brain stem responses to danger and fear. (p. 294)

The use-dependent nature of brain development underlies the lasting impact of traumatic events on homeostatic functioning (via the brain stem and locus coeruleus), memory (via the hippocampus, amygdala, and frontal cortex) and executive functioning (via the orbitofrontal cortex, cingulate, and dorsolateral prefrontal cortex; Perry, Pollard, Blakley, & Baker, 1995, cited in van der Kolk, 2003). It also affects changes in the neuroendrocrine system (via the hypothalamic–pituitary–adrenal axis and all neurotransmitter systems; Weiner, Lowe, & Levine, 1992; Stanton, Gutierrez, & Levine, 1988, cited in van der Kolk, 2003). Thus, as Perry *et al.* (1995) suggest, state becomes trait; adaptive responses to a chronically traumatic environment (e.g., states of hyperarousal and dissociation) lead to neurobiologically mediated difficulties with self-regulation, as well as alterations in memory functioning and executive planning.

Van der Kolk (2003) posits that difficulty regulating emotions "leads to problems with self-definition as reflected by (1) a lack of a continuous, predictable sense of self, with a poor sense of separateness and disturbances of body image, (2) poorly modulated affect and impulse control, including aggression against self and others, and (3) uncertainty about the reliability and predictability of others, leading to distrust, suspiciousness, and problems with intimacy (van der Kolk & Fisler, 1994; Cole & Putnam, 1992)" (p. 298). Dissociation, which disrupts the formation of a "continuous, predictable" sense of self, is thought to mediate the relationship between lack of emotional self-regulation and altered self-perceptions in those who have experienced chronic trauma. Dissociation and constriction proceed from increases in norepinephrine and endogenous opioids, which occur in response to the recognition of danger and decreases psychological and physical pain perception (van der Kolk & van der Hardt, 1991). They also reflect the imperative to ignore feelings of fear and anxiety in the absence of the ability or the resources to regulate them (Crittenden, 1985, cited in van der Kolk, 2003). Intrusion occurs because memories of traumatic events are encoded in a state of alarm and on an iconic level, as bodily sensations, images, and behavioral reactions, rather than on a symbolic level as a narrative located in space and time. When a trauma survivor experiences a state of alarm triggered by similar contextual cues, it activates the same pathways and retrieves the sensations, images, and behaviors of the trauma (van der Kolk & van der Hardt, 1991), the self schemas and RRMs. These neurobiological alterations also account for the attentional deficits and explosive anger often observed in stress response syndromes; increases in norepinephrine are associated with impaired functioning in the prefrontal cortex (Crittenden, 1997, cited in van der Kolk, 2003). The prefrontal cortex controls attention and is involved in planning, which can help moderate impulsive behavior.

The impact of trauma on interpersonal relationships

As noted above, the difficulty many trauma survivors experience with intimacy in relationships also relates to deficits or disruptions in self-regulation. This is particularly true of those who have experienced early trauma because the capacity to self-regulate develops within the context of early attachment relationships. Developmental research shows what clinical observations have long suggested: primary caretakers' attunement to their infants' over- and under-regulated states scaffolds the infant's development of self-regulatory functions (Beebe & Lachman, 2002; Cozolino, 2006; Fonagy, 2008; Hesse & Main, 2000; Schore, 1994; Siegel, 2007; Stern, 1985; Tronick, 2007; Wallin, 2007, cited in Ginot, 2012). As caretakers repeatedly help to regulate the infant's emotional experience by either attending to the infant or restraining from intrusive involvement with the infant, they create foundational experiences of mutually satisfying intimacy and autonomous regulation. These experiences of benign self–other configurations are internalized and form the basis of adaptive self schemas and RRMs. When a traumatic environment (e.g., war, famine, extreme poverty, domestic violence, abuse, neglect, or death) disrupts primary caretakers' ability to attune to the infant, self schemas and RRMs that result in dysregulated self states, particularly within the context of intimate relationships, may develop.

Schore and Schore (2008) summarize the findings of developmental and neurobiological research on the relationship between attachment, self-regulation, and interpersonal functioning:

> The essential task of the first year of human life is the creation of a secure attachment bond of emotional communication between the infant and the primary caregiver. In order to enter into this communication, the mother must be psychobiologically attuned to the dynamic shifts in the infant's bodily-based internal states of central and autonomic arousal. During the affective communications embedded in mutual gaze episodes the psychobiologically attuned sensitive caregiver appraises nonverbal expressions of the infant's arousal and then regulates these affective states, both positive and negative. The attachment relationship mediates the dyadic regulation of emotion, wherein the mother (primary caregiver) co-regulates the infant's postnatally developing central (CNS) and autonomic (ANS) nervous systems ... These adaptive capacities are central to self-regulation, i.e. the ability to flexibly regulate psychobiological states of emotions through interactions with other humans, interactive regulation in interconnected contexts, and without other humans, autoregulation in autonomous contexts. (p. 11)

Without the self-regulative capacities that develop within the context of a relatively attuned and non-threatening primary attachment relationship, individuals are unable to use relationships to achieve regulation, engage in dyadic attunement and mutual regulation, or achieve regulation autonomously. Thus, those who experience early and chronic trauma may be at once more dependent on others for comfort and unable to take comfort in intimate relationships with others.

The psychological, emotional, and behavioral implications of this are captured in the disorganized/disoriented attachment classification in children, marked by "an observed contradiction in movement pattern ... [and] a lack of orientation to the present environment" (Hesse & Main, 2000, p. 1099), and the unresolved/disorganized attachment classification in adults, reflected in "disorganization or disorientation in discourse or reasoning while attempting to discuss potentially traumatic events" (Hesse & Main, 2000, p. 1111). Although the disorganized attachment classification has been found in about 15% of low-risk samples (Lyons-Ruth, 2003), Carlson, Cicchetti, Barrett, and Grunewald (1989) and Lyons-Ruth (1996) have reported it at rates of 80% in children with a

history of maltreatment. Such fundamental failures in self-regulation signal dissociative tendencies and reinforce reliance on defenses such as splitting (e.g., idealization and denigration). These defenses may contribute to maladaptive self schemas and RRMs that interfere with the ability to form and maintain satisfying interpersonal relationships, including the therapeutic relationship. Reflection on the connection between self-regulation, self schemas, and interpersonal functioning is accordingly an important focus of psychotherapy with trauma survivors (Bromberg, 1998; Ginot, 2012; Horowitz, 2011, 2014).

General phases of self experiences after trauma

There are different challenges to a person's sense of identity during a stress response syndrome. These can be generalized into the following prototypical sequence.

Initial outcry phase: With a massive impact of bad news, some people experience an alarm reaction that includes an imperative impulse to protect both self and others. The primary identity question is, "Can I survive or will I succumb?"

Denial and avoidance phase: Next, a "business as usual" self state may replace the acute alarm reactions. A numbing of emotions and some disavowal of reality may lead to dissociative experiences: "This event does not affect me," "What happened does not seem real," or "I totally escaped harm."

Intrusive feelings and ideas phase: The person in this phase is jolted by reality reminders and the unbidden emergence of traumatic memories and fantasies. He or she may experience intense pangs of feelings associated with somatic components of threat appraisal. The person may become secondarily terrified of losing self-control.

Working through phase: As intrusive emotional ideations about the trauma become less intense, and the sense of episodic numbing decreases, the narrative work of trauma evaluation leads towards attitude revisions, including new plans for adaptation. A sense of self-competence may gradually reform. Enhanced harmony between various self-attitudes may develop.

Completion stage: When the work of adapting to stress has been mostly completed, narrations have been modified and the person has made adaptive and rational changes in his or her self-organization and self-judgmental attitudes.

Case example: massive trauma and work on self-reorganization

This vignette illustrates how working through trauma can lead to a greater sense of self-possession through self-reorganization that integrates past, present, and future self-schemas.

Sophia made an excellent living as a sought-after model until a sudden car accident resulted in severe injuries that caused permanent blindness and required amputation of one of her legs. She also emerged with severe facial scarring. Sophia spent weeks in the hospital and then months in a rehabilitation institution. Initially, she did not allow herself to be fully aware of the implications of her eye injuries. She would not discuss her blindness with medical staff. She did, however, think and talk about the loss of her leg. Her lack of recognition of her blindness was astonishing to team members because she had to be constantly assisted with many bodily functions.

Sophia's sense of self and her mental body image had not shifted to accommodate the terrible news of her physically altered body. She repeatedly asked staff members when she could again schedule her modeling appointments. Only after weeks passed did she communicate about being blind; the topic of her facial disfigurement and loss of a career was discussed even later. After three months passed, she accepted a recommendation for psychotherapy. In the context of this therapy, Sophia took two years to recover her psychological equilibrium and develop a sense of self that was coherent with her altered bodily functions and social opportunities. She learned new self-concepts through a variety of means, including identification with the effective roles and positive attitudes she observed in various health professionals. She trained as a rehabilitation therapist specializing in music therapy. Later she married.

Sophia's goal of total bodily restoration was not possible. A catastrophic mismatch of current and ideal body occurred, leading to a potential self state of feeling ugly, unwanted, and worthless. A compromise role as a completely isolated loner might have been used to avoid these dreaded experiences of self. Therapeutic intervention enabled Sophia to construct a more adaptive, desirable sense of a future self, which could be projected as a possible future for intimate relationships. Sophia continued activation of her pre-trauma body image long after her accident. Concurrently, she slowly and unconsciously formed a new body image that could accord with her drastic posttrauma changes. Her adaptation increased as her new body image gradually evolved, was matched with expectations, and evoked less horror and self-disgust because she slowly forged new role concepts for relationships.

A comparison between a desired and a dreaded body image can generate horrifying emotions. Defenses can attenuate distress. Cognitive controls can, for example, prevent use of emotionally evocative forms of representation – as when Sophia would not use conscious visual imagery to imagine her new body and how it would appear to others. Sophia had to change her expectations by re-schematizations of various self and other representations. Control processes that constantly inhibit information or that consistently distort reality numb emotion at the cost of impairing the processes of trauma mastery through re-schematization. This results in overmodulated states. Conversely, control processes that fail to regulate emotional arousals lead to undermodulated states that feel dangerously out of control. The aim in therapy is to foster, by attention-focusing, control processes that allow flexible appraisals of new realities. By fostering adaptive behavioral coping, therapeutic work can promote gradual identity re-schematization. This can result in well-modulated states, even when considering distressing new realities.

In adaptive coping, posttraumatic emotions are titrated by control processes to levels that are tolerable. A reduction of Sophia's defense against mental imagery (a function not impaired organically by her blindness) was approached gradually so that the fear, anger, and sorrow evoked in her felt manageable. In the short term, she appeared worse because of the unavoidable suffering of mourning her bodily losses. Over the long term, she improved because of the re-schematization of her sense of how she appeared to others. She was less apprehensive about their possible responses to seeing her. She gradually revised her own initial self-evaluation from an "I am disgustingly ugly" response to a later response of "This is how I look now, and both I and they can accept me as a worthwhile person."

Person schema theory (Horowitz, 2011, 2014) suggests that any traumatic event may be subsequently associated with multiple self and relationship concepts as a part of information processing in complex neural circuitries. Some meanings of the trauma may have implications that are in conflict with existing schemas and their intrinsic expectations and intentions. Understanding existing schemas and their level of coherence before the trauma enables a comprehensive formulation of what re-schematization of self concepts after the trauma will entail. This can aid in treatment planning and help the clinician accurately interpret the patient's behavior in treatment as well his/her responses to the patient, ultimately scaffolding the skills required to achieve a sense of posttraumatic growth in identity and relationship capacities.

Summary

Traumatic events often lead to a sense of self with traits of incompetence, inferiority, degradation, depersonalization, or identity diffusion. By facilitating the development of narrative structures about new aspects of self and how existing self-schemas are harmonized, clinicians can help patients master symptoms, improve their emotional regulation, and reorganize self-schemas in meaningful ways after trauma. Clinicians treating stress response syndromes may benefit from assessing level of self-organization pre- and posttrauma. Formulation and treatment planning that include these considerations may help clinicians stay with the comprehensive experience of the trauma survivor throughout the consultation and treatment process, while enabling identification of focused treatment goals. Attending to both the patient's and the clinician's own shifts in self states during sessions may enable perception of as yet unintegrated selves, which may underlie phenomena that would otherwise be misinterpreted (Bromberg, 1998; Horowtiz, 2014). It is also possible that the clinician's stance that trauma can lead to a greater sense of self-possession through reorganization involving increased access to multiple, potentially conflicting self states may implicitly communicate to the patient that it is safe to access these self states within the context of the therapeutic space, thereby facilitating internalization of this stance through identification with the clinician.

Notes

1 RRMs may be distinguished from supra-ordinate self schemas by their interpersonal focus and their scope. An overly simplified but explicit articulation of an RRM might be, "You are a caretaker in intimate relationships. You can expect others to be dependent and easily hurt. Others will have limited capacity to nurture you and will reject you if you hurt them or ask too much. Your ability to be loving and nurturing connects you to others and protects you from isolation." In contrast, a supra-ordinate self schema might link the sense of competence in intimate relationships with a sense of professional and athletic competence and give rise to an identity of a competent person. This may or may not be accessible to self schemas that acknowledge the individual's needs in intimate relationships, areas of less competence in relationships, and potential conflicts between these aspects of self.

2 Bender, Morey, and Skodol (2011) recommended a similar delineation of levels of personality functioning, operationalized in the Level of Personality Functioning Scale (LPFS), to be included in section II of the DSM-5 (American Psychiatric Association, 2013).

3 Self-regulation and a fundamental theory of mind are the necessary precursors to the development of the advanced reflective functioning Fonagy, Gergely, Jurist, and Target (2004) define as mentalization. However, mentalization also enables more effective self-regulation and a more sophisticated theory of mind; they become mutually reinforcing.

References

Agaibi, C. E., & Wilson, J. P. (2005). Trauma, PTSD, and resilience: A review of the literature. *Trauma, Violence, & Abuse*, 6(3), 195–216.

Aldwin, C. M., Sutton, K., & Lachman, M. (1996). The development of coping resources in adulthood. *Journal of Personality*, 64, 837–871.

American Psychiatric Association. (2013). *Diagnostic and Statistical Manual of Mental Disorders* (5th ed.). Washington, DC: American Psychiatric Association.

Bachar, E., Hadar, H., & Shalev, A. Y. (2005). Narcissistic vulnerability and the development of PTSD: A prospective study. *Journal of Nervous and Mental Disease*, 193, 762–765.

Baldwin, M. (1992). Relational schemas and the processing of social information. *Psychologiacl Bulletin*, 112, 461–484.

Beebe, B., & Lachmann, F. (2002). *Infant Research and Adult Treatment: Co-constructing Interactions*. Hillsdale, NJ: Analytic Press.

Beegly, M., & Cicchetti, D. (1994) Child maltreatment, attachment, and the self system: Emergence of an internal state lexicon in toddlers at high social risk. *Development and Psychopathology*, 6, 5–30.

Bender, D. S., Morey, L. C., & Skodol, A. E. (2011). Toward a model for assessing level of personality functioning in DSM-5, Part 1: A review of theory and methods. *Journal of Personality Assessment*, 93(4), 332–346.

Besser, A., Zeigler-Hill, V., Pincus, A. L., & Neria, Y (2013). Pathological narcissism and acute anxiety symptoms after trauma: A study of Israeli citizens exposed to war. *Psychiatry*, 76(4), 381–397.

Bowlby, J. (1969). *Attachment and Loss, Vol. 1: Attachment.* New York, NY: Basic Books.

Bromberg, P.M. (1998). Standing in the spaces: The multiplicity of self and the psychoanalytic relationship. In *Standing in the Spaces: Essays on Clinical Process, Trauma, and Dissociation* (pp. 291–316). New York, NY: Psychology Press. (Original work published 1996.)

Carlson, V., Cicchetti, D., Barrett, D., & Grunewald, K. (1989). Disorganized/disoriented attachment relationships in maltreated infants. *Developmental Psychology*, 25, 525–531.

Cole, P., & Putnam, F. (1992). Effect of incest on self and social functioning: A developmental psychopathology perspective. *Journal of Consulting and Clinical Psychology*, 60, 174–84.

Cozolino, L. (2006). *The Neuroscience of Human Relationships: Attachment and the Developing Brain.* New York, NY: Norton.

Crittenden, P. (1985). Maltreated infants: Vulnerability and resilience. *Journal of Child Psychology and Psychiatry*, 26, 85–96.

Crittenden P. (1997). Truth, error, omission, distortion, and deception: The application of attachment theory to the assessment and treatment of psychological disorder. In S. Dollinger & L. F. DiLalla (Eds.), *Assessment and Intervention Issues Across the Life Span* (pp. 35–76). Hillsdale, NJ: Erlbaum.

Fonagy, P. (2008). The mentalization-focused approach to social development. In F. N. Busch (Ed.), *Mentalization: Theoretical Considerations, Research Findings, and Clinical Implications* (pp. 3–56). New York, NY: The Analytic Press.

Fonagy, P., Gergely, G., Jurist, E. L., & Target, M. (2004). *Affect Regulation, Mentalization, and the Development of the Self.* New York, NY: Other Press.

Ginot, E. (2012). Self-narratives and dysregulated affective state: The neuropsychological links between self-narratives, attachment, affect, and cognition. *Psychoanalytic Psychology*, 29(1), 59–80.

Herman, J. L. (1992). *Trauma and Recovery.* New York, NY: Basic Books.

Hesse, E., & Main, M. (2000). Disorganized infant, child, and adult attachment: Collapse in behavioral and attentional strategies. *Journal of the American Psychoanalytic Association*, 48, 1097–1148.

Horowitz, M. J. (1991). *Person Schemas and Maladaptive Interpersonal Patterns.* Chicago, IL: University of Chicago Press.

Horowitz, M. J. (1998). *Cognitive Psychodynamics: From Conflict to Character.* New York, NY: John Wiley & Sons.

Horowitz, M. J. (2011). *Stress Response Syndromes* (5th ed.). Northvale, NJ: Jason Aronson.

Horowitz, M. J. (2014). *Identity and the New Psychoanalytic Explorations of Self-organization.* London: Routledge.

Kihlstrom, J. F. (1987). The cognitive unconscious. *Science*, 237(4821), 1445–1452.

Levenson, H. (1995). *Time-limited Dynamic Psychotherapy: A Guide to Clinical Practice.* New York, NY: Basic Books.

Levenson, H. (2003). Time-limited dynamic psychotherapy: An integrationist perspective. *Journal of Psychotherapy Integration*, 13(3/4), 300–333.

Lyons-Ruth, K. (1996). Attachment relationships among children with aggressive behavior problems. *Journal of Clinical and Consulting Psychology*, 64, 64–73.

Lyons-Ruth, K. (2003). Dissociation and the parent–infant dialogue: A longitudinal perspective from attachment research. *Journal of the American Psychoanalytic Association*, 51, 883–911.

Nadel, L. (1992). Multiple memory systems: What and why. *Journal of Cognitive Neuroscience*, 4, 179–88.

Park, C. L., Cohen, L., & Murch, R. (1996). Assessment of stress related growth. *Journal of Personality*, 64, 71–105.

Perry, B., Pollard, R., Blakley, T., & Baker, W. (1995). Childhood trauma, the neurobiology of adaptation and use-dependent development of the brain: How states become traits. *Infant Mental Health Journal*, 16(4), 271–291.

Piaget, J. (1962). *Play, Dreams, and Imitation in Childhood.* New York, NY: Norton.

Ryle, A. (1997). The structure and development of borderline personality disorder: A proposed model. *British Journal of Psychiatry*, 170, 82.

Schacht, T. E., Binder, J. L., & Strupp, H. H. (1984). The dynamic focus. In H. H. Strupp & J. L. Binder (Eds.), *Psychotherapy in a New Key: A Guide to Time-Limited Dynamic Psychotherapy* (pp. 65–109). New York, NY: Basic Books.

Schneider-Rosen, K., & Cicchetti, D. (1984). The relationship between affect and cognition in maltreated infants: Quality of attachment and the development of visual self-recognition. *Child Development*, 55, 648–658.

Schneider-Rosen, K., & Cicchetti, D. (1991). Early self-knowledge and emotional development: Visual self-recognition and affective reactions to mirror self-image in maltreated and non-maltreated toddlers. *Developmental Psychology*, 27, 481–488.

Schore, A. N. (1994). *Affect Regulation and the Origin of the Self: The Neurobiology of Emotional Development.* Hillsdale, NJ: Erlbaum.

Schore, J.R., & Schore, A.N. (2008) Modern attachment theory: The central role of affect regulation in development and trauma. *Clinical Social Work Journal*, 36, 9–20.

Siegel, D. J. (2007). *The Mindful Brain: Reflection and Attunement in the Cultivation of Well Being*. New York, NY: Norton.

Stanton M., Gutierrez Y., & Levine S. (1988). Maternal deprivation potentiates pituitary–adrenal stress responses in infant rats. *Behavioral Neuroscience*, 102, 692–700.

Stern, D. N. (1985). *The Interpersonal World of the Infant: A View from Psychoanalysis and Developmental Psychology*. New York, NY: Basic Books.

Teicher, M., Anderson, S., & Polcari, A. (2002). Developmental neurobiology of childhood stress and trauma. *Psychiatric Clinics of North America*, 25, 397–426.

Tronick, E. (2007). *The Neurobehavioral and Social-Emotional Development of Infants and Children*. New York, NY: Norton.

van der Kolk, B. A. (2003). The neurobiology of childhood trauma and abuse. *Child and Adolescent Psychiatric Clinics of North America*, 12, 293–317.

van der Kolk, B. A., & Fisler, R. (1994). Childhood abuse and neglect and loss of self-regulation. *Bulletin of the Menninger Clinic*, 58(2), 145–168.

van der Kolk, B. A., & van der Hart, O. (1991). The intrusive past: The flexibility of memory and the engraving of trauma. *American Imago*, 48(4), 425–454.

Wachtel, P. L. (1993). *Therapeutic Communication: Knowing What To Say When*. New York, NY: The Guilford Press.

Wallin, W. J. (2007). *Attachment in Psychotherapy*. New York, NY: The Guilford Press.

Weiner, S. G., Lowe, E. L., & Levine, S. (1992). Pituitary–adrenal response to weaning in infant squirrel monkeys. *Psychobiology*, 20(1), 65–70.

Young, J. E., Klosko, J. S., & Weishaar, M. E. (2003). *Schema Therapy: A Practitioner's Guide*. New York, NY: Guilford Press.

Chapter 12

Self processes in obsessive–compulsive disorder

Claire Ahern and Michael Kyrios

This chapter examines how "the self" is implicated in obsessive–compulsive disorder (OCD). The chapter begins by presenting the phenomenology of OCD and theoretical accounts that credit the involvement of self-processes in OCD, with emphasis given to Guidano and Liotti's (1983) theory of self-ambivalence. Then, empirical support for a relationship between obsessive–compulsive (OC) phenomena and various self constructs is reviewed. Ambivalence about moral self-worth, and burgeoning research into implicit self processes, are proposed to have particular relevance in our understanding of the development, maintenance and treatment of OCD.

Phenomenology of OCD

Both the DSM 5.0 (American Psychiatric Association [APA], 2013) and ICD 10 (World Health Organization, 2015) recognize the central feature of OCD to be the presence of obsessions and/or compulsions. Obsessions are defined as thoughts, images or impulses that are intrusive and occur repetitively. In contrast to the intrusive phenomena observed in other psychiatric disorders, obsessions are considered to be ego-dystonic, that is individuals with OCD recognize that the content of their obsessions is incongruent with their self-view or ideas about the world (Clark & Rhyno, 2004).

Individuals with OCD experience obsessions as unwanted, but such obsessions are hard to ignore and difficult to control; thus marked anxiety or distress ensues. In response, repetitive, rigid, and intentional behaviors or mental acts are performed in order to help prevent or reduce the anxiety or distress that follows an obsession, or to prevent the occurrence of some future

perceived threat (APA, 2013). While these compulsions are designed to reduce discomfort, they are maladaptive safety-seeking behaviors and recognized to be central to the persistence of obsessional problems; they alleviate discomfort in the short term but are associated with longer-term maintenance of discomfort and increases in the urge to engage in further neutralizing responses (Salkovskis, 1989; Salkovskis, Thorpe, Wahl, Wroe, & Forrester, 2003; Salkovskis, Westbrook, Davis, Jeavons, & Gledhill, 1997).

OCD is increasingly recognized to be a heterogeneous condition. Although the current diagnostic criteria suggest a discrete disorder, the manifestation of OCD symptoms can vary widely and variant symptoms can have differential responses to treatment (McKay *et al.*, 2004). The most popular basis for classification of OCD is based on overt symptom presentation, with common compulsive themes including checking, cleaning, counting, reassurance-seeking, repeating actions and acting out behavioral patterns in a specific order (Rasmussen & Eisen, 1994; Rasmussen & Tsuang, 1986). Hoarding, arranging, and counting compulsions are the least common but have been rated as the most distressing of the compulsions (Foa *et al.*, 1995). More recently, hoarding has been regarded as a separate disorder (APA, 2013) and is discussed by Moulding and colleagues in Chapter 13 of this book.

Theoretical discourse about self processes in OCD

Investigation into self-processes may be a logical extension of current cognitive accounts of OCD. In Rachman's (1997) influential cognitive theory of obsessions, he notes that one of the pivotal reasons that

The Self in Understanding and Treating Psychological Disorders, ed. Michael Kyrios, Richard Moulding, Guy Doron, Sunil S. Bhar, Maja Nedeljkovic, and Mario Mikulincer. Published by Cambridge University Press. © Cambridge University Press, 2016.

unwanted intrusions are so distressing to people with OCD is because these individuals believe they reveal something about the person's true self.

> [Patients with OCD] interpreted these thoughts, impulses or images as revealing important but usually hidden elements in their character, such as: these obsessions mean that deep down I am an evil person, I am dangerous, I am unreliable, I may become totally uncontrollable… I am weird, I am going insane (and will lose control), I am a sinful person, I am fundamentally immoral. (p. 794)

Along these lines, Purdon and Clark (1999) theorize that ego-dystonic intrusions are more likely to turn into obsessions because they represent a threat to the individual's self-view. Clark (2004) argues that individuals who are uncertain in their self-concept are vulnerable to perceiving their unwanted intrusions as a "threat to core personal values and ideals" (p. 139). Likewise, Doron and Kyrios (2005) propose that perceived incompetence in highly valued self-domains informs a "sensitive" self-concept, which is easily threatened by unwanted intrusions, and thus serves as a vulnerability to the development of OCD. Similarly, Aardema and O'Connor (2007) propose that an underdeveloped self-concept leads to self-doubt, excessive self-monitoring and distrust in an individual's self-concept, and consequent absorption in imaginary possibilities of self. This makes such individuals vulnerable to noticing intrusions and promotes discordance between a person's actual self and their feared possible self. The authors suggest that the resulting distress leads to compulsive attempts to correct or safeguard the self (Aardema & O'Connor, 2007). Certainly, there are a number of cognitive accounts that credit the involvement of self-processes in OCD (Bhar & Kyrios, 2007; Doron & Kyrios, 2005; Moulding, Aardema, & O'Connor, 2014; O'Neill, 1999; Rowa, Purdon, Summerfeldt, & Antony, 2005). Guidano and Liotti's (1983) model of self-ambivalence is an early influential model that directly addresses the self in OCD and its developmental prequelae.

Guidano and Liotti's (1983) theory of self-ambivalence

Following from the work of Bowlby (1969), and drawing from psychoanalytic, attachment, cognitive, developmental, and social frameworks, Guidano and Liotti (1983) developed a theoretical model expounding the etiology of obsessionality; early ambivalent attachment experiences and a broad focus on moral perfectionism lead towards the development of an ambivalent self-concept and predisposition towards developing OCD. As explained in the following paragraphs, their theory of self-ambivalence is based upon three related features: contradictory self-views, uncertainty about self-worth, and preoccupation in verifying one's self-worth.

Guidano and Liotti (1983) postulated that during the developmental period, children begin to structure a self-image through interaction with the people closest to them. They contend that the reciprocity within the attachment relationship of self-ambivalent individuals is poor, where parental behavior toward the child is perceived to give plausible but competing interpretations by the child about their worth and loveability. For example, the parent may constantly care for and show interest in the child, but be unaffectionate and undemonstrative. This leads towards development of a self-concept based on contradictory and competing views about self-worth; such children perceive themselves to be concurrently "worthy" and "unworthy." The experience of recurrent oscillations between contradictory feelings makes it difficult for the individual to be certain about evaluations of the self.

In order to achieve clarification of their self-worth, Guidano and Liotti (1983) proposed, self-ambivalent individuals are in constant pursuit of certainty in self-worth. They vigilantly monitor their thoughts and behaviors as a meaningful measure of self, such that their "sense of personal worth is intertwined with omnipotence of thought" (Guidano, 1987, p. 178). In this way, self-ambivalent individuals are particularly predisposed to notice unwanted intrusions. Unwanted intrusions that challenge the reliability of one's self-worth arouse excessive alarm, partly due to their uncontrollable nature, but mostly because they threaten the self-ambivalent individual's rigid standards of moral perfectionism (Guidano & Liotti, 1983).

As obsessions develop from excessive attention to intrusions that threaten valued self-views, the self-ambivalent individual seeks to reinstate their self-worth. Thus, as Guidano and Liotti (1983) suggested, neutralization strategies, such as compulsions, become solutions for self-ambivalent individuals to control their mixed feelings. For instance, an individual may compulsively recite prayers in order to resolve blasphemous thoughts. Another individual may engage in compulsive checking in order to avoid feelings of personal irresponsibility. Doing so provides the individual with evidence that they are adhering to their moral values, and thus their moral self-worth is temporarily reinstated. So, rather than acknowledging their limitations, the self-ambivalent individual strives for total control, believing that there is a need to be more vigilant, to try harder; "the solution is to become more perfect, and thus even more obsessional" (Guidano, 1987, p. 186).

Guidano and Liotti's model has received renewed interest as researchers from both psychoanalytic (Kempke & Luyten, 2007) and cognitive (Bhar & Kyrios, 2007) frameworks recognize the importance of an ambivalent self in the etiology of OC phenomena. Although direct examination of the theoretical model proposed by Guidano and Liotti (1983) has received little empirical attention, the following section outlines mounting support for the self-constructs implied in their theory, and in their relationship with OCD phenomena.

Empirical support for self processes in OCD

Self-esteem

The reciprocal relationship of self-esteem to personal goals, self-beliefs, and interactions with others means that it is fundamentally related to our experience of daily life (Crocker & Park, 2004). Consequently, it is not surprising that a relationship between low self-esteem and psychopathology has been widely implicated in both the expression and development of psychological disorders (see Zeigler-Hill, 2011 for a review). In their retrospective examination into prodromal symptoms, Fava, Savron, Rafanelli, Grandi, and Canestrari (1996) found that low self-esteem was one of the common symptoms preceding the onset of OCD, suggesting that it may be a vulnerability factor for OCD. However, it is perhaps a non-specific predisposing factor because other disorders also demonstrate pre-morbid signs of low self-esteem (e.g., depression; Orth, Robins, & Meier, 2009). Furthermore, although a wealth of research shows that OCD symptoms have an association with low self-esteem, it appears that it cannot distinguish OCD from other mental disorders (Bhar & Kyrios, 2007; Ehntholt, Salkovskis, & Rimes, 1999; Teachman & Clerkin, 2007). For instance, Ehntholt et al. (1999) showed that depressive, anxious, and obsessive symptoms all had significant correlations with self-esteem.

It is likely, however, that examination of self-esteem in isolation from other variables is not specific enough to detect differences between disorders. For instance, Wu, Clark, and Watson (2006) found that the combination of low self-esteem and low entitlement was able to distinguish OCD patients from other psychiatric outpatients. Similarly, Ehntholt et al. (1999) showed that compared to anxious controls, low self-esteem of individuals in an OCD group was characterized by specific concerns about criticism from others. Although low self-esteem appears to have an association with mental distress in general, we next discuss how it is the concurrent endorsement of both positive and negative self-esteem that may have more relevance to OCD phenomena.

Self-ambivalence

According to Guidano and Liotti (1983), the self-concept in self-ambivalent individuals is structured in such a way that they concurrently endorse positive and negative self-evaluations. The resultant uncertainty in self-beliefs then leads self-ambivalent individuals to look to their environment for confirming evidence of either of their self-views, and this way they are predisposed to attending to their unwanted intrusions and vulnerable to threats to self. Along these lines, Riketta and Zeigler (2007) showed that contradictory self-beliefs and feelings (experienced ambivalence) and the co-presence of positive and negative self-views (structural ambivalence) lead to a labile self-esteem that varies according to the environmental context. In an experiment following explicit success or failure feedback, the self-esteem of unambivalent individuals remained constant. In contrast, the self-esteem of highly ambivalent individuals became more positive or negative following success or failure, respectively. Later related work using subtle priming methods showed similar results (DeMarree, Morrison, Wheeler, & Petty, 2011), suggesting that self-ambivalence can lead to interpreting both explicit and implicit self-relevant information in a way that is associated with greater negative effects on self-esteem.

Drawing from Guidano and Liotti's (1983) work, Bhar and Kyrios (2007) developed the Self-Ambivalence Measure (SAM) to assess the three features central to the theory of self-ambivalence: dichotomous self-views, uncertainty about self-worth, and preoccupation with verifying self-worth. After controlling for anxious and depressive symptoms, the

SAM significantly predicted OCD symptoms (Bhar & Kyrios, 2000, 2007), with this relationship fully mediated by OC beliefs identified as being of particular relevance to OCD (e.g., an inflated sense of personal responsibility, threat overestimation, importance and need to control thoughts, perfectionism and intolerance for uncertainty [Obsessive-Compulsive Cognitions Working Group, 1997, 2005]). Individuals with OCD also reported higher SAM scores than a non-clinical control cohort, but not an anxious group. While there was no significant difference between the clinical groups, this potentially reflected a sampling issue as the anxious group endorsed specific OC beliefs at the same levels of the OCD group. Alternatively, self-ambivalence may have greater relevance to a broader range of disorders. There is now a small but growing amount of empirical literature to demonstrate that self-ambivalence, as measured by the SAM, has been implicated in OC-related disorders such as compulsive hoarding (Frost, Kyrios, McCarthy, & Matthews, 2007), body dysmorphic disorder and social anxiety (Labuschagne, Castle, Dunai, Kyrios, & Rossell, 2010; Phillips, Moulding, Kyrios, Nedeljkovic, & Mancuso, 2011).

As the SAM total score relates to general ambivalence in self-worth, it does not capture specific notions regarding the multidimensional and contingent nature of self-worth (Harter & Whitesell, 2003; Marsh, Parada, & Ayotte, 2004), particularly relating to Guidano and Liotti's (1983) focus on compliance with moral rules. In line with their theoretical predictions and a multidimensional view of self, Bhar and Kyrios (2007) created a subscale of the SAM to assess ambivalence about morality. Like the total SAM score, the moral ambivalence subscale significantly predicted OC beliefs and symptoms and even outperformed the SAM in predicting OC beliefs of inflated self-worth. As will be discussed, the idea that morality has relevance to the self-worth of individuals with OCD is not unique to these researchers.

Self-concept

Obsessions as ego-dystonic

Some of the prominent cognitive models of OCD suggest that the very reason that obsessions are distressing is because they are ego-dystonic; contradictory to one's sense of self (Clark, 2004; Purdon & Clark, 1999; Rachman, 1997). This idea stemmed from the landmark work by Rachman and de Silva (1978), where

they demonstrated that the intrusions reported by a cohort with OCD were more alien to individuals' sense of self than the intrusions of a non-clinical sample. Subsequent empirical research further supports this notion. For instance, Clark, Purdon, and Byers (2000) showed that sexually anxious and erotophobic students reported feeling more disapproval and more distress about sexual intrusions, and a greater desire to avoid sexual intrusions, than students with a positive disposition toward sexuality. Similarly, Rowa and colleagues (Rowa & Purdon, 2003; Rowa et al., 2005) compared the most and least upsetting current obsessions in both non-clinical and clinical OCD samples and found that distress ratings were best explained by the degree to which intrusions contradicted the individual's sense of self.

Recent related work suggests that the distress associated with intrusions may not only be due to their ego-dystonic nature, but also because individuals fear these intrusions reflect an undesired facet of themselves. In their assessment of the intrusive images in an OCD and anxious control cohorts, Lipton, Brewin, Linke, and Halperin (2010) found that imagery of an OCD cohort was distinct in being more likely to contain unacceptable themes of harm, and in making inferences of the self as dangerous. Similarly, Aardema et al. (2013) created a questionnaire measuring fear of self and found that it significantly predicted obsessions and cognitions related to OCD. This measure also had strong relationships with measures of self-ambivalence and distrust of self, which the authors contend supports the notion that obsessions are distressing to those individuals with high self-doubt as they fear that the intrusion represents a possibility for who they are, or could become (Aardema & O'Connor, 2007).

Moral self in OCD

Research supports that a contingent self-worth is associated with specific attachment styles, where inconsistent feedback from parents, such as fluctuations in approval and disapproval, provide conflicting messages to the child (Crocker & Park, 2004; Harter & Whitesell, 2003). When combined with pressures to feel or behave in specific ways, often very high and unrealistic standards, the individual is vulnerable to developing an unstable sense of self-worth that is dependent on perceived competence in personally important domains.

In line with Guidano and Liotti's (1983) theory, a self-worth that is highly contingent upon moral standards may have particular relevance to OCD. Rachman

(1997) argued that those individuals who strive for moral perfectionism are more prone to obsessions as they view all of their actions and thoughts as significant markers of their moral standing. Similarly, Shafran, Thordarson, and Rachman (1996) propose that individuals with OCD have a tendency to view their unacceptable thoughts as morally equivalent to unacceptable actions, an appraisal process that has predicted thought suppression, which in turn predicted OCD symptoms on an undergraduate sample (Rassin, Muris, Schmidt, & Merckelbach, 2000). In later work comparing an OCD cohort with anxious and community controls, Ferrier and Brewin (2005) demonstrated that individuals with OCD were significantly more likely to make negative moral inferences about themselves based on their intrusions, and that their "feared self" traits were significantly more likely to consist of being bad and immoral. Additionally, in a culturally diverse non-clinical sample, García-Soriano, Clark, Belloch, del Palacio, and Castañeiras (2012) demonstrated a relationship between OCD symptoms and a measure of self-worth contingent upon meeting life domains relevant to obsessionality (including morality, responsibility, and saving/collecting). Finally, Doron, Szepsenwol, Elad-Strenger, Hargil, and Bogoslavsky (2013) showed that perceptions of morality and character as a stable and fixed trait was associated with increased severity of OC symptoms, and that this relationship was mediated by OC beliefs about the importance and control of thoughts, and inflated responsibility/overestimation of threat. The authors propose that these individuals have high desire to maintain positive self-evaluations and are vulnerable to experiences that challenge moral competence, such as unwanted intrusions.

A self-worth contingent on moral standards may not be in and of itself an etiological factor for OCD, but that concurrent uncertainty or ambivalence about morality has more relevance to the disorder. For instance, Ahern, Kyrios, and Mouding (2015) found no association between moral contingent self-worth and OCD symptoms in a non-clinical sample, but an interaction with self-ambivalence was significant, whereby individuals who were concurrently self-ambivalent and endorsed high moral standards reported the highest levels of OCD symptoms. Moreover, for individuals who were not ambivalent, there was no relationship between endorsement of OCD symptoms and adherence to morality-contingent self-worth. Related work by Doron and colleagues (Doron, Kyrios, & Moulding, 2007; Doron, Moulding, Kyrios, & Nedeljkovic, 2008)

demonstrates a relationship between OCD phenomena and sensitivity in moral self-worth. Students who had a "sensitive" moral self-concept, conceptualized as highly valuing morality yet concurrently feeling incompetent in that domain, demonstrated significantly greater levels of all OC beliefs and symptoms than students not sensitive in moral self-concept, or sensitive in other domains (e.g., sport; Doron *et al.*, 2007). A follow-up study with a clinical sample confirmed that moral self-sensitivity was related to higher severity of OCD symptoms (specifically, obsessional thoughts of harm, contamination, and checking) and OCD cognitions within the OCD cohort, while anxious and non-clinical control samples did not show sensitivity in moral self-worth (Doron *et al.*, 2008).

In addition, there is now some experimental support for the relationship between moral ambivalence and OC phenomena. In a series of experiments on nonclinical samples, Doron, Sar-El, and Mikulincer (2012) developed a subtle priming task to induce high versus low competence in the self-concept domains of either morality or sport. The authors showed that priming moral incompetence increased participants' reported urge to engage, and likelihood of engaging in, contamination-related behaviors. Moreover, in a follow-up study using similar methodology, Abramovitch (2013) demonstrated that inducing negative moral self-perceptions led to greater endorsement of the OC belief that thoughts are important and must be controlled. Finally, as an analogue to OC symptoms, Perera-Delcourt, Nash, and Thorpe (2014) examined the deliberative behavior of non-clinical individuals (length and time taken to respond to moral dilemmas) after experimental priming of either moral self-ambivalence, general uncertainty, or neither. Individuals who received the moral self-ambivalence prime and reported pre-existing high levels of moral self-ambivalence displayed significantly more deliberative behavior than the control conditions.

Overall, the theoretical and empirical studies provide mounting evidence that self-ambivalence and uncertainty about moral self-worth have a particular association with OC phenomena. However, this research is primarily based on self-report data, which are problematic because self-report measures of self-concept and self-esteem are vulnerable to response distortions and difficulty with introspection (Bosson, 2006; Dijksterhuis, Albers, & Bongers, 2009; Olson, Fazio, & Hermann, 2007). As the next section illustrates, our understanding of OCD may be enhanced through use of methodologies that capture implicit self-processes.

Implicit self and OCD

When one considers that implicit measures have demonstrated they can outperform explicit measures in predicting specific aspects of psychopathology that are involved in OCD (see Egloff & Schmukle, 2002; Spalding & Hardin, 1999; Van Bockstaele *et al.*, 2011), it is surprising that few OCD studies have included measures of implicit cognitive processes. Nonetheless, research by Nicholson and colleagues (Nicholson & Barnes-Holmes, 2012; Nicholson, Dempsey, & Barnes-Holmes, 2014; Nicholson, McCourt, & Barnes-Holmes, 2013) showed that implicit appraisals of disgust and contamination predicted self-reported OCD tendencies, OC-related beliefs and behavioral avoidance. Using an experimental design, Teachman and colleagues (Teachman, 2007; Teachman, Woody, & Magee, 2006) examined how aspects of the cognitive theory of OCD relate to implicit self. Teachman *et al.* (2006) experimentally manipulated appraisals of the importance of intrusive thoughts, giving participants either no information or informing them that their intrusions were either important or meaningless. For individuals with high convictions on OCD beliefs, information that their intrusions were important led to implicit appraisals of themselves as more dangerous than harmless. In a related study that manipulated the moral meaning of intrusions, Teachman and Clerkin (2007) showed that for individuals who had a high need for certainty, the moral condition related to implicit ratings of self as dangerous. The authors suggested that these results are in line with the cognitive model of OCD and mood-state dependent hypotheses; when under conditions that induce stress, OCD beliefs may serve as a cognitive vulnerability to negative implicit self-judgments (Teachman *et al.*, 2006).

These findings provide an initial indication of how implicit measurement tools can enhance our understanding of OCD. They do not, however, elucidate what type of pre-existing self-profile makes one vulnerable to making negative self-appraisals in the context of unwanted intrusions. Given that research into the self in OCD primarily focuses on known, or explicit, processes (Aardema & O'Connor, 2007; Bhar & Kyrios, 2007; Doron *et al.*, 2007, 2008; Ferrier & Brewin, 2005), and Guidano and Liotti's notion of contrasting and competing self-views, questions are raised as to whether self-reported ambivalent self-esteem and sensitivity in moral self-concept may involve a discrepancy between implicit and explicit self-views.

Self-discrepancy and OCD

A growing body of research supports the notion that, regardless of the direction, discordance between implicit and explicit self-esteem is associated with a variety of negative affective experiences (Lupien, Seery, & Almonte, 2010; Petty, Briñol, Tormala, Blair, & Jarvis, 2006; Rudolph, Schröder-Abé, Riketta, & Schütz, 2010; Schröder-Abé, Rudolph, & Schütz, 2007; Vater *et al.*, 2013). Briñol, Petty, and Wheeler (2006) further show that individuals with these discrepancies engage in a greater elaboration of discrepancy-related information, presumably in an effort to reduce the discrepancy. Although implicit–explicit discrepancies can take two forms (Zeigler-Hill, 2006), it is the discrepant low self-esteem (high implicit–low explicit) that may have particular relevance to OCD phenomena. Zeigler-Hill and Terry (2007) contend that high implicit self-esteem in the context of a low explicit self-esteem provides individuals with an inner optimism, and a sense that they only need to "try harder" and persevere. Unrealistically high and rigid perfectionistic standards may then be adopted in an effort to raise levels of explicit self-esteem and resolve their inconsistent self-attitudes (Guidano & Liotti, 1983). Indeed, this self-discrepancy profile show the highest levels of maladaptive perfectionism (Zeigler-Hill & Terry, 2007).

Recent research from our own research group has lent preliminary support that it is not implicit self-processes *per se* that are most closely related to OC phenomena, but their concurrent discrepancy with explicit self-esteem. Specifically, in a combined clinical OCD and non-clinical sample, discrepant low self-esteem (high implicit self-esteem, low explicit self-esteem) significantly predicted self-ambivalence, and OCD symptom scores, while implicit moral self-worth did not. When comparing non-clinical and OCD cohorts, not surprisingly, individuals with OCD held the highest levels of OCD symptoms. Of the non-clinical participants, however, individuals with this particular self-profile reported the highest level of OC symptoms (Ahern, 2013). These results add to the growing literature on the internal discomfort or conflict associated with a discrepant explicit and implicit self-esteem (Briñol *et al.*, 2006; Lupien *et al.*, 2010; Schröder-Abé *et al.*, 2007; Vater, Schröder-Abé, Schütz,

Lammers, & Roepke, 2010), and suggests that findings of low self-esteem in OCD in previous research (Fava *et al.*, 1996; Wu *et al.*, 2006) may need to be interpreted in the context of a high implicit self-esteem. Within Guidano and Liotti's (1983) model, these findings suggest that individuals with OCD have an internal conflict between explicit beliefs that they are not yet worthy or good and an inner optimism that they can or should be.

The self in the treatment of OCD

As outlined in section 2 of this book, a number of treatment approaches target the self or self-related cognitions. Even when self construals are not targeted directly or explicitly, maladaptive self constructs can be modified by psychological treatment. For instance, Bhar and colleagues have demonstrated that self-ambivalence not only resolves as a result of individual CBT for OCD, but that the extent of resolution is implicated in the extent of positive therapeutic outcome (Bhar, Kyrios, & Hordern, 2015). By further understanding the role of self-ambivalence in treatment, we might be able increase the specificity and effectiveness of therapeutic interventions for OCD.

Guidano and Liotti (1983) suggest that self-ambivalence has developed from an anxious ambivalent attachment relationship whereby as a child the individual receives contradictory messages on acceptability and rejection. Individuals with high attachment insecurity are vigilant to subtle cues about rejection by others (Foster, Kernis, & Goldman, 2007). Thus, in a clinical setting, therapists should be mindful that OCD clients might be sensitive to rejection, possibly as a result of their sense of shame. A consistent, supportive and open manner on behalf of the therapist will provide the ambivalent client with a contrast to their previous attachment experiences. An experience of validation will help the client to feel understood in a manner that mirrors one's appraisals of self. So, with a sound therapeutic alliance, the client can use the therapist as a secure base to explore alternate views of self. New ways of reflecting on the self can be openly negotiated, experienced, and internalized into the client's self-system (Moretti & Higgins, 1999).

As explicated by Clark in this book (Chapter 5), these ideas are commensurate with broad CBT approaches to OCD, which aim to help clients restructure faulty appraisals and accept more adaptive explanations for obsessions (see also Clark, 2004). However, it is also possible that more traditional CBT approaches to treating OCD (e.g., Exposure with Response Prevention, Cognitive Therapy) may benefit in being more direct in the management of self-concept for individuals with OCD (Doron & Moulding, 2009). For instance, this chapter highlights the importance of morality as a contingent domain in supporting overall self-esteem. Therapy may benefit from recognition and explanation for how this domain became an important indicator of self-worth for affected individuals (Guidano & Liotti, 1983). An understanding that their focus on morality may be an internalized form of what significant others expected of them can be a starting point to encourage the development of individuals' own standpoint (Higgins, 1987). Cognitive techniques, such as activity planning, could help to increase investment in additional domains, thereby expanding the limited self contingencies of those with OCD and broadening opportunities to develop self-worth. The rigid boundaries of maladaptive beliefs of being moral and personally responsible or perfectionistic may be modified by challenging clients about the personal meaning and origins of these constructs, and by inviting them to consider other behaviors and attitudes that could be included in this domain.

If intrusions can represent unwanted aspects of self, then clients may benefit from understanding that their symptoms derive from a feared self that is not based on reality, but due to their conflicting internal feelings. Collaboration with the client on their positive qualities and asking them to record thought diaries of positive self-related thoughts may enable the client to develop a more balanced self-view. Alternatively, discussing the impact of discrepancies between perceived–ideal or implicit–explicit self construals can lead to the more direct processing of information that closes the dissonance. When combined with behavioral experiments that test the exaggerated importance of beliefs of unworthiness (e.g., the client could confide in a friend about an action or thought that they perceived as evidence of their "unworthiness," thereby provoking an opportunity for feared consequences to come about), or that helps to confirm new adaptive beliefs (e.g., asking the client to behave as a "worthy person" and note any differences to previous behavior), the client can learn to pay less attention to feelings of self-worth but give more credence to objective measures of worth (e.g., roles in their life), thereby allowing clients to discover alternative perceptions of themselves. Such a strategy would have a direct impact on resolving the dissonance and, hence, resolving self-ambivalence. Finally, clients can be helped to see that they can live a life that is consistent with their values but using a more flexible framework rather than the rigid and highly perfectionistic or intolerant patterns in which they have been engaging. Such techniques are consistent with narrative, as well as CBT, psychodynamic, schema-based, and ACT-based strategies as outlined in Section 2 of this volume.

Conclusion

This chapter outlines the theoretical and empirical context for understanding how self-processes are implicated in OCD, whereby Guidano and Liotti's (1983) theory of self-ambivalence is considered a useful framework for incorporating the possible developmental origins of the disorder. These authors contend that OCD is characterized by ambivalent attachments derived from parenting styles experienced as rejecting but camouflaged under an outward mask of absolute devotion. This can lead to the development of dichotomous self-views, and because these views are not securely attained they can fluctuate, subsequently leading to self-uncertainty and a preoccupation with verifying self-standing. Ultimately, the individual becomes overattentive to their thoughts, becoming liable to notice and feel threatened by unwanted intrusions. In order to protect a valued self-view, individuals develop rigid beliefs in morality and perform compulsions in an effort to assert that they are indeed inherently worthy. Empirical evidence for a relationship between OC phenomena and self-processes were reviewed. An ambivalent self-worth, particularly one contingent on meeting high moral standards, was proposed to have particular relevance to OCD. Although the majority of OCD research supporting such notions has focused on explicit self-views, this chapter outlines the new but growing field of implicit processes in OCD and suggests that a discrepancy between implicit and explicit self-processes, specifically a discrepant low self-esteem, may also have relevance to OC phenomena. This chapter then outlines how this literature may enhance our understanding of the phenomenology of OCD, and the possible etiological origins and maintenance of this disorder, and in turn translate into useful treatment approaches.

References

Aardema, F., Moulding, R., Radomsky, A. S., *et al.* (2013). Fear of self and obsessionality: Development and validation of the Fear of Self Questionnaire. *Journal of Obsessive–Compulsive and Related Disorders*, 2(3), 306–315. doi: 10.1016/j.jocrd.2013.05.005

Aardema, F., & O'Connor, K. (2007). The menace within: Obsessions and the self. *Journal of Cognitive Psychotherapy*, 21, 182–197. doi: 10.1891/088983907781494573

Abramovitch, A. , Doron, G., Sar-El, D., & Altenburger, E.(2013). Subtle threats to moral self-perceptions trigger obsessive–compulsive related cognitions. *Cognitive Therapy & Research*, 37(6), 1132–1139. doi: 10.1007/s10608-013-9568-6

Ahern, C. (2013). *The role of self-construals in obsessive–compulsive disorder*. Unpublished PhD Dissertation. Swinburne University of Technology.

Ahern, C., Kyrios, M., & Mouding, R. (2015). Self-based concepts and obsessive-compulsive phenomena. *Psychopathology*.

American Psychiatric Association [APA]. (2013). *Diagnostic and Statistical Manual of Mental Disorders* (5th ed.). Arlington, VA: American Psychiatric Publishing.

Bhar, S., & Kyrios, M. (2000). Ambivalent self-esteem as meta-vulnerability for obsessive–compulsive disorder. In R. G. Craven & H. W. Marsh (Eds.), *Self-Concept Theory, Research and Practice: Advances from the New Millennium*, Proceedings of the Inaugural International Conference, University of Western Sydney, Sydney, Australia, October 5–6, 2000 (pp. 143–156) Parramatta, NSW: SELF Research Centre, University of Western Sydney.

Bhar, S., & Kyrios, M. (2007). An investigation of self-ambivalence in obsessive–compulsive disorder. *Behaviour Research and Therapy*, 45(8), 1845–1857. doi: 10.1016/j.brat.2007.02.005

Bhar, S., Kyrios, M., & Hordern, C. (2015). Self-ambivalence in the cognitive-behavioral treatment of obsessive–compulsive disorder. *Psychopathology*.

Bosson, J. K. (2006). Conceptualization, measurement, and functioning of nonconscious self-esteem. In M. Kernis (Ed.), *Self-esteem Issues and Answers: A Sourcebook of Current Perspectives* (pp. 53–59). London: Psychology Press.

Bowlby, J. (1969). *Attachment* (Vol. 1). New York, NY: Basic Books.

Briñol, P., Petty, R. E., & Wheeler, S. C. (2006). Discrepancies between explicit and implicit self-concepts: Consequences for information processing. *Journal of Personality and Social Psychology*, 91, 154–170. doi: 10.1037/0022-3514.91.1.154

Clark, D. A. (2004). *Cognitive-Behavioural Therapy for OCD*. New York, NY: Guilford Press.

Clark, D. A., Purdon, C., & Byers, E. S. (2000). Appraisal and control of sexual and non-sexual intrusive thoughts in university students. *Behaviour Research and Therapy*, 38(5), 439–455.

Clark, D. A., & Rhyno, S. (2004). Unwanted intrusive thoughts in nonclinical individuals: Implications for clinical disorders. In D. A. Clark (Ed.), *Intrusive Thoughts in Clinical Disorders: Theory, Research, and Treatment*. New York, NY: Guilford Publications.

Crocker, J., & Park, L. E. (2004). The costly pursuit of self-esteem. *Psychology Bulletin*, 130(3), 392–414. doi: 10.1037/0033-2909.130.3.392

DeMarree, K. G., Morrison, K. R., Wheeler, S. C., & Petty, R. E. (2011). Self-ambivalence and resistance to subtle self-change attempts. *Personality and Social Psychology Bulletin*, 37(5), 674–686. doi: 10.1177/0146167211400097

Dijksterhuis, A., Albers, L. W., & Bongers, K. (2009). Digging for the real attitude: Lessons from research on implicit and explicit self-esteem. In R. Petty, R. Fazio, & P. Brinol (Eds.), *Attitudes: Insights from the New Wave of Implicit Measures* (pp. 229–250). New York, NY: Psychology Press.

Doron, G., & Kyrios, M. (2005). Obsessive compulsive disorder: A review of possible specific internal representations within a broader cognitive theory. *Clinical Psychology Review*, 25(4), 415–432. doi: 10.1016/j.cpr.2005.02.002

Doron, G., Kyrios, M., & Moulding, R. (2007). Sensitive domains of self-concept in obsessive–compulsive disorder (OCD): Further evidence for a multidimensional model of OCD. *Journal of Anxiety Disorders*, 21(3), 433–444. doi: 10.1016/j.janxdis.2006.05.008

Doron, G., & Moulding, R. (2009). Cognitive behavioral treatment of obsessive compulsive disorder: A broader framework. *The Israel Journal of Psychiatry and Related Sciences*, 46(4), 257–263.

Doron, G., Moulding, R., Kyrios, M., & Nedeljkovic, M. (2008). Sensitivity of self-beliefs in obsessive compulsive disorder. *Depression and Anxiety*, 25(10), 874–884. doi: 10.1002/da.20369

Doron, G., Sar-El, D., & Mikulincer, M. (2012). Threats to moral self-perceptions trigger obsessive compulsive contamination-related behavioral tendencies. *Journal of Behavior Therapy and Experimental Psychiatry*, 43(3), 884–890.

Doron, G., Szepsenwol, O., Elad-Strenger, J., Hargil, E., & Bogoslavsky, B. (2013). Entity perceptions of morality and character are associated with obsessive compulsive phenomena. *Journal of Social and Clinical Psychology*, 32(7), 733–752. doi: 10.1521/jscp.2013.32.7.733

Egloff, B., & Schmukle, S. C. (2002). Predictive validity of an Implicit Association Test for assessing anxiety. *Journal of Personality and Social Psychology*, 83(6), 1441–1455.

Ehntholt, K. A., Salkovskis, P. M., & Rimes, K. A. (1999). Obsessive–compulsive disorder, anxiety disorders, and self-esteem: An exploratory study. *Behaviour Research and Therapy*, 37(8), 771–781.

Fava, G. A., Savron, G., Rafanelli, C., Grandi, S., & Canestrari, R. (1996). Prodromal symptoms in obsessive–compulsive disorder. *Psychopathology*, 29(2), 131–134.

Ferrier, S., & Brewin, C. R. (2005). Feared identity and obsessive–compulsive disorder. *Behaviour Research and Therapy*, 43(10), 1363–1374. doi: 10.1016/j.brat.2004.10.005

Foa, E. B., Kozak, M. J., Goodman, W. K., *et al.* (1995). DSM-IV field trial: Obsessive–compulsive disorder. *American Journal of Psychiatry*, 152(1), 90–96. doi: 10.1176/ajp.152.1.90

Foster, J. D., Kernis, M. H., & Goldman, B. M. (2007). Linking adult attachment to self-esteem stability. *Self and Identity*, 6(1), 64–73. doi: 10.1080/15298860600832139

Frost, R. O., Kyrios, M., McCarthy, K. D., & Matthews, Y. (2007). Self-ambivalence and attachment to possessions. *Journal of Cognitive Psychotherapy*, 21(3), 232–242. doi: 10.1891/088983907781494582

García-Soriano, G., Clark, D. A., Belloch, A., del Palacio, A., & Castañeiras, C. (2012). Self-worth contingencies and obsessionality: A promising approach to vulnerability? *Journal of Obsessive–Compulsive and Related Disorders*, 1(3), 196–202. doi: http://dx.doi.org/10.1016/j.jocrd.2012.05.003

Guidano, V., & Liotti, G. (1983). *Cognitive Processes and Emotional Disorders*. New York, NY: Guilford Press.

Harter, S., & Whitesell, N. R. (2003). Beyond the debate: Why some adolescents report stable self-worth over time and situation, whereas others report changes in self-worth. *Journal of Personality*, 71(6), 1027–1058.

Higgins, E. T. (1987). Self-discrepancy: A theory relating self and affect. *Psychology Review*, 94(3), 319–340. doi: 10.1037/0033-295X.94.3.319

Kempke, S., & Luyten, P. (2007). Psychodynamic and cognitive-behavioral approaches of obsessive–compulsive disorder: Is it time to work through our ambivalence? *Bulletin of the Menninger Clinic*, 71(4), 291–311.

Labuschagne, I., Castle, D. J., Dunai, J., Kyrios, M., & Rossell, S. L. (2010). An examination of delusional thinking and cognitive styles in body dysmorphic disorder. *Australian and New Zealand Journal of Psychiatry*, 44(8), 706–712. doi: 10.3109/00048671003671007

Lipton, M. G., Brewin, C. R., Linke, S., & Halperin, J. (2010). Distinguishing features of intrusive images in obsessive–compulsive disorder. *Journal of*

Anxiety Disorders, 24(8), 816–822. doi: 10.1016/j.janxdis.2010.06.003

Lupien, S. P., Seery, M. D., & Almonte, J. L. (2010). Discrepant and congruent high self-esteem: Behavioral self-handicapping as a preemptive defensive strategy. *Journal of Experimental Social Psychology*, 46(6), 1105–1108. doi: 10.1016/j.jesp.2010.05.022

Marsh, H. W., Parada, R. H., & Ayotte, V. (2004). A multidimensional perspective of relations between self-concept (Self Description Questionnaire II) and adolescent mental health (Youth Self-Report). *Psychological Assessment*, 16(1), 27–41. doi: 10.1037/1040-3590.16.1.27

McKay, D., Abramowitz, J. S., Calamari, J. E., *et al.* (2004). A critical evaluation of obsessive-compulsive disorder subtypes: Symptoms versus mechanisms. *Clinical Psychology Review*, 24(3), 283–313. doi: 10.1016/j.cpr.2004.04.003

Moretti, M. M., & Higgins, E. T. (1999). Internal representations of others in self-regulation: A new look at a classic issue. *Social Cognition*, 17(2), 186–208.

Moulding, R., Aardema, F., & O'Connor, K. P. (2014). Repugnant obsessions: A review of the phenomenology, theoretical models, and treatment of sexual and aggressive obsessional themes in OCD. *Journal of Obsessive–Compulsive and Related Disorders*, 3(2), 161–168. doi: 10.1016/j.jocrd.2013.11.006

Nicholson, E., & Barnes-Holmes, D. (2012). Developing an implicit measure of disgust propensity and disgust sensitivity: Examining the role of implicit disgust propensity and sensitivity in obsessive–compulsive tendencies. *Journal of Behavior Therapy and Experimental Psychiatry*, 43, 922–930. doi: 10.1016/j.jbtep.2012.02.001

Nicholson, E., Dempsey, K., & Barnes-Holmes, D. (2014). The role of responsibility and threat appraisals in contamination fear and obsessive–compulsive tendencies at the implicit level. *Journal of Contextual Behavioral Science*, 3(1), 31–37. doi: 10.1016/j.jcbs.2013.11.001

Nicholson, E., McCourt, A., & Barnes-Holmes, D. (2013). The Implicit Relational Assessment Procedure (IRAP) as a measure of obsessive beliefs in relation to disgust. *Journal of Contextual Behavioral Science*, 2(1–2), 23–30. doi: 10.1016/j.jcbs.2013.02.002

Obsessive–Compulsive Cognitions Working Group. (1997). Cognitive assessment of Obsessive-Compulsive Disorder, *Behaviour Research & Therapy*, 35, 667–681.

Obsessive–Compulsive Cognitions Working Group. (2005) Psychometric validation of the obsessive belief questionnaire and interpretation of intrusions inventory: Part 2, factor analyses and testing of a brief version. *Behaviour Research & Therapy*, 43, 1527–1542.

Olson, M. A., Fazio, R. H., & Hermann, A. D. (2007). Reporting tendencies underlie discrepancies between implicit and explicit measures of self-esteem. *Psychological Science*, 18(4), 287–291. doi:10.1111/j.1467-9280.2007.01890.x

O'Neill, S. A. (1999). Living with obsessive–compulsive disorder: A case study of a woman's construction of self. *Counselling Psychology Quarterly*, 12(1), 73.

Orth, U., Robins, R. W., & Meier, L. L. (2009). Disentangling the effects of low self-esteem and stressful events on depression: Findings from three longitudinal studies. *Journal of Personality and Social Psychology*, 97(2), 307–321. doi: 10.1037/a0015645

Perera-Delcourt, R., Nash, R. A., & Thorpe, S. J. (2014). Priming moral self-ambivalence heightens deliberative behaviour in self-ambivalent individuals. *Behaviour and Cognitive Psychotherapy*, 42(6), 682–692. doi: 10.1017/S1352465813000507

Petty, R. E., Briñol, P., Tormala, Z. L., Blair, W., & Jarvis, G. (2006). Implicit ambivalence from attitude change: An exploration of the PAST model. *Journal of Personality and Social Psychology*, 90(1), 21–41. doi: 10.1037/0022-3514.90.1.21

Phillips, B., Moulding, R., Kyrios, M., Nedeljkovic, M., & Mancuso, S. (2011). The relationship between body dysmorphic disorder symptoms and self-construals. *Clinical Psychologist*, 15(1), 10–16. doi: 10.1111/j.1742-9552.2011.00004.x

Purdon, C., & Clark, D. A. (1999). Metacognition and obsessions. *Clinical Psychology and Psychotherapy*, 6(2), 102–110.

Rachman, S. (1997). A cognitive theory of obsessions. *Behaviour Research and Therapy*, 35(9), 793–802. doi: 10.1016/S0005-7967(97)00040-5

Rachman, S., & de Silva, P. (1978). Abnormal and normal obsessions. *Behaviour Research and Therapy*, 16(4), 233–248. doi: 10.1016/0005-7967(78)90022-0

Rasmussen, S. A., & Eisen, J. L. (1994). The epidemiology and differential diagnosis of obsessive compulsive disorder. *Journal of Clinical Psychiatry*, 55(Suppl.), 5–10; discussion 11–14.

Rasmussen, S. A., & Tsuang, M. T. (1986). Clinical characteristics and family history in DSM-III obsessive–compulsive disorder. *American Journal of Psychiatry*, 143(3), 317–322.

Rassin, E., Muris, P., Schmidt, H., & Merckelbach, H. (2000). Relationships between thought–action fusion, thought suppression and obsessive–compulsive symptoms: A structural equation modeling approach. *Behaviour Research and Therapy*, 38(9), 889–897.

Riketta, M., & Ziegler, R. (2007). Self-ambivalence and reactions to success versus failure. *European Journal of Social Psychology*, 37(3), 547–560. doi: 10.1002/ejsp.376

Rowa, K., & Purdon, C. (2003). Why are certain intrusive thoughts more upsetting than others? *Behavioural and Cognitive Psychotherapy*, 31(1), 1–11. doi: 10.1017/S1352465803001024

Rowa, K., Purdon, C., Summerfeldt, L. J., & Antony, M. M. (2005). Why are some obsessions more upsetting than others? *Behaviour Research and Therapy*, 43(11), 1453–1465. doi: 10.1016/j.brat.2004.11.003

Rudolph, A., Schröder-Abé, M., Riketta, M., & Schütz, A. (2010). Easier when done than said! Implicit self-esteem predicts observed or spontaneous behavior, but not self-reported or controlled behavior. *Journal of Psychology*, 218(1), 12–19. doi: 10.1027/0044-3409/a000003

Salkovskis, P. (1989). Cognitive-behavioural factors and the persistence of intrusive thoughts in obsessional problems. *Behaviour Research and Therapy*, 27(6), 677–682; discussion 683–674.

Salkovskis, P., Thorpe, S. J., Wahl, K., Wroe, A. L., & Forrester, E. (2003). Neutralizing increases discomfort associated with obsessional thoughts: An experimental study with obsessional patients. *Journal of Abnormal Psychology*, 112(4), 709–715. doi: 10.1037/0021-843x.112.3.709

Salkovskis, P., Westbrook, D., Davis, J., Jeavons, A., & Gledhill, A. (1997). Effects of neutralizing on intrusive thoughts: An experiment investigating the etiology of obsessive–compulsive disorder. *Behaviour Research and Therapy*, 35(3), 211–219. doi: 10.1016/s0005-7967(96)00112-x

Schröder-Abé, M., Rudolph, A., & Schütz, A. (2007). High implicit self-esteem is not necessarily advantageous: Discrepancies between explicit and implicit self-esteem and their relationship with anger expression and psychological health. *European Journal of Personality*, 21(3), 319–339. doi: 10.1002/per.626

Shafran, R., Thordarson, D. S., & Rachman, S. (1996). Thought–action fusion in obsessive compulsive disorder. *Journal of Anxiety Disorders*, 10(5), 379–391.

Spalding, L. R., & Hardin, C. D. (1999). Unconscious unease and self-handicapping: Behavioral consequences of individual differences in implicit and explicit self-esteem. *Psychological Science*, 10(6), 535–539.

Teachman, B. A. (2007). Linking obsessional beliefs to OCD symptoms in older and younger adults. *Behaviour Research and Therapy*, 45(7), 1671–1681. doi: 10.1016/j.brat.2006.08.016

Teachman, B. A., & Clerkin, E. M. (2007). Obsessional beliefs and the implicit and explicit morality of intrusive thoughts. *Cognition and Emotion*, 21(5), 999–1024. doi: 10.1080/02699930600985576

Teachman, B. A., Woody, S. R., & Magee, J. C. (2006). Implicit and explicit appraisals of the importance of intrusive thoughts. *Behaviour Research and Therapy*, 44(6), 785–805. doi: 10.1016/j.brat.2005.05.005

Van Bockstaele, B., Verschuere, B., Koster, E. H. W., *et al.* (2011). Differential predictive power of self report and implicit measures on behavioural and physiological fear responses to spiders. *International Journal of Psychophysiology*, 79(2), 166–174. doi: 10.1016/j.ijpsycho.2010.10.003

Vater, A., Ritter, K., Schröder-Abé, M., *et al.* (2013). When grandiosity and vulnerability collide: Implicit and explicit self-esteem in patients with narcissistic personality disorder. *Journal of Behavior Therapy and Experimental Psychiatry*, 44(1), 37–47. doi: 10.1016/j.jbtep.2012.07.001

Vater, A., Schröder-Abé, M., Schütz, A., Lammers, C. H., & Roepke, S. (2010). Discrepancies between explicit and implicit self-esteem are linked to symptom severity in borderline personality disorder. *Journal of Behavior Therapy and Experimental Psychiatry*, 41(4), 357–364. doi: 10.1016/j.jbtep.2010.03.007

World Health Organization. (2015). Obsessive–Compulsive Disorder. In *International Statistical Classification of Diseases and Related Health Problems* (10th ed.). http://apps.who.int/classifications/icd10/browse/2015/en#ssssss/F42.0

Wu, K. D., Clark, L. A., & Watson, D. (2006). Relations between Obsessive–Compulsive Disorder and personality: Beyond Axis I–Axis II comorbidity. *Journal of Anxiety Disorders*, 20(6), 695–717. doi: 10.1016/j.janxdis.2005.11.001

Zeigler-Hill, V. (2006). Discrepancies between implicit and explicit self-esteem: Implications for narcissism and self-esteem instability. *Journal of Personality*, 74(1), 119–144. doi: 10.1111/j.1467-6494.2005.00371.x

Zeigler-Hill, V. (2011). The connections between self-esteem and psychopathology. *Journal of Contemporary Psychotherapy*, 41(3), 157–164. doi: 10.1007/s10879-010-9167-8

Zeigler-Hill, V., & Terry, C. (2007). Perfectionism and explicit self-esteem: The moderating role of implicit self-esteem. *Self and Identity*, 6(3–4), 137–153. doi: 10.1080/15298860601118850

Chapter

13

The self in the obsessive–compulsive-related disorders: hoarding disorder, body dysmorphic disorder, and trichotillomania

Richard Moulding, Serafino G. Mancuso, Imogen Rehm, and Maja Nedeljkovic

The most recent DSM saw a reclassification of obsessive–compulsive disorder (OCD) as the prototypical disorder within a separate grouping that also includes hoarding disorder, body dysmorphic disorder (BDD), trichotillomania (TTM; hair pulling disorder), and skin-picking disorder (American Psychiatric Association [APA], 2013). This followed a long-standing debate over whether there is a spectrum of disorders sharing etiological underpinnings or phenomenology with OCD (Abramowitz, McKay, & Taylor, 2011; Moulding, Nedeljkovic, & Kyrios, 2011). While much research has highlighted the role of self in the symptomatology and treatment of OCD *per se* (see Ahern & Kyrios, Chapter 12 in this volume; Aardema *et al.*, 2013; Bhar & Kyrios, 2007; Doron, Moulding, Kyrios, & Nedeljkovic, 2008; Moulding, Aardema, & O'Connor, 2014), less has considered the role of self in the OCD spectrum. This chapter aims to address this gap – specifically with reference to hoarding disorder, BDD, and TTM.

Hoarding disorder

In hoarding disorder, the individual accumulates a large amount of possessions due to psychological difficulty in discarding them, regardless of the value that others apply to these possessions (APA, 2013). Individuals typically hoard the same kinds of items as are collected by individuals without hoarding, albeit more of them, but they also often collect idiosyncratic items that they find of particular interest or importance (Mogan, Kyrios, Schweitzer, Yap, & Moulding, 2012). Concepts related to self-concept often saturate therapeutic

conversations with individuals who hoard – it has been suggested that this reflects a "fusion" between identity and possessions, which itself is a normative process. For example, Steketee and Frost (2010) note that people seem to value possessions more if they are connected to a celebrity (e.g., Jerry Seinfeld's pirate shirt), as if the laws of sympathetic contagion apply to objects and identity (i.e., where objects become similar through touching each other). Such notions are not new – in 1890 William James stated that "… it is clear that between what a man calls me and what he simply calls mine the line is difficult to draw … a man's Self is the sum-total of all that he can call his …" (p. 291). Belk (1988) discusses such notions in terms of the "extended self," whereby objects partially form part of, and determine, one's identity. Belk suggests that the extended self comprises not just the body and internal processes, but also the person's ideas and experiences, and the persons, places, and things to which they feel attached; albeit that the self also is hierarchically composed such that some possessions are more central to self.

Steketee and Frost (2010) suggest that the same issues apply to hoarding, as when discussing their client "Irene," whose possessions "… connected her to something bigger than herself. They gave her an expanded identity, a more meaningful life. It wasn't the objects themselves that she valued, but the connections they symbolised" (p. 45). The efforts of individuals with hoarding to "rehouse" their possessions to a good (and known) home, and acquiring objects to give to others, can be seen as an extension of this idea. Belk (1988) discusses Sartre's notion that such gift-giving is part of the process of self-expansion – "A gift continues to be

The Self in Understanding and Treating Psychological Disorders, ed. Michael Kyrios, Richard Moulding, Guy Doron, Sunil S. Bhar, Maja Nedeljkovic, and Mario Mikulincer. Published by Cambridge University Press. © Cambridge University Press, 2016.

associated with the giver so that the giver's identity is extended to include the recipient" (p. 151). This dovetails with our own observations of individuals with hoarding who keep relationships alive (in a symbolic sense) through buying gifts for friends and relatives; while sometimes these are active relationships, at other times these relationships are estranged or fractured and the individual may not have seen the potential recipient for many years.

This emotional attachment to objects, as an extension of self and social identity, is a key cognition within Steketee and Frost's influential hoarding model (Kyrios, 2014; Steketee & Frost, 2007; Steketee, Frost, & Kyrios, 2003). Endorsement of items comprising this subscale in Steketee et al.'s Savings Cognitions Inventory, such as "Throwing away this possession is like throwing away a part of me," and "Losing this possession is like losing a friend" relate to higher hoarding symptoms in both non-clinical and clinical samples (Kyrios, Mogan, Moulding, Frost, & Yap, in preparation; Steketee et al., 2003). Similarly, through a qualitative study, Kellett, Greenhalgh, Beail, and Ridgway (2010) identified individuals' relationships with hoarded items as a key theme – with emotional relationships characterized by anthropomorphizing of objects and a sense of object–person fusion. For example, one participant reported acquiring an object because "I think that that thing will be really lonely left on the shelf" (p. 146), while another reported that "The person that has all this stuff, it's theirs, it's a part of them, even ridiculous year old newspapers" (p. 146). Non-clinical studies have related the tendency to anthropomorphize to hoarding behaviors (Neave, Jackson, Saxton, & Hönekopp, 2015; Timpano & Shaw, 2013). Anthorpomorphizing (at least with regard to non-human agents) has generally been linked to an unfulfilled desire for human connection (Epley, Waytz, & Cacioppo, 2007), which may be a factor in some individuals who hoard who have disrupted family or social relationships or a traumatic social history.

Such "self"-involvement in stuff is likely exacerbated by other beliefs in individuals who hoard. Perceived or real deficits in memory are common in hoarding, along with a need to have possessions "in view," and character traits of extreme perfectionism (Steketee & Frost, 2003, 2007). Such factors are likely to contribute to the need in hoarding to maintain objects as "reminders" or diaries of experience (indeed, individuals often seem to "hoard" their experiences in the same way as their objects). If the objects are part of the

extended self as suggested by Belk (1988), then they also help maintain one's identity over time, which is perceived as necessary if one doubts one's memory. At the other extreme, clinical experience suggests that to individuals who hoard, objects also seem to represent possible future selves – whom one might become, what one might do, opportunities one has. Therapeutic discussions commonly include letting possible selves go, or even "die," when discarding the related items (e.g., to let go of crochet needles is to let go of the improved future self that has learnt to crochet).

However, such a discussion prompts the question as to why individuals feel such an excessive need to focus on their extended self as manifested through objects. Unfortunately, few studies have directly examined self-concept in hoarding as an underlying dimension. Building on work in OCD, Frost, Kyrios, McCarthy, and Matthews (2007) suggested that there may be an underlying difficulty with self-concept in hoarding, in the form of an ambivalent self-concept characterized by a preoccupation with a dichotomous and reactive self (i.e., self as both good and bad). Related work on compulsive buying (which is distinguished by the lack of value given to possessions once acquired) has drawn on the idea of material possessions substituting for an underlying negative self-view (Dittmar, 2005; Kyrios, Frost, & Steketee, 2004). Alternatively, when considering that individuals with hoarding also often use terms such as "building a cocoon," "nesting," and "building a wall" (see Steketee & Frost, 2010), there is the idea that to these individuals, their "stuff" represents safety or a "secure base" (see attachment theory; Bowlby, 1988; Mikulincer and Doron, Chapter 3 in this volume). Such ideas regarding objects imply a self-concept characterized by vulnerability associated with insecure attachment relationships (see Mikulincer & Doron, this volume) and perceptions of the world as a dangerous place (this is also consistent with high levels of comorbid generalized anxiety disorder in hoarding; e.g., Moulding, Nedeljkovic, Kyrios, Osbourne, & Mogan, in preparation). Steketee and Frost (2010) reported that after a stressful day, "Irene" spoke of wanting to go home in order to "gather my treasures around me." This notion is not surprising, given the background of trauma that is highly prominent in many – but not all – individuals with hoarding (Cromer, Schmidt, & Murphy, 2007; Hartl, Duffany, Allen, Steketee, & Frost, 2005). In their qualitative study, Kellett et al. (2010) similarly report childhood factors as a key theme, for example, "Well as a kid I had a cupboard full of toys and that was where I retreated from the hostile world …" (p. 145). More generally, a study linking anxious attachment with materialism was taken to suggest that relationships with objects can sometimes serve as a substitute for relationships with people when the individual finds it hard to form such relationships (Norris, Lambert, DeWall, & Fincham, 2012). These speculations suggest that further research on the function of the wider attachment construct in hoarding may be useful (cf. Kellett et al., 2010; Kellett & Holden, 2013).

Finally, and somewhat orthogonally, notions of self-regulation are also prominent in hoarding. Individuals with hoarding commonly experience comorbid attention deficit hyperactivity disorder, implying difficulties with goal-setting that are reflected in their problems in organization and carrying through with discarding tasks (cf. Lynch, McGillivray, Moulding, & Byrne, 2015). Examining this notion, Timpano and Schmidt (2013) found that (a) questionnaire-based self-control deficits were associated with hoarding symptoms in a non-clinical sample; (b) such deficits were similarly pronounced in hoarding vs. samples with OCD, GAD or SAD; and (c) that experimental tasks in non-clinical participants designed to deplete self-regulation resources resulted in fewer objects discarded. Conversely, individuals with hoarding often acquire impulsively, although such deficits seem particularly pronounced when the individual is experiencing emotions, particularly negative emotions. Hoarding tendencies are strongly linked to anxiety sensitivity and poor distress tolerance (Coles, Frost, Heimberg, & Steketee, 2003; Timpano, Buckner, Richey, Murphy, & Schmidt, 2009; Timpano, Shaw, Cougle, & Fitch, 2014). Hoarding (Phung, Moulding, Taylor, & Nedeljkovic, 2015; Timpano et al., 2013) and compulsive buying tendencies (Alemis & Yap, 2013) have been linked to negative urgency – impulsivity as a way of avoiding or reducing negative emotions.

Turning to treatment implications, the dominant treatment for hoarding is derived from the cognitive-behavioral model of Steketee and Frost (2007; Tolin, Frost, & Steketee, 2007), with the limited available evidence suggesting it is effective (Tolin, Frost, Steketee, & Muroff, 2015). Components of this approach could be conceptualized as influencing self-concept, in particular, the restructuring of beliefs such that items are implicitly or explicitly viewed as things external to the self; this potential is hardly surprising, given the acknowledgment given by Steketee and Frost to self-concept (e.g., Steketee & Frost, 2010).

For example, it is suggested to clients that *making* art is the defining characteristic of an artist, rather than *owning* art resources.

However, consideration of self-themes may open therapy up to a broader consideration of "how to define self," to the use of exercises such as activity scheduling, and to values-exercises emphasized within acceptance and commitment therapy (e.g., Zettle, Chapter 6, this volume). Equally, being aware of the "self" implied by items makes the therapist more mindful of the potential difficulties in discarding. After CBT strategies have been introduced, there may be a need for more specific work on self-concept. Given the normalcy of self-concept expanding to comprise one's "stuff," it could be said that an issue with hoarding clients is not that they extend the self to include possessions, but the *extent* to which they do so, the lack of recognition of hierarchies of importance of objects, and the extent to which objects are privileged over other parts of the extended self. Finally, we and others have noted the particular value of group-based work, which seem particularly useful in alleviating the common sense of shame in hoarding (itself reflected in the way individuals with hoarding often "hide" their hoards or refuse visitors) – that the very act of hoarding itself makes one defective – which could work in a vicious cycle if the hoarding is acting partially to alleviate an initial underlying negative self-concept (Moulding et al., submitted; Schmalisch, Bratiotis, & Muroff, 2010).

Body dysmorphic disorder

BDD is characterized by a preoccupation with one or more perceived defects in physical appearance that are not observable or appear slight to others (APA, 2013). The importance of physical appearance is considered an idealized value in BDD – individuals with BDD typically equate their self-worth or sense of self almost exclusively in terms of their physical appearance (Didie, Kuniega-Pietrzak, & Phillips, 2010; Hrabosky et al., 2009; Phillips, Moulding, Kyrios, Nedeljkovic, & Mancuso, 2011; Veale, 2002a). This overvalued ideation, however, reinforces the processing of the self as an aesthetic object (Neziroglu, Khemlani-Patel, & Veale, 2008; Veale, 2004).

The self as an aesthetic object is key to Veale's cognitive-behavioral model of BDD (Neziroglu et al., 2008; Veale, 2001, 2004; Veale & Neziroglu, 2010). An impression of the self is constructed by an individual with BDD using somatic sensations, thoughts, and feelings about their physical appearance. This impression is usually experienced as visual, negative, recurrent, and viewed from the perspective of an observer (Osman, Cooper, Hackmann, & Veale, 2004). In the absence of a discrete visual image, the individual may instead experience a "felt impression" of the constructed self as a combination of physical sensations, verbal thoughts, and feelings of shame or anxiety (Neziroglu et al., 2008; Veale, 2004). However, this mental image or "felt impression" is distorted and inaccurate (Cooper & Osman, 2007; Veale, 2004).

Due to excessive self-focused attention in non-social situations, the "felt impression" is compared to an internalized appearance ideal (Neziroglu et al., 2008), but there is a marked discrepancy between the two (Veale, Kinderman, Riley, & Lambrou, 2003; Veale & Riley, 2001). As a result, individuals with BDD may experience increased self-consciousness, negative self-judgments about their appearance, and negative emotions including distress, anxiety, internal shame, and depression (Cooper & Osman, 2007; Neziroglu et al., 2008; Osman et al., 2004; Veale, 2002b, 2004; Veale et al., 2003). Distraction, checking behaviors, camouflaging, avoidance, and reassurance-seeking behaviors may then be performed in an attempt to alleviate these emotions (Cooper & Osman, 2007; Neziroglu et al., 2008).

An individual with BDD may also use the "felt impression" to check how they appear or compare to others during social situations (Neziroglu et al., 2008). This self-focused attention has two main consequences. First, feelings of external shame are triggered when the individual rates their appearance as more unattractive than others (Veale, 2002b). Second, attention to the environment is reduced so that an individual is unable to disconfirm fears of negative evaluation (Neziroglu et al., 2008; Veale & Neziroglu, 2010), which may in turn elicit feelings of external shame (Veale, 2002b).

In addition to self-focused attention, self as an aesthetic object contributes to the lack of a self-serving bias in relation to self-judgments of attractiveness (Neziroglu et al., 2008; Veale & Neziroglu, 2010). Individuals with BDD, for example, rate their own facial attractiveness as significantly lower than do independent evaluators (Buhlmann, Etcoff, & Wilhelm, 2008). Veale and Neziroglu (2010) suggest that selective attention to disliked appearance features produces more accurate self-evaluations of such features in persons with BDD. However, the lack of the self-serving bias to compensate or override this increased accuracy results in pronounced negative appraisals of their appearance. It has been suggested that these negative appraisals result in lower self-esteem observed among individuals with BDD (Labuschagne, Castle, Dunai, Kyrios, & Rossell, 2010). In addition to lower self-esteem, Labuschagne et al. found that BDD patients have higher levels of self-ambivalence relative to matched controls (see also Phillips et al., 2011). According to the authors, the high self-ambivalence results in continuous re-evaluation of their self-concept, which would serve to further increase ambivalence. Consistent with psychological theories about the etiology of OCD (see Ahern and Kyrios, Chapter 12 in this volume), sensitivities relating to the self in BDD (e.g., appearance, social rejection) could lead to rituals or neutralizing aimed at "alleviating" underlying negative self-perceptions by avoiding situations or "fixing" perceived appearance-related deficits (Buhlmannn, Teachman, Naumann, Fehlinger, & Rieg, 2009).

While the dominant treatment for BDD is based on cognitive-behavioral interventions (e.g., Veale, 2010; Wilhelm, Phillips, Fama, Greenberg, & Steketee, 2011), these approaches may be ineffective in addressing the problematic overidentification of appearance with the self in BDD (Jarry & Ip, 2005). Neziroglu et al. (2008) suggested that acceptance and commitment therapy (ACT; Hayes, Strosahl, & Wilson, 1999) may have potential utility as an intervention for BDD, particularly in relation to experiencing the self from a first-person perspective as well as the idealized value placed on appearance. The central tenet of ACT is that psychological distress and functional impairment are caused by experiential avoidance (Hayes, Wilson, Gifford, Follette, & Strosahl, 1996), which occurs when an individual is unwilling to remain in contact with unwanted private events (i.e., thoughts, emotions, memories, and bodily sensations). An ACT approach for BDD would therefore focus on the dysfunctional processes of overinvestment in physical appearance and avoidance by directly targeting psychological inflexibility related to body image; or the capacity to experience the perceptions, sensations, feelings, thoughts, and beliefs about the body fully and intentionally (Sandoz, Wilson, Merwin, & Kellum, 2013).

ACT for BDD commences with the identification of unwanted private events and experiential avoidance strategies, with examination of the effectiveness of these strategies (Hayes et al., 1999). Values clarification is conducted in conjunction with this phase (Hayes et al., 1999). Individuals with BDD may have difficulty in defining and articulating their values (Mancuso, Knoesen, Chamberlain, Cloninger, & Castle, 2009) and may give the impression that they value appearance above all else (Didie et al., 2010; Hrabosky et al., 2009; Neziroglu et al., 2008; Silver, Reavey, & Fineberg, 2010). Merwin and Wilson (2009), however, suggest that core values may be hidden in layers of language for persons who overvalue their appearance. Therefore, values may be identified by asking the individual with BDD why their appearance is important (e.g., "What does looking attractive promise?"), with their answer reflecting valued life directions.

Cognitive defusion, the next phase of an ACT intervention, helps individuals to observe their appearance-related thoughts dispassionately and without attempts to control or change them (Hayes et al., 1999). Mindfulness techniques help the person shift focus from thought-content (e.g., "I am unattractive") to thought-process (e.g., "I notice I am having the thought that 'I am unattractive'"; Blackledge, 2007). The final phase of an ACT intervention involves committed action, where the individual commits to pursuing values-consistent behavior instead of engaging in behaviors that interfere with movement towards their values (Fletcher & Hayes, 2005; Hayes et al., 1999). Therefore, a person with BDD may commit to reducing their safety seeking and avoidance behaviors and increasing their values-consistent behavior (Merwin & Wilson, 2009).

Trichotillomania (hair pulling disorder)

TTM is characterized by the repetitive removal of hair causing hair loss, typically from the scalp, eyebrows, and eyelashes (APA, 2013). Hair can symbolically express one's social status and conformity to the norms of a social group; gender identity (i.e., femininity/masculinity) and sexuality; racial and cultural identity; and can even be perceived as a reflection of personality traits (Basow & Braman, 1998; Cash, 2001; Hunt & McHale, 2005; Synnott, 1987). As such, it is understandable that hair loss for both men and women has been found to adversely impact upon one's self-concept, including body image and self-worth (Alfonso, Richter-Appelt, Tosti, Viera, & García, 2005; Cash, 1999; Hilton, Hunt, Emslie, Salinas, & Ziebland, 2008; Münstedt, Manthey, Sachsse, & Vahrson, 1997). When physical appearance is a source of self-esteem, hair loss resulting from

androgenic alopecia (i.e., male-/female-pattern baldness) has been found to have a greater negative impact upon one's psychological well-being (Cash, 2001).

Surprisingly, there is a dearth of research that has investigated the impact of TTM on self-concept, despite most afflicted females having 30%–70% of hair missing from their hairpulling site(s) at any stage of the lifespan (Flessner, Woods, Franklin, Keuthen, & Piacentini, 2009). Individuals with TTM are secretive about their disorder, go to great lengths to hide their hair loss (e.g., with make-up, wigs, clothes), avoid activities that may reveal their hair loss, and are selective about whom they disclose their hairpulling to (Casati, Toner, & Yu, 2000; Stemberger, Thomas, Mansueto, & Carter, 2000). This is understandable given that negative social evaluation is greater when hair loss is attributed to TTM as opposed to when it is attributed to genetic reasons (Ricketts, Brandt, & Woods, 2012). Arguably, this may be due to others' perceptions that individuals with TTM lack self-control (Ricketts et al., 2012). Women with TTM report having very limited control over their hairpulling (Casati et al., 2000), which may contribute to perceptions of self as weak, flawed or inept (Diefenbach, Tolin, Hannan, Crocetto, & Worhunsky, 2005).

The aforementioned experiences associated with hair loss and TTM symptoms – personal weakness, vulnerability, self-consciousness – have all been implicated in definitions of shame (Blum, 2008; H. B. Lewis, 1971; M. Lewis, 1995; Weingarden & Renshaw, 2014). Blum suggested that shame is comprised of intense pain, discomfort or anger directed at the self for being "no good, inadequate, and unworthy," accompanied by a desire to hide and reduce "any further painful exposure of the self and end the discomfort" (p. 94). Much of the secretive and avoidant behaviors of individuals with TTM can be understood in the context of shame (Noble, 2012). Weingarden and Renshaw (2014) recently reviewed the evidence for symptom-based shame (i.e., shame related to hairpulling behaviors; see Noble, 2012) and body shame (i.e., shame resulting from changes to one's physical appearance) in TTM. Although research regarding shame in TTM is scant, they concluded that both types of shame are likely to perpetuate TTM symptoms.

Symptom-based shame and body shame are intuitively appealing concepts in relation to TTM, but fail to acknowledge the negative *self*-evaluations that are core to the experience of shame (Blum, 2008; H. B. Lewis, 1971; M. Lewis, 1995). Shame arises when one interprets one's actions as a failure of the *whole self* as opposed to interpreting the *actions/behaviors* themselves as failings (H. B. Lewis, 1971; M. Lewis, 1995). Hence, cognitive appraisals of self are essential to the emotional experience of shame, yet the relevance of cognition to the etiology and phenomenology of TTM appears to have been underestimated due to the automaticity of hairpulling behavior (e.g., Mansueto, Townsley-Stemberger, McCombs-Thomas, & Goldfinger-Golomb, 1997). In their biopsychosocial model, Franklin and Tolin (2007) proposed that negative self-evaluations associated with low self-esteem or perceived low control over hairpulling are initially consequences of TTM symptoms, but become triggers of hairpulling episodes over time. As per the roles of symptom-related and body shame (Weingarden & Renshaw, 2014), negative self-evaluations were seen as secondary to or stemming from TTM. However, the content of these negative self-evaluations was not speculated upon, nor has this model been tested.

Our own research has identified a range of cognitions that contribute to the onset and maintenance of hairpulling episodes in TTM, including negative self-beliefs (Rehm, Nedeljkovic, Moulding, & Thomas, 2013). Qualitative interviews with eight women with TTM identified that all participants endorsed negative self-beliefs comprising two core themes: (1) a sense of worthlessness, and (2) a sense of being "abnormal." As a 23-year-old woman who pulled her eyelashes and eyebrows stated, "It makes me feel crazy […] no one could ever love someone with a hairpulling syndrome." Participants' descriptions of themselves as worthless, "bad," or incapable implicated shameful self-evaluations that often precipitated hairpulling episodes. All participants believed that hairpulling helped them cope with these self-judgments and associated negative emotions (e.g., anger, guilt, anxiety). For instance, several participants experienced a "trance-like" dissociative state while pulling that helped them distract from, minimize, or avoid their unpleasant internal experiences. For some, this included a near-total absence of awareness of such experiences, while for others this involved facilitating positive emotions and cognitions in place of the negative ones (Rehm *et al.*, 2013). Similarly, among African-American women with TTM, participants with negative perceptions of their racial identity were more likely to experience happiness, calmness, or relief during and after hairpulling episodes compared to those with positive perceptions of their racial identity (Neal-Barnett & Stadulis, 2006). This

suggests that self-construals may influence the type of emotion-regulation function that hairpulling serves.

The interrelated roles of shame and self-concept pose questions about the directionality of their relationship to TTM development. The cognitive-affective experience of shame has long been suggested to play a predisposing role in the development of psychopathology (H. B. Lewis, 1971; Tangney, Wagner, & Gramzow, 1992). Tangney *et al.* suggested that individuals who are prone to experiencing shame may be more likely to experience repeated threats to their self-concept, and as such, are vulnerable to developing psychological maladjustment. In turn, the resulting psychological symptoms may elicit symptom-related shame, triggering further shame and maladjustment (Tangney *et al.*, 1992).

Indeed, shame proneness is associated with dissociative behavior (Irwin, 1998; Talbot, Talbot, & Tu, 2004), a phenomenon that is increasingly being recognized in TTM (Gupta, 2013; Lochner *et al.*, 2004; Lochner, Simeon, Niehaus, & Stein, 2002). Experiential avoidance has also been implicated in TTM (Begotka, Woods, & Wetterneck, 2004; Houghton *et al.*, 2014; Norberg, Wetterneck, Woods, & Conelea, 2007). Norberg *et al.* reported that experiential avoidance mediated the relationships between TTM severity and shame, fear of negative evaluation, and dysfunctional beliefs about appearance. What this may suggest is not that these cognitions are irrelevant to TTM, but that they may be so threatening to the self-concept that the individual is compelled to engage in hairpulling as a means to distract from or avoid the negative emotions that arise from such cognitions. This process has been termed "shame bypassing" (H. B. Lewis, 1971; M. Lewis, 1995), which may be the function of dissociation in shame-prone individuals (Talbot *et al.*, 2004). As one of our participants explained, "You're also thinking about how bad you are … I guess that's a feeling you want away, so you want to pull and take that feeling away" (Rehm *et al.*, 2013). Empirical evaluation of the bypassed shame model is, however, very limited (Platt, 2014), and the single study that evaluated the role of shame dimensions in TTM reported that characterological shame was not associated with TTM severity (Noble, 2012). However, using a newly validated measure of TTM-relevant beliefs with a large internet-based sample of individuals with TTM symptoms, our research group have found that the negative-self beliefs identified in our qualitative study (Rehm *et al.*, 2013) did indeed account for a small but significant portion of the variance in TTM severity, even after controlling for depression (Rehm, Nedeljkovic, Moulding, & Thomas, 2014).

Research on the interrelationships between shame, self-concept, avoidance-based emotion regulation strategies, and TTM remains preliminary. Models of TTM do not acknowledge that hair makes an important contribution to identity, and underestimate the influence of cognitions, including-self evaluations, in the onset and maintenance of hairpulling episodes. Furthermore, shame is typically viewed as a psychological consequence of TTM (e.g., Stemberger et al., 2000), with shame-related self-construals rarely considered as potential vulnerability factors. These oversights flow on to psychological treatments for TTM (e.g., adjunctive ACT or dialectical behavior therapy [DBT]), which currently omit the role of shame and self-concept in TTM (e.g., Crosby, Dehlin, Mitchell, & Twohig, 2012; Keuthen & Sprich, 2012). As Noble (2012) advocated, addressing shame and negative self-evaluation could be highly beneficial for TTM treatments. One, formulating hairpulling as a coping behavior that serves an important emotion regulation function (i.e., "something I do to cope") may help clients detach TTM from their sense of self, and reduce the presence or impact of negative self-evaluations (e.g., "I'm worthless, I'm abnormal, I'm weak") that may be perpetuating their symptoms. Two, by reducing the impact of shame, clients may be more inclined to disclose other "shameful" but risky and relatively common behaviors associated with their hairpulling, such as trichophagia (hair-eating; Grant & Odlaug, 2008). Both ACT and DBT could help clients to identify the influence that shame and negative self beliefs have upon their symptoms, and importantly, to establish a sense of self that is not constrained to the impact of TTM.

Conclusions

The preceding discussion indicates that self-concept seems important across the OCD spectrum disorders, albeit with differing emphases tied to their differing phenomenology. However, there is a common thread of identification of self with what is normally just a component of self (i.e., possessions, appearance, or hair), along with strong elements of shame, a lack of acceptance of negative experience, and limited emotional regulation strategies to deal with challenges to these self-concepts. Concepts of attachment and

ambivalence are important factors to examine across these disorders, as are concepts of self-regulation, but these issues have received limited research to date in terms of phenomenology, conceptual models or treatment. Such concepts are important to our understanding of the etiology and maintenance of disorders. For example, the rituals associated with each disorder may all help to alleviate negative self-concept or shame, and this itself may be implicated in the onset of disorders – especially given that symptoms tend to begin during adolescence or childhood for these disorders, a sensitive period for identity formation. Across all these disorders, it is therefore suggested that examination of self and identity is important, along with therapeutic strategies and emotional regulation work across a range of treatment frameworks. Overall, it is hoped that this examination may expand the conceptualization of, and treatment related to, these debilitating and understudied disorders, as well as providing future directions for research.

References

Aardema, F., Moulding, R., Radomsky, A. S., et al. (2013). Fear of self and obsessionality: Development and validation of the Fear of Self Questionnaire. Journal of Obsessive–Compulsive and Related Disorders, 2(3), 306–315.

Abramowitz, J. S., McKay, D., & Taylor, S. (Eds.). (2011). Obsessive–Compulsive Disorder: Subtypes and Spectrum Conditions. New York, NY: Elsevier.

Alemis, M. C., & Yap, K. (2013). The role of negative urgency impulsivity and financial management practices in compulsive buying. Australian Journal of Psychology, 65(4), 224–231.

Alfonso, M., Richter-Appelt, H., Tosti, A., Viera, M. S., & García, M. (2005). The psychosocial impact of hair loss among men: A multinational European study. Current Medical Research and Opinion, 21(11), 1829–1836.

American Psychiatric Association. (2013). Diagnostic and Statistical Manual of Mental Disorders, DSM-5. Washington, DC: American Psychiatric Publishing.

Basow, S. A., & Braman, A. C. (1998). Women and body hair: Social perceptions and attitudes. Psychology of Women Quarterly, 22, 637–645.

Begotka, A. M., Woods, D. W., & Wetterneck, C. T. (2004). The relationship between experiential avoidance and the severity of trichotillomania in a nonreferred sample. Journal of Behavior Therapy and Experimental Psychiatry, 35(1), 17–24.

Belk, R. W. (1988). Possessions and the extended self. The Journal of Consumer Research, 15, 139–168.

Bhar, S. S., & Kyrios, M. (2007). An investigation of self-ambivalence in obsessive–compulsive disorder. *Behaviour Research and Therapy*, 45(8), 1845–1857.

Blackledge, J. (2007). Disrupting verbal processes: Cognitive defusion in acceptance and commitment therapy and other mindfulness-based psychotherapies. *Psychological Record*, 57(4), Article 6.

Blum, A. (2008). Shame and guilt, misconceptions and controversies: A critical review of the literature. *Traumatology*, 14(3), 91–102.

Bowlby, J. (1988). *A Secure Base: Parent–Child Attachment and Healthy Human Development*. New York, NY: Basic Books.

Buhlmann, U., Etcoff, N. L., & Wilhelm, S. (2008). Facial attractiveness ratings and perfectionism in body dysmorphic disorder. *Journal of Anxiety Disorders*, 22(3), 540–547.

Buhlmann, U., Teachman, B. A., Naumann, E., Fehlinger, T., & Rieg, W. (2009). The meaning of beauty: Implicit and explicit self-esteem and attractiveness beliefs in BDD. *Journal of Anxiety Disorders*, 23, 694–702.

Casati, J., Toner, B. B., & Yu, B. (2000). Psychosocial issues for women with trichotillomania. *Comprehensive Psychiatry*, 41(5), 344–351.

Cash, T. F. (1999). The psychosocial consequences of androgenetic alopecia: A review of the research literature. *British Journal of Dermatology*, 141, 398–405.

Cash, T. F. (2001). The psychology of hair loss and its implications for patient care. *Clinics in Dermatology*, 19(2), 161–166.

Coles, M. E., Frost, R. O., Heimberg, R. G., & Steketee, G. (2003). Hoarding behaviors in a large college sample. *Behaviour Research and Therapy*, 41(2), 179–194.

Cooper, M., & Osman, S. (2007). Metacognition in body dysmorphic disorder: A preliminary exploration. *Journal of Cognitive Psychotherapy*, 21(2), 148–155.

Cromer, K. R., Schmidt, N. B., & Murphy, D. L. (2007). Do traumatic events influence the clinical expression of compulsive hoarding? *Behaviour Research and Therapy*, 45(11), 2581–2592.

Crosby, J. M., Dehlin, J. P., Mitchell, P. R., & Twohig, M. P. (2012). Acceptance and commitment therapy and habit reversal training for the treatment of trichotillomania. *Cognitive and Behavioral Practice*, 19(4), 595–605.

Didie, E. R., Kuniega-Pietrzak, T., & Phillips, K. A. (2010). Body image in patients with body dysmorphic disorder: Evaluations of and investment in appearance, health/illness, and fitness. *Body Image*, 7(1), 66–69.

Diefenbach, G. J., Tolin, D. F., Hannan, S., Crocetto, J., & Worhunsky, P. (2005). Trichotillomania: Impact on psychosocial functioning and quality of life. *Behaviour Research and Therapy*, 43(7), 869–884.

Dittmar, H. (2005). A new look at "compulsive buying": Self-discrepancies and materialistic values as predictors of compulsive buying tendency. *Journal of Social and Clinical Psychology*, 24(6), 832–859.

Doron, G., Moulding, R., Kyrios, M., & Nedeljkovic, M. (2008). Sensitivity of self-beliefs in obsessive compulsive disorder. *Depression and Anxiety*, 25(10), 874–884.

Epley, N., Waytz, A., & Cacioppo, J. T. (2007). On seeing human: A three-factor theory of anthropomorphism. *Psychological Review*, 114(4), 864.

Flessner, C. A., Woods, D. W., Franklin, M. E., Keuthen, N. J., & Piacentini, J. (2009). Cross-sectional study of women with trichotillomania: A preliminary examination of pulling styles, severity, phenomenology, and functional impact. *Child Psychiatry and Human Development*, 40(1), 153–167.

Fletcher, L., & Hayes, S. (2005). Relational Frame Theory, Acceptance and Commitment Therapy, and a functional analytic definition of mindfulness. *Journal of Rational-Emotive & Cognitive-Behavior Therapy*, 23(4), 315–336.

Franklin, M. E., & Tolin, D. F. (2007). *Treating Trichotillomania: Cognitive-behavioral Therapy for Hairpulling and Related Problems*. Dordrecht: Springer.

Frost, R. O., Kyrios, M., McCarthy, K. D., & Matthews, Y. (2007). Self-ambivalence and attachment to possessions. *Journal of Cognitive Psychotherapy*, 21(3), 232–242.

Grant, J. E., & Odlaug, B. L. (2008). Clinical characteristics of trichotillomania with trichophagia. *Comprehensive Psychiatry*, 49(6), 579–584.

Guidano, V. (1987). *Complexity of the Self*. New York, NY: Guilford Press.

Gupta, M. A. (2013). Emotional regulation, dissociation, and the self-induced dermatoses: Clinical features and implications for treatment with mood stabilisers. *Clinics in Dermatology*, 31(1), 110–117.

Hartl, T. L., Duffany, S. R., Allen, G. J., Steketee, G., & Frost, R. O. (2005). Relationships among compulsive hoarding, trauma, and attention-deficit/hyperactivity disorder. *Behaviour Research and Therapy*, 43(2), 269–276.

Hayes, S., Wilson, K., Gifford, E., Follette, V., & Strosahl, K. (1996). Experiential avoidance and behavioral disorders: A functional dimensional approach to diagnosis and treatment. *Journal of Consulting and Clinical Psychology*, 64(6), 1152–1168.

Hayes, S. C., Strosahl, K. D., & Wilson, K. G. (1999). *Acceptance and Commitment Therapy: An Experiential Approach to Behavior Change*. New York, NY: Guilford.

Hilton, S., Hunt, K., Emslie, C., Salinas, M., & Ziebland, S. (2008). Have men been overlooked? A comparison of young men and women's experiences of chemotherapy-induced alopecia. *Psycho-Oncology*, 17, 577–583.

Houghton, D. C., Compton, S. N., Twohig, M. P., *et al.* (2014). Measuring the role of psychological inflexibility in trichotillomania. *Psychiatry Research*, 220(1–2), 356–361.

Hrabosky, J. I., Cash, T. F., Veale, D., *et al.* (2009). Multidimensional body image comparisons among patients with eating disorders, body dysmorphic disorder, and clinical controls: A multisite study. *Body Image*, 6(3), 155–163.

Hunt, N., & McHale, S. (2005). The psychological impact of alopecia. *British Medical Journal (Online)*, 331, 951–953.

Irwin, H. J. (1998). Affective predictors of dissociation II: Shame and guilt. *Journal of Clinical Psychology*, 54, 237–245.

James, W. (1890/1950). *The Principles of Psychology* (Vol. 1). New York, NY: Dover.

Jarry, J. L., & Ip, K. (2005). The effectiveness of stand-alone cognitive-behavioural therapy for body image: A meta-analysis. *Body Image*, 2(4), 317–331.

Kellett, S., Greenhalgh, R., Beail, N., & Ridgway, N. (2010). Compulsive hoarding: An interpretative phenomenological analysis. *Behavioural and Cognitive Psychotherapy*, 38(2), 141–155.

Kellett, S., & Holden, K. (2013). Emotional attachment to objects in hoarding: A critical review of the evidence. In G. Steketee (Ed.), *The Oxford Handbook of Hoarding and Acquiring* (pp. 120–138). Oxford: Oxford University Press.

Keuthen, N. J., & Sprich, S. E. (2012). Utilizing DBT skills to augment traditional CBT for trichotillomania: An adult case study. *Cognitive and Behavioral Practice*, 19(2), 372–380.

Kyrios, M. (2014). Psychological models of compulsive hoarding. In R. O. Frost & G. Steketee (Eds.), *The Oxford Handbook of Hoarding and Acquiring* (pp. 206–220). Oxford: Oxford University Press.

Kyrios, M., Frost, R. O., & Steketee, G. (2004). Cognitions in compulsive buying and acquisition. *Cognitive Therapy and Research*, 28(2), 241–258.

Kyrios, M., Mogan, C., Moulding, R., *et al.* (in preparation). The cognitive-behavioral model of Hoarding Disorder: Evidence from clinical and non-clinical cohorts. Paper in preparation.

Labuschagne, I., Castle, D. J., Dunai, J., Kyrios, M., & Rossell, S. L. (2010). An examination of delusional thinking and cognitive styles in body dysmorphic disorder. *Australian and New Zealand Journal of Psychiatry*, 44, 706–712.

Lewis, H. B. (1971). *Shame and Guilt in Neurosis*. New York, NY: International Universities Press.

Lewis, M. (1995). *Shame: The Exposed Self*. New York, NY: The Free Press.

Lochner, C., Seedat, S., Hemmings, S. M. J., *et al.* (2004). Dissociative experiences in obsessive–compulsive disorder and trichotillomania: Clinical and genetic findings. *Comprehensive Psychiatry*, 45(5), 384–391.

Lochner, C., Simeon, D., Niehaus, D. J. H., & Stein, D. J. (2002). Trichotillomania and skin-picking: A phenomenological comparison. *Depression and Anxiety*, 15(2), 83–86.

Lynch, F. A., McGillivray, J. A., Moulding, R., & Byrne, L. K. (2015). Hoarding in attention deficit hyperactivity disorder: Understanding the comorbidity. *Journal of Obsessive–Compulsive and Related Disorders*, 4, 37–46.

Mancuso, S. G., Knoesen, N. P., Chamberlain, J. A., Cloninger, C. R., & Castle, D. J. (2009). The temperament and character profile of a body dysmorphic disorder outpatient sample. *Personality and Mental Health*, 3, 284–294.

Mansueto, C. S., Townsley Stemberger, R. M., McCombs Thomas, A., & Goldfinger Golomb, R. (1997). Trichotillomania: A comprehensive behavioral model. *Clinical Psychology Review*, 17(5), 567–577.

Merwin, R., & Wilson, K. (2009). Understanding and treating eating disorders: An ACT perspective. In J. T. Blackledge, J. V. Ciarrochi & F. P. Deane (Eds.), *Acceptance and Commitment Therapy: Contemporary Theory Research and Practice* (pp. 87–117). Bowen Hills, Queensland: Australian Academic Press.

Mogan, C., Kyrios, M., Schweitzer, I., Yap, K., & Moulding, R. (2012). Phenomenology of hoarding – What is hoarded by individuals with hoarding disorder? *Journal of Obsessive–Compulsive and Related Disorders*, 1(4), 306–311.

Moulding, R., Aardema, F., & O'Connor, K. P. (2014). Repugnant obsessions: A review of the phenomenology, theoretical models, and treatment of sexual and aggressive obsessional themes in OCD. *Journal of Obsessive–Compulsive and Related Disorders*, 3(2), 161–168.

Moulding, R., Nedeljkovic, M., & Kyrios, M. (2011). Obsessive compulsive disorder in the DSM. In G. Murray (Ed.), *A Critical Introduction to DSM*. New York, NY: Nova.

Moulding, R., Nedeljkovic, M., Kyrios, M., Osbourne, D., & Mogan, C. (submitted). Short-term cognitive-behavioral group treatment for Hoarding Disorder: A naturalistic treatment outcome study.

Münstedt, K., Manthey, N., Sachsse, S., & Vahrson, H. (1997). Changes in self-concept and body image during alopecia induced cancer chemotherapy. *Supportive Care in Cancer*, 5(2), 139–143.

Neal-Barnett, A., & Stadulis, R. (2006). Affective states and racial identity among African-American women with trichotillomania. *Journal of the National Medical Association*, 98(5), 753–757.

Neave, N., Jackson, R., Saxton, T., & Hönekopp, J. (2015). The influence of anthropomorphic tendencies on human hoarding behaviours. *Personality and Individual Differences*, 72, 214–219.

Neziroglu, F., Khemlani-Patel, S., & Veale, D. (2008). Social learning theory and cognitive behavioral models of body dysmorphic disorder. *Body Image*, 5(1), 28–38.

Noble, C. L. (2012). *The relationships among multidimensional perfectionism, shame and trichotillomania symptom severity.* Doctoral dissertation, Georgia State University, Georgia. Retrieved from http://scholarworks.gsu.edu/cps_diss/78

Norberg, M. M., Wetterneck, C. T., Woods, D. W., & Conelea, C. A. (2007). Experiential avoidance as a mediator of relationships between cognitions and hair-pulling severity. *Behavior Modification*, 31(4), 367–381.

Norris, J. I., Lambert, N. M., DeWall, C. N., & Fincham, F. D. (2012). Can't buy me love? Anxious attachment and materialistic values. *Personality and Individual Differences*, 53(5), 666–669.

Osman, S., Cooper, M., Hackmann, A., & Veale, D. (2004). Spontaneously occurring images and early memories in people with body dysmorphic disorder. *Memory*, 12(4), 428–436.

Phillips, B., Moulding, R., Kyrios, M., Nedeljkovic, M., & Mancuso, S. G. (2011). The relationship between body dysmorphic disorder symptoms and self-construals. *Clinical Psychologist*, 15, 10–16.

Phung, P., Moulding, R., Taylor, J.K., & Nedeljkovic, M. (2015). Emotional regulation, attachment to possessions and hoarding symptoms. *Scandinavian Journal of Psychology*, 56, 573–581.

Platt, M. G. (2014). *Feelings of shame and dissociation in survivors of high and low betrayal traumas.* Doctoral dissertation, University of Oregon, Oregon. Retrieved from http://pages.uoregon.edu/dynamic/jjf/theses/platt13.pdf

Rehm, I. C., Nedeljkovic, M., Moulding, R., & Thomas, A. (2013). *The role of self-beliefs in episodes of chronic hairpulling: Informing cognitive-behavioural models of trichotillomania.* Paper presented at the 7th Annual World Congress of Behavioural and Cognitive Therapies, Lima, Peru.

Rehm, I. C., Nedeljkovic, M., Moulding, R., & Thomas, A. (2014). *The qualitative development of a measure of cognitions and beliefs in trichotillomania.* Paper presented at the 28th International Conference of Applied Psychology, Paris.

Ricketts, E. J., Brandt, B. C., & Woods, D. W. (2012). The effects of severity and causal explanation on social perceptions of hair loss. *Journal of Obsessive–Compulsive and Related Disorders*, 1(4), 336–343.

Sandoz, E. K., Wilson, K. G., Merwin, R. M., & Kellum, K. K. (2013). Assessment of body image flexibility: The body image-acceptance and action questionnaire. *Journal of Contextual Behavioral Science*, 2(1), 39–48.

Schmalisch, C. S., Bratiotis, C., & Muroff, J. (2010). Processes in group cognitive and behavioral treatment for hoarding. *Cognitive and Behavioral Practice*, 17, 414–425.

Silver, J., Reavey, P., & Fineberg, N. A. (2010). How do people with body dysmorphic disorder view themselves? A thematic analysis. *International Journal of Psychiatry in Clinical Practice*, 14(3), 190–197.

Steketee, G., & Frost, R. (2003). Compulsive hoarding: Current status of the research. *Clinical Psychology Review*, 23(7), 905–927.

Steketee, G., & Frost, R. (2007). *Compulsive Hoarding and Acquiring – Therapist Guide.* Oxford: Oxford University Press.

Steketee, G., & Frost, R. (2010). *Stuff: Compulsive Hoarding and the Meaning of Things*: Boston, MA: Houghton Mifflin Harcourt.

Steketee, G., Frost, R., & Kyrios, M. (2003). Cognitive aspects of compulsive hoarding. *Cognitive Therapy and Research*, 27(4), 463–479.

Stemberger, R. M. T., Thomas, A. M., Mansueto, C. S., & Carter, J. G. (2000). Personal toll of trichotillomania: Behavioral and interpersonal sequelae. *Journal of Anxiety Disorders*, 14(1), 97–104.

Synnott, A. (1987). Shame and glory: A sociology of hair. *The British Journal of Sociology*, 38(3), 381–413.

Talbot, J. A., Talbot, N. L., & Tu, X. (2004). Shame-proneness as a diathesis for dissociation in women with histories of childhood sexual abuse. *Journal of Traumatic Stress*, 17(5), 445–448.

Tangney, J. P., Wagner, P., & Gramzow, R. (1992). Proneness to shame, proneness to guilt, and psychopathology. *Journal of Abnormal Psychology*, 101(3), 469–478.

Timpano, K. R., Buckner, J. D., Richey, J. A., Murphy, D. L., & Schmidt, N. B. (2009). Exploration of anxiety sensitivity and distress tolerance as vulnerability factors for hoarding behaviors. *Depression and Anxiety*, 26(4), 343–353.

Timpano, K. R., Rasmussen, J., Exner, C., Rief, W., Schmidt, N. B., & Wilhelm, S. (2013). Hoarding and the multi-faceted construct of impulsivity: A cross-cultural investigation. *Journal of Psychiatric Research*, 47(3), 363–370.

Timpano, K. R., & Schmidt, N. B. (2013). The relationship between self-control deficits and hoarding: A multimethod investigation across three samples. *Journal of Abnormal Psychology*, 122(1), 13–25.

Timpano, K. R., & Shaw, A. M. (2013). Conferring humanness: The role of anthropomorphism in hoarding. *Personality and Individual Differences*, 54(3), 383–388.

Timpano, K. R., Shaw, A. M., Cougle, J. R., & Fitch, K. E. (2014). A multifaceted assessment of emotional tolerance and intensity in hoarding. *Behavior Therapy*, 45(5), 690–699.

Tolin, D. F., Frost, R., & Steketee, G. (2007). *Buried in Treasures*. Oxford: Oxford University Press.

Tolin, D. F., Frost, R., Steketee, G., & Muroff, J. (2015). Cognitive behavioral therapy for hoarding disorder: A meta-analysis. *Depression and Anxiety*, 32(3), 158–166.

Veale, D. (2001). Cognitive-behavioural therapy for body dysmorphic disorder. *Advances in Psychiatric Treatment*, 7(2), 125–132.

Veale, D. (2002a). Over-valued ideas: A conceptual analysis. *Behaviour Research and Therapy*, 40(4), 383–400.

Veale, D. (2002b). Shame in body dysmorphic disorder. In P. Gilbert & J. Miles (Eds.), *Body Shame: Conceptualisation, Research, and Treatment* (pp. 267–282). New York, NY: Routledge.

Veale, D. (2004). Advances in a cognitive behavioural model of body dysmorphic disorder. *Body Image*, 1, 113–125.

Veale, D. (2010). Cognitive behavioral therapy for body dysmorphic disorder. *Psychiatric Annals*, 40(7), 333–340.

Veale, D., Kinderman, P., Riley, S., & Lambrou, C. (2003). Self-discrepancy in body dysmorphic disorder. *British Journal of Clinical Psychology*, 42(2), 157–169.

Veale, D., & Neziroglu, F. (2010). *Body Dysmorphic Disorder: A Treatment Manual*. Chichester: Wiley-Blackwell.

Veale, D., & Riley, S. (2001). Mirror, mirror on the wall, who is the ugliest of them all? The psychopathology of mirror gazing in body dysmorphic disorder. *Behaviour Research and Therapy*, 39(12), 1381–1393.

Weingarden, H., & Renshaw, K. D. (2014). Shame in the obsessive compulsive related disorders: A conceptual review. *Journal of Affective Disorders*, 171, 74–84.

Wilhelm, S., Phillips, K. A., Fama, J. M., Greenberg, J. L., & Steketee, G. (2011). Modular cognitive–behavioral therapy for body dysmorphic disorder. *Behavior Therapy*, 42(4), 624–633.

Chapter

14

Self-regulation in disordered gambling: a comparison with alcohol and substance use disorders

Simone N. Rodda, Kate Hall, Petra K. Staiger, and Nicki A. Dowling

Introduction

Pathological gambling was classified as a disorder of impulse control in the third and fourth editions of the *Diagnostic and Statistical Manual of Mental Disorders* (DSM; American Psychiatric Association [APA], 1987, 1994). In the DSM-IV, impulse control disorders were characterized by a "failure to resist an impulse, drive, or temptation to perform an act that is harmful to the person or to others" (APA, 1994, p. 609). This classification placed pathological gambling in the same category as kleptomania, pyromania, and intermittent explosive disorder. In contrast, the DSM-5 (APA, 2013) has reclassified pathological gambling as an addiction and related disorder, and renamed it gambling disorder. In this edition, gambling disorder is defined as persistent and recurrent problematic gambling behavior leading to clinically significant impairment or distress.

Locating gambling disorder with alcohol and substance use disorders reflects research findings that this disorder is similar to substance-related disorders in clinical expression, brain origin, comorbidity, physiology, and treatment (APA, 2013). The conceptualization of gambling disorder as a behavioral addiction is consistent with contemporary models of addiction that emphasize impairment of control, rather than biochemical or molecular changes, physiological dependence, and neuroadaptation resulting from the ingestion of an exogenous psychoactive agent (Grant, Potenza, Weinstein, & Gorelick, 2010). Behavioral addictions may involve gambling, internet use, video games, shopping, exercise, work, eating, and sex. Gambling disorder is, however, the only behavioral addiction to be included in the DSM-5, as it is the only disorder with sufficient evidence to establish diagnostic criteria and course descriptions (APA, 2013).

The standardized past-year prevalence of gambling disorder internationally ranges from 0.5% to 7.6%, with an average rate of 2.3% (Williams, Volberg, & Stevens, 2012). Gambling disorder prevalence rates are generally higher in jurisdictions with greater accessibility to gambling products (Productivity Commission, 2010). Although population prevalence estimates of gambling disorder are generally stable across time, longitudinal studies reveal that gambling problems at the individual level seem to be characterized by instability, fluidity, and multidirectionality (LaPlante, Nelson, LaBrie, & Shaffer, 2008). The incidence of gambling disorder (i.e. new cases) is estimated to be 0.36% (Victorian Department of Justice, 2011).

In terms of treatment for disordered gambling, most of the research efforts have been focused on cognitive or behavioral therapies and to a lesser extent motivational interviewing or brief therapies (Thomas *et al.*, 2011; Cowlishaw *et al.*, 2012). However, only between 8% and 17% of people with gambling problems seek help (Productivity Commission, 2010). Most people with gambling disorder who recover do so without formal assistance. While the evidence is limited, this suggests that a range of strategies and actions assist the person to regulate their time and money and regain control over their gambling (Hing, Nuske, & Gainsbury, 2011; Moore, Thomas, Kyrios, & Bates, 2012; Lubman *et al.*, 2015). However, little is known of the processes associated with losing control over gambling behaviors or regaining it. In keeping with the focus of this book on self constructs in psychological disorders, this chapter aims to describe a model of self-regulation and related ideas as they apply to disordered gambling.

The Self in Understanding and Treating Psychological Disorders, ed. Michael Kyrios, Richard Moulding, Guy Doron, Sunil S. Bhar, Maja Nedeljkovic, and Mario Mikulincer. Published by Cambridge University Press. © Cambridge University Press, 2016.

Self-regulation

Self-regulation is a broad term to describe how thoughts, actions, or feelings are controlled across a range of environments. Specifically, it refers to planned or unplanned comparisons of the self against internal standards and a process of overriding innate or learned responses when the self and standards are not in alignment (Baumeister, Heatherton, & Tice, 1994; Baumeister & Vohs, 2007). This may involve many adjustments and attempts through a process of self-monitoring. How readily the individual is able to bring the self and their standards into alignment is determined in part by their strength and determination as well as motivation to change (Baumeister, Vohs, & Tice, 2007).

However, self-regulation appears to be a limited resource. It appears individuals are relatively successful at exerting restraint for short-term gains, but less successful in maintaining self-regulation over the long term (Hagger, Wood, Stiff, & Chatzisarantis, 2010). For example, a series of experiments by Muraven, Tice, and Baumeister (1998) found that participants who engaged in different self-regulatory tasks (e.g., emotional control or thought suppression) were less capable of self-regulating in subsequent tasks (compared to participants who were not initially required to self-regulate), because resources to self-regulate had become depleted. However, the influence of depletion is not inevitably a loss of self-regulatory behavior. When individuals are sufficiently motivated, they are capable of overriding the effects of depletion, even when motivation is limited (Oaten & Cheng, 2006). This suggests that self-regulatory success may be jointly determined by depletion and motivation.

In terms of addictive behaviors, self-regulation also plays a role in initially restricting or limiting access to the substance or behavior and then later maintaining thoughts and behaviors associated with change (Baumeister & Vonasch, 2014). There is a surprising absence of research investigating the role of self-regulation in gambling disorder. Baumeister *et al.* (1994) were the first to briefly discuss self-regulation as applied to gambling disorder. The evidence, however, for this examination was based almost exclusively on males engaged in wagering and casino gambling in the USA. Since this time, there has been an exponential increase in accessibility of gambling opportunities due to the creation and distribution of the modern gaming machine (called slots, fruit machines, or electronic gaming machines) and also due to internet-enabled betting. Moreover, although gambling has traditionally been a masculine activity (Dowling, 2013), the increased availability of gambling in many countries has narrowed the gender gap, with women now comprising approximately one-third of problem gamblers in some jurisdictions (e.g., Christensen, Dowling, Jackson, & Thomas, 2014).

The remainder of this chapter will describe each major component of self-regulation. Given the absence of literature applying the self-regulation model to gambling, the literature available for the more advanced field of research into alcohol/drug use will be explored, followed by a review of the problem gambling literature.

Standards and goals

Standards include a range of goals, values, or guides that represent what the individual believes is an ideal way of being (Baumeister & Vonasch, 2014). Standards develop through experience and can be informed or imposed by others (e.g., community, family) or via a comparison against one's own past self. Effective standards and goals are those that are clear and well-defined. When self-regulation fails, it is often due to standards and goals that are unrealistic or overly optimistic, confusing, ambiguous, inconsistent, or conflicting (Baumeister & Vohs, 2007).

Externally imposed standards for alcohol and gambling consumption vary. Standards for alcohol consumption have been developed via the examination of the dose–response relationship between frequency of alcohol consumption and risk of adverse consequences (Babor, 2010; Bondy *et al.*, 1998; Room, 1996). This has allowed the identification of alcohol intake that distinguishes low- and high-risk behavior, known as responsible drinking limits (also known as behavioral indicators for low-risk drinking, low-risk limits, low-risk cut-offs, or low-risk thresholds), which are consistent behavioral patterns associated with alcohol-related harm (Wechsler, Dowdall, Davenport, & Castillo, 1995). These limits have served as the basis for quantitative behavioral guidelines incorporating the concept of a "standard drink" that can be promoted to the public.

In contrast, standards for gambling consumption have only recently been developed under the banner of "responsible gambling guidelines." These guidelines, which are recommended in many jurisdictions, include behaviors such as avoiding drinking alcohol while gambling, avoiding taking credit/debit cards to the gambling venue, and setting limits on the amount of money gambled (Lostutter, Lewis, Cronce, Neighbors, & Larimer, 2014). Most of these guidelines fail to include quantitative behavioral indicators of harmful gambling that gamblers can use to guide their gambling behavior. The development of such quantitative gambling guidelines is limited to several studies conducted in Canada and the USA (Currie, Hodgins, Casey, & El-Guebaly, 2012; Currie *et al.*, 2006, 2008). These analyses identified similar, although not identical, responsible gambling limits: gambling no more than 2–5 times per month; spending no more than $11–$85 (Canadian) per month on gambling; spending no more than 1–3% of gross household income on gambling activities; gambling for no longer than 60 minutes per session; and gambling on no more than 4 types of gambling activities per year.

The goals for adjusting alcohol or gambling consumption involve limiting or controlling the behavior or abstaining altogether. An abstinence approach is typically advocated for those who are highly substance-dependent and is grounded in the assumption that any alcohol or drug use will inevitably result in loss of control for dependent individuals. While this may be an important approach for some individuals, established treatments for alcohol dependence aimed at full abstinence require further evaluation. For example, a Cochrane review of Alcoholics Anonymous and other 12-step programs that require a goal of full abstinence found limited evidence for the effectiveness of these programs (Ferri, Amato, & Davoli, 2006). However, these findings should be taken with a great deal of caution given that the review also identified a lack of quality and quantity of research in this area.

Historically, total abstinence has also been viewed as the only legitimate and acceptable outcome of gambling disorder treatment, but this is changing. Research conducted in Australian services for gambling disorder (Dowling & Smith, 2007) suggests that one-quarter to one-third of clients select controlled or reduced gambling as a goal of treatment when it is available. This research indicates that most clients who select abstinence do so because they believe that it is not possible to control their gambling behavior. In contrast, clients who select controlled gambling do so because gambling retains some enjoyment, they believe that abstinence is unrealistic or overwhelming, or they want to successfully manage social situations involving gambling. Controlled gambling is most

likely to be selected by older clients with lower psychological distress, lower gambling disorder severity, and higher social support. A limited literature suggests that the selection of abstinence and controlled gambling results in equivalent problem gambling treatment outcomes (Dowling, Smith, & Thomas, 2009; Ladouceur, Lachance, & Fournier, 2009).

The importance of setting clear and unambiguous standards and goals for consumption of gambling products cannot be underestimated. To date, gamblers have been provided limited guidelines in terms of frequency of use and the risk of adverse consequences. Where advice has been provided, this is most often in terms of behavioral strategies (e.g., setting limits). To reduce the development of gambling problems, there is an urgent need to develop and disseminate a set of quantitative guidelines for gambling consumption (i.e., amount spent per month). For people with disordered gambling, the uptake and effectiveness of these measures as a means of controlling gambling also needs to be evaluated.

Monitoring

Self-monitoring refers to keeping track of behavior against standards and goals (Baumeister & Vohs, 2007). This central component of self-regulation, originally developed by Carver and Scheier (1982), proposes a feedback loop between standards and self-monitoring. When monitoring identifies that the self does not align with standards, the developing self-awareness can be uncomfortable for the individual and there is an attempt to change some aspect of the self. In terms of addictive behaviors, monitoring for the most part has been in relation to internet-based self-assessments and tracking consumption against the goal of limiting, controlling or abstaining.

Internet-based self-assessments are widely offered as a means of helping people assess their consumption. These screens provide immediate feedback on how consumption compares to the broader (normal) population and can assist in making the person aware of a discrepancy between the self and various standards. These screens may be especially helpful for those who perceive alcohol use as a defining characteristic of their personal identity and who are more likely to engage in greater alcohol consumption (Foster, Neighbors, & Young, 2014; Foster, Yeung, & Neighbors, 2014) and risky drinking behavior (Gray, LaPlante, Bannon, Ambady, & Shaffer, 2011).

If comparison of the self to the broader population evokes dissonance, behavioral change may occur. There is now a substantial body of evidence on the effectiveness of internet-based self-assessments for alcohol use (Cunningham, Wild, Cordingley, Van Mierlo, & Humphreys, 2010; Kypri et al., 2009; White, 2006) and other substances, such as cannabis (Tait, Spijkerman, & Riper, 2013).

In contrast, the results for screening and personalized feedback for disordered gambling are mixed. In an early pilot study, Cunningham, Hodgins, Toneatto, Rai, and Cordingley (2009) applied a brief online screening tool for severity of gambling problems and found short-term reductions in money spent gambling. In a follow-up study employing a more rigorous design, Cunningham, Hodgins, Toneatto, and Murphy (2012) provided gamblers with personalized feedback on the results of a gambling screen and gambling cognitions questionnaire compared to others of the same gender and gambling activity. In this study, screening with feedback did not have an impact on gambling behavior.

In addition to completing a tool that provides a snapshot of alignment with standards, tracking can occur over a period of time. Momentary, or real-time, assessment increases the effectiveness of education and treatment programs for reducing alcohol consumption, even though for many years this was in the form of paper and pencil diaries (Mullen et al., 1997). The internet has made monitoring more sophisticated and smart phones now offer unprecedented options for monitoring a range of behaviors against multiple standards. For example, smart phone applications can use GPS monitoring and initiate an intervention if standards such as avoidance of certain locations are breached (Gustafson et al., 2014).

In gambling disorder, much of the focus has been on the implementation of actions to reduce or manage gambling disorder rather than monitoring the self against standards and goals. For example, Hodgins and El-Guebaly (2000) found that problem gamblers who recovered without formal assistance endorsed stimulus control or avoidance, new activities, cognitive strategies and social support as important to their recovery. Similarly, Moore et al. (2012) investigated the types of strategies gamblers regularly use to manage their gambling. These include cognitive approaches (e.g., think about the negative consequences of gambling), direct action (e.g., seek professional help), social experience (e.g., go to venues that have other activities), avoidance (e.g., keep busy) and limit setting (e.g., setting a budget on

time or money). However, self-monitoring is generally included as a component of cognitive-behavior therapy treatment programs (e.g., Ladouceur et al., 2009), albeit with limited focus on its effectiveness. A recent interesting development that is aligned with the self-regulation model is real-time tracking while gambling. Tracking tools are now offered in land-based (Wohl, Gainsbury, Stewart, & Sztainert, 2013) and online (Griffiths, Wood, & Parke, 2009) gambling venues.

Even though there are significantly more opportunities to consume alcohol than there are to consume gambling products, there has been very limited research conducted with gamblers on the use of tracking and self-monitoring. The limited research involving internet-based self-assessment for disordered gambling has not produced the same good outcomes in terms of reduced consumption as demonstrated with the administration of alcohol screens. In addition, despite a growing number of gambling consumption applications becoming available there is currently no research that has evaluated whether this can assist people in self-regulation. Further research is needed to determine the most effective self-assessment tools and tracking devices so that these can be integrated into prevention and treatment programs. In addition, the range of strategies and actions gamblers use to change their gambling once a discrepancy between standards and behavior has been detected (e.g., thinking about the negative consequences of gambling) also needs to be evaluated in terms of uptake and helpfulness.

Self-control strength

Self-control strength (also known as goal strength) literally refers to the ability to persist or continue to self-monitor against standards, despite an impulse or desire to do otherwise (Baumeister et al., 2007). This strength is believed to be a limited resource that uses substantial amounts of blood glucose such that time is required to replenish resources following a self-regulation attempt. This means that strength is generally weakest when individuals are tired or under stress. Self-control strength can also be hampered by multiple or conflicting standards and also depletion of internal resources. Baumeister and Heatherton (1996) suggest that self-regulation fails when the actions of a lower standard or goal override those of a higher standard or goal. This is a common feature of gambling and substance use disorders, such that the individual has repeated and unsuccessful attempts to change.

Alcohol can have a significant impact on self-control strength such that it can lower self-awareness. At times, this may be intentional. Research has found that self-aware individuals consume more alcohol following negative feedback regarding personal failure than those who receive positive feedback regarding personal success, or who display low self-awareness (Hull & Young, 1983). Additionally, a study conducted by Hull, Young, and Jouriles (1986) demonstrated that highly self-aware individuals who had experienced negative self-relevant life events were significantly more likely to relapse to alcohol use following detoxification.

In relation to gambling disorder, venues in which gambling is available pose a special challenge for those attempting to control or limit their gambling behavior. In most Western countries, gambling has become available outside of casinos, at both land-based venues or via online platforms. This increase in accessibility means gambling need no longer be a planned event but an activity that can be engaged in anytime of the day or night. In both land-based and online gambling venues, a range of measures has been introduced to assist gamblers in self-regulation. Examples of measures for land-based venues include the collection of winnings over a certain amount, limits on cash machine access, and environmental changes such as increased natural light or visible clocks. Similarly, measures for online gambling venues include self-assessment, self-exclusion, and self-imposed spending and time limits (Griffiths *et al.*, 2009). Although these measures have face appeal, there is only limited evidence that these measures are helpful to people in reducing or limiting their time or money spent gambling (Blaszczynski *et al.*, 2011; Gainsbury, Blankers, Wilkinson, Schelleman-Offermans, & Cousijn, 2014).

Addictive behaviors by their very nature involve impairment to self-control, yet self-control is required in order to overcome the disorder. We know that alcohol consumption can have a significant impact on self-control and this can lead to a failure of self-regulation. To date, however, there has been limited research that has investigated the impact of gambling on self-control or how gambling may impact on the ability to stick to standards and goals. Given that gambling venues have been especially developed to keep people gambling for more time and money than planned, there is an urgent need to determine the features of the environment most responsible when there is a failure in self-regulation (e.g., venue size, ready access to cash). This should also include further

evaluation of measures that could be introduced to support self-regulation and adherence to standards and goals (i.e., technology to support limit-setting).

Motivation

Even with clear standards, effective self-monitoring and sufficient strength or willpower, self-regulation can fail if change is not deemed important. Motivation has recently been included as an important ingredient of the self-regulation model, mostly because of the role it plays in self-regulation failure. However, it can also make up for a lack of monitoring or strength, especially when resources are depleted and self-awareness is low (Baumeister & Vohs, 2007).

The transtheoretical model (Prochaska, DiClemente, & Norcross, 1992) aims to explain how people change and proposes five stages of change that include precontemplation, contemplation, preparation, action and maintenance. This model suggests that people progress through the continuum a number of times before the problem is resolved. In addition, the transtheoretical model proposes 10 processes that describe how people change.

The transtheoretical model has been widely applied to addictive behaviors. In terms of clinical practice, it forms the theoretical basis of Motivational Interviewing, and this is one of the most common therapeutic techniques applied across all of the addictive behaviors. While the model was originally formulated to describe the readiness of people engaged in smoking cessation, DiClemente and Hughes (1990) reported similar distinct profiles of readiness to change in people seeking treatment for alcohol use. In this study, the amount of alcohol consumed, temptation to drink, and self-efficacy were found to be distinctly different at each stage of change.

The transtheoretical model has also been applied in several studies examining gambling disorder. In a survey of 234 gamblers initiating treatment, Petry (2005) found most clients in treatment were actively involved or initiating change, with fewer clients ambivalent or uninvolved. Importantly, the stage of change at baseline impacted client outcomes at two months follow-up. Hodgins (2001) tested these processes with 37 recovered disordered gamblers and found the most frequently used processes for change were self-re-evaluation (feeling upset or shame about self-image and gambling), environmental re-evaluation (effects of gambling on others), dramatic relief (strong negative feelings about gambling), and self-liberation (commitment and belief that success is possible).

While the transtheoretical model has been widely accepted by clinicians and researchers across a range of fields, there is now a growing consensus that there are problems with the model. Robert West, the Editor-in-Chief of the prestigious peer-reviewed journal *Addiction*, argues that the model does not have stages with clear delineation and would be better described as a state of change model rather than a stage (i.e., current motivation or readiness to change; West, 2005). In addition, he suggests it might be better to simply ask people about their desire and ability to change while taking into account personal and situational factors.

To this end, multiple studies have applied a series of readiness rulers to illicit drug users and smokers who were not currently attempting to change their behavior (Abar, Baumann, Rosenbaum, Boyer, & Boudreaux, 2012; Abar et al., 2013). These studies found a pattern of high readiness and low confidence. Similarly, Rodda, Lubman, Iyer, Gao, and Dowling (2015) applied these rulers to over 1000 gamblers accessing a brief intervention via an online help service. They found four out of five gamblers were ready to change their gambling but reported co-occurring low confidence to manage an urge. Gamblers typically reported lower confidence at session commencement, with levels significantly lower than the high scores reported for importance and readiness. This research is important in capturing motivation in a moment in time. However, we know that motivation fluctuates throughout the change process and although motivation can peak and propel the person to take action it can also dissipate, especially when standards and goals are in conflict. To better understand the impact of fluctuating motivation, more research conducted in real-time settings is needed (i.e., when the person is faced with a situation requiring self-regulation).

Clinical applications

The self-regulation model has important clinical applications across substance misuse and disordered gambling. Given the applicability of its component parts to disordered gambling, it is perhaps surprising that only one comprehensive treatment manual has been published (Ciarrocchi, 2001). This manual applies the self-regulation model to problem gambling and describes a range of relevant clinical interventions. For the most part, the interventions involve motivational

interviewing (MI)/motivational enhancement therapies (MET) and cognitive-behavioral therapies (CBT) with a focus on goal-setting and resolving conflict between goals (i.e., abstinence/reduction, work, family, relationship, health, financial, recreational, and spiritual), gambling triggers, and relapse, as well as emotional regulation. CBT and MI have been found to be the most effective in the treatment of gambling disorder in a Cochrane review (Cowlishaw et al., 2012) and are recommended in the only available evidence-based clinical practice guideline for the treatment of gambling disorder (Thomas et al., 2011).

Many brief interventions for gambling disorder are based on MI or MET. MI is a client-centered, directive counseling method that helps resolve ambivalence about change. It is underpinned by a series of principles, described as MI Spirit, that honors the self as vitally important in the change process (Miller & Rollnick, 2012). The autonomy of the self is respected and the client's intrinsic resources for change are elicited by the therapist. Within MI, the therapist is viewed as a facilitator rather than an expert who evokes the client's intrinsic values, standards, and goals to motivate change. MI highlights the discrepancy between valued standards and gambling behaviors through tools such as readiness rulers or screening and feedback. The resulting dissonance is theorized to be one of the mechanisms for behavior change (Miller & Rollnick, 2012). Strategies such as comparing where you are now versus where you would like to be in 5 years' time highlight any inconsistencies between current behaviors and standards. Motivation is also enhanced through supporting "self-efficacy" or the belief that one has the capacity to change. Related to both strength and also motivation to self-regulate, a goal of MI is to enhance the client's confidence in his or her capacity to change and to overcome any barriers that may prevent change from occurring. Enhancing self-efficacy in MI is a key element in motivating someone to change self-destructive behaviors such as substance use or gambling disorder. In practical terms, self-efficacy is promoted through a focus on past successful behavior change, strengths, and affirmation regarding any efforts to change.

In contrast, the cognitive behavioral model, pioneered by Aaron T. Beck, proposes that dysfunctional or distorted thinking (which in turn influences mood and behavior) are common to all psychological disturbances, including gambling disorder. Used across many areas of psychopathology, CBT interventions therefore use a variety of strategies to produce cognitive change in order to bring about enduring emotional and behavioral change. Core beliefs about the self and how one relates to others and the world are proposed to be the enduring cognitive phenomena that underpin all cognitions (Beck, 1976). CBT for gambling can assist the individual to identify and challenge beliefs that are global, rigid, or overgeneralized, and those that may be getting in the way of being able to set clear and realistic standards (Ciarrocchi, 2001). For example, gamblers develop complex belief systems aimed at getting the edge over luck and to predict uncertain and random outcomes (e.g., illusion of control; Toneatto, 2002). Derived from early experiences, core beliefs are enduring and influence all interpretations of the self (Beck, 1995). Indeed, for some, luck is viewed as a personal attribute that can be controlled (Wohl, Young, & Hart, 2005), and this can mean a delay in realizing a failure of self-regulation. CBT can be helpful in addressing self-regulation failure by identifying and challenging permission-granting beliefs, expectancies, and permissive thinking that can undermine self-monitoring. Behavioral strategies such as graded exposure to high-risk situations or triggers and behavioral experiments to practice effective coping responses similarly provide opportunity for cognitive disputation of beliefs about the self and can increase self-control strength and build self-efficacy.

Marlatt and Gordon's (1985) Relapse Prevention model applies a cognitive and behavioral model to addictive behaviors that incorporates both a conceptual model of relapse and a set of cognitive and behavioral strategies to prevent or limit relapse episodes. Relapse prevention has been described as a self-control program and focuses on changing cognitions and behaviors in order to manage the precipitants of relapse (e.g. high-risk situations, lack of coping skills, urges and cravings, outcome expectancies, and the abstinence violation effect (AVE)). Relapse prevention focuses on changing cognitions and behaviors in order to manage high-risk situations and avoid relapse. This can be especially helpful in developing clear and non-ambiguous standards and addressing the implementation of goals. For example, even though complete abstinence is a common goal for people changing their addictive behavior, this goal can make people vulnerable to the abstinence violation effect (AVE). The AVE occurs when an individual who has made a commitment to abstain has an initial lapse (engaging in a one-off use of a substance or behavior). If the person attributes the cause of this initial lapse to aspects of the self that are internal, global, and stable (e.g., lack of

strength or willpower) then a full relapse will likely follow (Marlatt & Gordon, 1985). Furthermore, the AVE can mean that self-monitoring of behavior against standards is abandoned. More recently, elements of Relapse Prevention have been integrated with mindfulness-based cognitive therapies in Mindfulness-Based Relapse Prevention (MBRP) (Bowen et al., 2010). In the treatment of addictive behaviors, MBRP has a foundation in formal meditation principles that fosters awareness of cognitions and emotions, triggers, destructive habitual patterns, and "automatic" reactions that are not aligned with standards and may lead to a failure of self-regulation.

Conclusion

Gambling disorder, now classified as an addiction and related disorder, shares many similarities with alcohol and substance misuse. This includes a similar course of persistent and recurrent problems that lead to significant impairment or harm to the individual. There are several models that explain the development and maintenance of disordered gambling, but these models are limited in terms of understanding the specific role of the self in gambling disorder. However, the self-regulation model can explain how gambling can develop into a problem through the lack of clear or defined standards, self-awareness and attention to monitoring, as well as insufficient self-control strength. Similar to alcohol and substance use, disordered gambling can be treated with MI and CBT approaches that can increase alignment between standards and the self and improve strength and willpower by improving self-efficacy and skills to manage relapse. There is promising initial evidence that targeting self-regulation can improve outcomes for alcohol and substance use, but more work is needed to understand how this model explains and predicts the development and recovery from disordered gambling.

References

Abar, B., Baumann, B. M., Rosenbaum, C., Boyer, E., & Boudreaux, E. D. (2012). Readiness to change alcohol and illicit drug use among a sample of emergency department patients. *Journal of Substance Use*, 17, 260–268.

Abar, B., Baumann, B. M., Rosenbaum, C., *et al.* (2013). Profiles of importance, readiness and confidence in quitting tobacco use. *Journal of Substance Use*, 18, 75–81.

American Psychiatric Association. (1987). *Diagnostic and Statistical Manual, 3rd Edition, Revised*. Washington, DC: American Psychiatric Association.

American Psychiatric Association. (1994). *Diagnostic and Statistical Manual of Mental Disorders (DSM-IV)*. Washington, DC: American Psychiatric Association.

American Psychiatric Association. (2013). *DSM 5*. Washington, DC: American Psychiatric Association.

Babor, T. (2010). *Alcohol: No Ordinary Commodity: Research and Public Policy*. Oxford: Oxford University Press.

Baumeister, R. F., & Heatherton, T. F. (1996). Self-regulation failure: An overview. *Psychological Inquiry*, 7(1), 1–15.

Baumeister, R. F., Heatherton, T. F., & Tice, D. M. (1994). *Losing Control: How and Why People Fail at Self-Regulation*. New York, NY: Academic Press.

Baumeister, R. F., & Vohs, K. D. (2007). Self-regulation, ego depletion, and motivation. *Social and Personality Psychology Compass*, 1, 115–128.

Baumeister, R. F., Vohs, K. D., & Tice, D. M. (2007). The strength model of self-control. *Current Directions in Psychological Science*, 16, 351 355.

Baumeister, R. F., & Vonasch, A. J. (2014). Uses of self-regulation to facilitate and restrain addictive behavior. *Addictive Behaviors*, 44, 3–8.

Beck, A. T. (1976). *Cognitive Therapy and the Emotional Disorders*. New York, NY: International Universities Press.

Beck, J. S. (1995). *Cognitive Therapy*: Chichester: Wiley Online Library.

Blaszczynski, A., Collins, P., Fong, D., *et al.* (2011). Responsible gambling: General principles and minimal requirements. *Journal of Gambling Studies*, 27, 565–573.

Bondy, S. J., Rehm, J., Ashley, M. J., *et al.* (1998). Low-risk drinking guidelines: The scientific evidence. *Canadian Journal of Public Health/Revue canadienne de sante publique*, 90, 264–270.

Bowen, S., Chawla, N., & Marlatt, G. A. (2010). *Mindfulness-Based Relapse Prevention for Addictive Behaviors: A Clinician's Guide*. New York, NY: Guilford Press.

Carver, C. S., & Scheier, M. F. (1982). Control theory: A useful conceptual framework for personality–social, clinical, and health psychology. *Psychological Bulletin*, 92, 111.

Christensen, D. R., Dowling, N. A., Jackson, A. C., & Thomas, S. A. (2014). Gambling participation and problem gambling severity in a stratified random survey: Findings from the Second Social and Economic Impact Study of Gambling in Tasmania. *Journal of Gambling Studies*, 1–19.

Ciarrocchi, J. W. (2001). *Counseling Problem Gamblers: A Self-Regulation Manual for Individual and Family Therapy*. New York, NY: Academic Press.

Cowlishaw, S., Merkouris, S., Dowling, N., *et al.* (2012). Psychological therapies for pathological and problem gambling. *Cochrane Database of Systematic Reviews*, 11, CD008937.

Cunningham, J. A., Hodgins, D. C., Toneatto, T., & Murphy, M. (2012). A randomized controlled trial of a personalized feedback intervention for problem gamblers. *PLoS ONE*, 7, e31586.

Cunningham, J. A., Hodgins, D. C., Toneatto, T., Rai, A., & Cordingley, J. (2009). Pilot study of a personalized feedback intervention for problem gamblers. *Behavior Therapy*, 40, 219 224.

Cunningham, J. A., Wild, T. C., Cordingley, J., Van Mierlo, T., & Humphreys, K. (2010). Twelve-month follow-up results from a randomized controlled trial of a brief personalized feedback intervention for problem drinkers. *Alcohol and Alcoholism*, 45, 258–262.

Currie, S. R., Hodgins, D. C., Casey, D. M., & El-Guebaly, N. (2012). Examining the predictive validity of low-risk gambling limits with longitudinal data. *Addiction*, 107, 400–406.

Currie, S. R., Hodgins, D. C., Wang, J., *et al.* (2006). Risk of harm among gamblers in the general population as a function of level of participation in gambling activities. *Addiction*, 101, 570–580.

Currie, S. R., Hodgins, D. C., Wang, J., *et al.* (2008). Replication of low-risk gambling limits using Canadian provincial gambling prevalence data. *Journal of Gambling Studies*, 24, 321–335.

DiClemente, C. C., & Hughes, S. O. (1990). Stages of change profiles in outpatient alcoholism treatment. *Journal of Substance Abuse*, 2, 217–235.

Dowling, N. (2013). Treatment of female problem gambling. In D. Richard, A. Blaszczynski, & L. Nower (Eds.), *The Wiley-Blackwell Handbook of Disordered Gambling* (pp. 225–250). Chichester: John Wiley and Sons, Ltd.

Dowling, N., & Smith, D. (2007). Treatment goal selection for female pathological gambling: A comparison of abstinence and controlled gambling. *Journal of Gambling Studies*, 23, 335–345.

Dowling, N., Smith, D., & Thomas, T. (2009). A preliminary investigation of abstinence and controlled gambling as self-selected goals of treatment for female pathological gambling. *Journal of Gambling Studies*, 25, 201–214.

Ferri, M., Amato, L., & Davoli, M. (2006). Alcoholics Anonymous and other 12-step programmes for alcohol dependence. *The Cochrane Library of Systematic Reviews*, 3, CD005032.

Foster, D. W., Neighbors, C., & Young, C. M. (2014). Drink refusal self-efficacy and implicit drinking identity: An evaluation of moderators of the relationship between self-awareness and drinking behavior. *Addictive Behaviors*, 39, 196–204.

Foster, D. W., Yeung, N., & Neighbors, C. (2014). I think I can't: Drink refusal self-efficacy as a mediator of the relationship between self-reported drinking identity and alcohol use. *Addictive Behaviors*, 39, 461–468.

Gainsbury, S. M., Blankers, M., Wilkinson, C., Schelleman-Offermans, K., & Cousijn, J. (2014). Recommendations for international gambling harm-minimisation guidelines: Comparison with effective public health policy. *Journal of Gambling Studies*, 30, 771–788.

Grant, J. E., Potenza, M. N., Weinstein, A., & Gorelick, D. A. (2010). Introduction to behavioral addictions. *The American Journal of Drug and Alcohol Abuse*, 36, 233–241.

Gray, H. M., LaPlante, D. A., Bannon, B. L., Ambady, N., & Shaffer, H. J. (2011). Development and validation of the Alcohol Identity Implicit Associations Test (AI-IAT). *Addictive Behaviors*, 36, 919–926.

Griffiths, M. D., Wood, R. T., & Parke, J. (2009). Social responsibility tools in online gambling: A survey of attitudes and behavior among internet gamblers. *Cyberpsychology & Behavior*, 12, 413–421.

Gustafson, D. H., Mctavish, F. M., Chih, M.-Y., et al. (2014). A smartphone application to support recovery from alcoholism: A randomized clinical trial. *JAMA Psychiatry*, 71, 566–572.

Hagger, M. S., Wood, C., Stiff, C., & Chatzisarantis, N. L. (2010). Ego depletion and the strength model of self-control: A meta-analysis. *Psychological Bulletin*, 136, 495.

Hing, N., Nuske, E., & Gainsbury, S. (2011). Gamblers at-risk and their help-seeking behaviour. Retrieved from http://www.gamblingresearch.org.au/home/research/gra+research+reports/ gamblers+at+risk+and+their+help+seeking+behaviour+(2011)

Hodgins, D. C. (2001). Processes of changing gambling behavior. *Addictive Behaviors*, 26, 121–128.

Hodgins, D. C., & El-Guebaly, N. (2000). Natural and treatment-assisted recovery from gambling problems: A comparison of resolved and active gamblers. *Addiction*, 95, 777–789.

Hull, J. G., & Young, R. D. (1983). Self-consciousness, self-esteem, and success–failure as determinants of alcohol consumption in male social drinkers. *Journal of Personality and Social Psychology*, 44, 1097.

Hull, J. G., Young, R. D., & Jouriles, E. (1986). Applications of the self-awareness model of alcohol consumption: Predicting patterns of use and abuse. *Journal of Personality and Social Psychology*, 51, 790.

Kypri, K., Hallett, J., Howat, P., et al. (2009). Randomized controlled trial of proactive web-based alcohol screening and brief intervention for university students. *Archives of Internal Medicine*, 169, 1508–1514.

Ladouceur, R., Lachance, S., & Fournier, P. (2009). Is control a viable goal in the treatment of pathological gambling? *Behaviour Research and Therapy*, 47, 189–197.

LaPlante, D. A., Nelson, S. E., Labrie, R. A., & Shaffer, H. J. (2008). Stability and progression of disordered gambling: Lessons from longitudinal studies. *The Canadian Journal of Psychiatry*, 53, 52–60.

Lostutter, T. W., Lewis, M. A., Cronce, J. M., Neighbors, C., & Larimer, M. E. (2014). The use of protective behaviors in relation to gambling among college students. *Journal of Gambling Studies*, 30, 27–46.

Lubman, D. I., Rodda, S. N., Hing, N., et al. (2015). *Gambler Self-Help Strategies: A Comprehensive Assessment of Self-Help Strategies and Actions*. Melbourne: Gambling Research Australia.

Marlatt, G., & Gordon, J. (Eds.). (1985). *Relapse Prevention: A Self-Control Strategy for the Maintenance of Behavior Change*. (pp. 85–101). New York, NY: Guilford.

Miller, W. R., & Rollnick, S. (2012). *Motivational Interviewing: Helping People Change*. New York, NY: Guilford Press.

Moore, S. M., Thomas, A. C., Kyrios, M., & Bates, G. (2012). The self-regulation of gambling. *Journal of Gambling Studies*, 28, 405–420.

Mullen, P. D., Simons-Morton, D. G., Ramírez, G., et al. (1997). A meta-analysis of trials evaluating patient education and counseling for three groups of preventive health behaviors. *Patient Education and Counseling*, 32, 157–173.

Muraven, M., Tice, D. M., & Baumeister, R. F. (1998). Self-control as a limited resource: Regulatory depletion patterns. *Journal of Personality and Social Psychology*, 74, 774.

Oaten, M., & Cheng, K. (2006). Longitudinal gains in self-regulation from regular physical exercise. *British Journal of Health Psychology*, 11, 717–733.

Petry, N. M. (2005). Stages of change in treatment-seeking pathological gamblers. *Journal of Consulting and Clinical Psychology*, 73(2), 312.

Prochaska, J. O., Diclemente, C. C., & Norcross, J. C. (1992). In search of how people change: Applications to addictive behaviors. *American Psychologist*, 47, 1102.

Productivity Commission. (2010). Gambling, report no. 50. Canberra.

Rodda, S. N., Lubman, D. I., Iyer, R., Gao, C., & Dowling, N. (2015). Subtyping based on readiness and confidence: The identification of help-seeking profiles for gamblers accessing web-based counselling. *Addiction*, 110, 494–501.

Room, R. (1996). Drinking patterns and drinking problems: From specifying the relationship to advising the public. *Addiction*, 91, 1441–1444.

Tait, R. J., Spijkerman, R., & Riper, H. (2013). Internet and computer based interventions for cannabis use: A meta-analysis. *Drug and Alcohol Dependence*, 133, 295–304.

Thomas, S. A., Merkouris, S. S., Radermacher, H. L., *et al.* (2011). An Australian guideline for treatment in problem gambling: An abridged outline. *Medical Journal of Australia*, 195(11), 664–665.

Toneatto, T. (2002). Cognitive therapy for problem gambling. *Cognitive and Behavioral Practice*, 9, 191–199.

Victorian Department of Justice. (2011). *The Victorian Gambling Study: A Longitudinal Study of Gambling and Public Health – Wave Two Findings.* Melbourne: Victorian Department of Justice.

Wechsler, H., Dowdall, G. W., Davenport, A., & Castillo, S. (1995). Correlates of college student binge drinking. *American Journal of Public Health*, 85, 921–926.

West, R. (2005). Time for a change: Putting the Transtheoretical (Stages of Change) Model to rest. *Addiction*, 100, 1036–1039.

White, H. R. (2006). Reduction of alcohol-related harm on United States college campuses: The use of personal feedback interventions. *International Journal of Drug Policy*, 17, 310–319.

Williams, R. J., Volberg, R. A., & Stevens, R. M. (2012). The population prevalence of problem gambling: Methodological influences, standardized rates, jurisdictional differences, and worldwide trends. Ontario Problem Gambling Research Centre.

Wohl, M. J., Gainsbury, S., Stewart, M. J., & Sztainert, T. (2013). Facilitating responsible gambling: The relative effectiveness of education-based animation and monetary limit setting pop-up messages among electronic gaming machine players. *Journal of Gambling Studies*, 29, 703–717.

Wohl, M. J., Young, M. M., & Hart, K. E. (2005). Untreated young gamblers with game-specific problems: Self-concept involving luck, gambling ecology and delay in seeking professional treatment. *Addiction Research & Theory*, 13, 445–459.

Chapter

15

The self in autism

Istvan Molnar-Szakacs and Lucina Q. Uddin

Introduction

Individuals with autism spectrum disorder (ASD) can exhibit profound social deficits which often manifest as difficulty with social interaction and communication with others, or *interpersonal* interaction. However, recent work has revealed increasing evidence for altered self-representation, or *intrapersonal* cognition in ASD. In this chapter we review recent studies of the self in ASD, with an emphasis on paradigms examining "physical" aspects of the self, including self-recognition, agency, and perspective-taking, and "psychological" aspects of the self, including self-knowledge and autobiographical memory. An emerging consensus is that psychological aspects of self-representation are altered in ASD to a greater extent than are physical aspects. A brain region that may be a potential locus of self-related deficits in ASD is the medial prefrontal cortex, part of the default mode network. Another brain system implicated in self-related processing in ASD is the mirror neuron system. Collectively, this body of neuroimaging work demonstrates that: (i) taking a systems-based approach to the study of brain disorders such as ASD can be informative beyond traditional localizationist approaches, and (ii) examining atypical self-related processing in ASD can provide a more comprehensive framework for understanding the complex social, cognitive, and affective symptomatology of the disorder.

ASD is a neurodevelopmental condition, which at its very core involves atypical self-representation. The term "autism" is derived from the Greek word "autos," meaning "self" or "directed from within." Kanner's early report describes how he was particularly struck by the solitary nature of the children he observed, whom he subsequently labeled with the term autism, which is still used today. Kanner's work describes several examples of extreme self-focus in children with autism. One child he observed "behaved as if people as such did not matter or even exist," and another gave "the impression of being self-absorbed." Of another child he wrote: "he got happiest when left alone, almost never cried to go to his mother, did not seem to notice his father's homecomings, and was indifferent to visiting relatives ... he seems to be self-satisfied ... to get his attention almost requires one to break down a mental barrier between his inner consciousness and the outside world" (Kanner, 1943). In more recent work, Frith and colleagues refer to this self-absorption as naïve egocentrism, and describe how it can be a source of difficulty in social interchange for individuals with ASD (U. Frith & de Vignemont, 2005).

Subsequent descriptions of ASD have emphasized social and communicative deficits, restricted interests, and repetitive behaviors (Lord *et al.*, 2000; Lord, Rutter, & Le Couteur, 1994). According to the recent DSM-5 diagnostic criteria, ASD is specifically characterized by deficits in social–emotional reciprocity, non-verbal communicative behaviors, and the ability to maintain relationships, along with stereotyped or repetitive motor movements, insistence on sameness, and fixated interests (APA, 2013). Surprisingly, nowhere in the current DSM-5 diagnostic criteria for ASD is the term "self" mentioned, although it is becoming increasingly evident that self-related cognition in individuals with ASD may be altered. In this chapter, we summarize recent empirical contributions providing insights into the nature

The Self in Understanding and Treating Psychological Disorders, ed. Michael Kyrios, Richard Moulding, Guy Doron, Sunil S. Bhar, Maja Nedeljkovic, and Mario Mikulincer. Published by Cambridge University Press. © Cambridge University Press, 2016.

of self-representation in autism, focusing primarily on studies that used neuroscientific approaches. We begin by briefly discussing what is meant by the multifaceted term "self" as used in neuroscience and psychology, and go on to review different aspects of the self that have been investigated in individuals with ASD.

The self in cognitive neuroscience and psychology

While the self is a hot topic in cognitive neuroscience and psychology, the term may be used to describe multiple different cognitive phenomena. William James wrote in *The Principles of Psychology* that the self is not a single primordial entity (James, 1983). This early conceptualization set the stage for examination of multiple facets of the self. Recently, cognitive neuroscientists and neuropsychologists, facilitated by developments in brain imaging technology, have undertaken the task of linking the self to its neural substrates. Researchers are asking which brain regions and systems are critical to different forms of self-related processing (for reviews see Molnar-Szakacs & Arzy, 2009; Molnar-Szakacs & Uddin, 2012, 2013; Uddin, 2011; Uddin, Iacoboni, Lange, & Keenan, 2007). The majority of modern theories of the self focus on one particular aspect, such as visual self-recognition or agency, and attempt to uncover the neural basis of that process (Jeannerod, 2003; Kelley *et al.*, 2002; Lieberman, 2007).

A particularly useful distinction first proposed by Gillihan and Farah (2005) is between *physical* and *psychological* aspects of the self. Physical aspects of the self are related to embodied cognition, and are typically examined in studies of self-face recognition, agency, and perspective-taking. Psychological aspects of the self tend to be operationalized with studies of autobiographical memory and self-knowledge in the form of personality traits. This conceptual distinction is borne out in neuroimaging work, which suggests that physical or embodied self-related processes and psychological or evaluative self-related processes rely on distinct but interacting, large-scale fronto-parietal brain networks (Lieberman, 2007; Uddin *et al.*, 2007). If the distinction of the self from others is a key aspect of social behavior and is a precursor of later conceptual self-development, it is of interest to investigate these functions in individuals with ASD. As a complete review of the concept of self and its various manifestations in psychological

literature is beyond the scope of this review, we will focus primarily on the paradigms mentioned above and highlight the current status of research examining these processes in individuals with ASD.

The physical and embodied self in autism

Self-face recognition

Face-processing abilities have been quite extensively characterized in behavioral studies of ASD (Jemel, Mottron, & Dawson, 2006). However, most neuroimaging studies of face perception in ASD have focused on emotion recognition, using unfamiliar faces, or faces of famous individuals, as stimuli. These early studies focused on the role of the fusiform gyrus, a cortical area specialized for face-processing (Kanwisher, McDermott, & Chun, 1997), and reported reductions in activity in the fusiform in individuals with ASD (Pierce, Muller, Ambrose, Allen, & Courchesne, 2001; Schultz *et al.*, 2000). However, subsequent studies did not replicate this finding of fusiform hypoactivity during face perception in autism (Hadjikhani *et al.*, 2004; Hadjikhani, Joseph, Snyder, & Tager-Flusberg, 2007).

While the aforementioned studies revealed possible alterations in facial information processing in individuals with ASD and in the associated neuronal circuitry, this early literature reflects a relatively strong focus on studying emotion recognition (Dawson, Webb, Carver, Panagiotides, & McPartland, 2004), rather than recognition of facial identity *per se*. Furthermore, some of the early results have not been replicated in later studies. Little empirical work has been devoted to examining brain responses to the self and close familiar others in autism, making it difficult to determine exactly to what extent this form of self-representation is altered in the disorder, and whether it is related more generally to other-face processing.

The ability to recognize oneself in the mirror has only been demonstrated in humans, chimpanzees (G. G. Gallup, 1970; Povinelli & Gallup, 1997), orangutans (Lethmate & Ducker, 1973), elephants (Plotnik, de Waal, & Reiss, 2006), and the bottlenose dolphin (Reiss & Marino, 2001). Evidence of the capacity for self-face recognition is thought to be indicative of an underlying self-concept (G. G. Gallup, Jr., 1977). Around two years of age, typically developing infants begin to show behavior indicating that they recognize themselves in the mirror (Amsterdam, 1972). Children with autism exhibit a developmental delay in the acquisition of this ability, although the majority of children that have been tested do eventually show evidence of self-recognition (Dawson & McKissick, 1984; Lind & Bowler, 2009; Spiker & Ricks, 1984).

The neural mechanisms subserving self-face recognition in ASD have recently been investigated in several imaging studies. An event-related potential (ERP) study examined brain responses to self, familiar, and unfamiliar faces in children with pervasive developmental disorder (PDD; this includes ASD). They found that children with PDD did not show significant differences in the early posterior negativity (EPN) or P300 components during viewing of self, familiar, or unfamiliar faces, whereas both the EPN and P300 responses in typically developing (TD) participants were enhanced in the self-face condition in comparison to the familiar-face condition (Gunji, Inagaki, Inoue, Takeshima, & Kaga, 2009). This work provides evidence for a reduced or even absent self-reference effect (i.e., enhanced memory for information encoded with reference to oneself) in patients with ASD.

One may hypothesize that this reduced sensitivity to "self" is related to the impaired attentional processing of self-referential stimuli. To test this hypothesis, a recent study investigated the neural correlates of face and name detection in ASD. Four categories of face/name stimuli were used: own, close-other, famous, and unknown. TD participants clearly showed a significant self-reference effect: higher P300 amplitude to the presentation of own face and own name than to the close-other, famous, and unknown categories, indicating preferential processing of self-related information. In contrast, detection of both own and close-other's face and name in the group with ASD was associated with enhanced P300, suggesting similar attention allocation for self and close-other related information. These findings suggest that the self-reference effect is absent in the participants with ASD when self is compared to close-other, indicating that attention allocation in this group is modulated by personal significance (Cygan, Tacikowski, Ostaszewski, Chojnicka, & Nowicka, 2014).

Using event-related functional magnetic resonance imaging (fMRI) to measure brain responses to images of the subjects' own face morphed with the faces of others, it was shown that while both TD children and children with ASD activated right inferior frontal gyrus when identifying images containing a greater percentage of their own face, TD children showed activation of this system during both self- and other-face processing. The groups did not demonstrate behavioral differences on the task, as both could perform the self–other discrimination and there were no significant group differences in reaction time. As children with ASD only recruited this system while viewing images containing mostly their own face, the authors concluded that children with ASD lack the shared neural representations for self and others that TD children possess (Uddin et al., 2008).

A near-infrared spectroscopy (NIRS) study also identified the right inferior frontal gyrus as being activated in response to self-faces in a group of children with ASD and TD males. This study additionally reported that children with the most severe symptoms showed lower activity in the right inferior frontal gyrus. These findings suggest that dysfunction in the right inferior frontal gyrus region, implicated across studies of self-face recognition (Devue & Bredart, 2011), may be one of the crucial neural substrates underlying ASD symptomatology (Kita et al., 2011).

Interestingly, the region of the inferior frontal gyrus is one of the anchors of the human mirror neuron system (MNS; for reviews see Iacoboni & Dapretto, 2006; Iacoboni & Mazziotta, 2007; Rizzolatti & Craighero, 2004; Uddin et al., 2007). The human MNS contains neurons with special properties that link what we see (perception) with what we do (action) and connect us to those around us by providing a neural substrate for meaningful social interaction (Gallese, Keysers, & Rizzolatti, 2004). Mirror neurons are active when we perform an action, and when we see that action being performed (Rizzolatti & Sinigaglia, 2010). By extension, when we observe the emotional states of others, we can feel the same emotion in empathy (Carr, Iacoboni, Dubeau, Mazziotta, & Lenzi, 2003; Gazzola, Aziz-Zadeh, & Keysers, 2006; Molnar-Szakacs & Overy, 2006). Based on this unique property of mirror neurons to internally simulate actions performed by others, it has been proposed that the MNS may provide the link between physical representations of the self and others (Molnar-Szakacs & Uddin, 2012, 2013; Uddin et al., 2007). Discussions of the human MNS generally refer to a network of regions, including the inferior frontal gyrus (IFG)/premotor cortex (PMC), the insular cortex (IC), primary sensory and primary motor cortices, the inferior parietal lobule (IPL), and the superior temporal sulcus (STS) (Iacoboni & Dapretto, 2006; Rizzolatti & Craighero, 2004).

Due to intense interest and study, the MNS in humans has already been associated with a wide variety of higher-level functions in addition to action representation, including imitation and imitation learning (Buccino et al., 2004; Iacoboni et al., 1999; Koski, Iacoboni, Dubeau, Woods, & Mazziotta, 2003; Molnar-Szakacs, Iacoboni, Koski, & Mazziotta, 2005), intention understanding (Gallese & Goldman, 1998; Iacoboni et al., 2005), empathy and theory of mind (ToM; Carr et al., 2003; Leslie, Johnson-Frey, & Grafton, 2004; J. H. Williams, Whiten, Suddendorf, & Perrett, 2001), self-representation (Molnar-Szakacs & Arzy, 2009; Uddin, Kaplan, Molnar-Szakacs, Zaidel, & Iacoboni, 2005; Uddin, Molnar-Szakacs, Zaidel, & Iacoboni, 2006), and the evolution of language (Arbib, 2005; Rizzolatti & Arbib, 1998). Interestingly, these cognitive functions subserved at least in part by the MNS – including imitation (Charman et al., 1997; J. H. Williams et al., 2001), empathy and ToM (Charman et al., 1997), self-representation (Lombardo, Barnes, Wheelwright, & Baron-Cohen, 2007), and language (Baltaxe & Simmons, 1977) – are all impaired to some extent in autism. In fact, dysfunction of the MNS has been proposed as a possible cause of autism (Iacoboni & Dapretto, 2006; Oberman & Ramachandran, 2007; J. H. Williams et al., 2001).

Aside from the studies described here, we have found no reports of the brain basis of self-face recognition abilities in autism, despite the strong emphasis on face perception in the autism neuroimaging literature. One recent behavioral study investigated the implicit access to physical self representation in children with ASD and in TD children. Participants were submitted to a visual matching-to-sample task with stimuli depicting their own or other people's body or face parts and were required to decide which of the two vertically aligned images matched the central target stimulus. The researchers found that children with ASD were less accurate compared to TD children. Interestingly, children with ASD performed the task better when they visually matched their own, compared to others', stimuli, showing the self-advantage effect, as well as TD children (Gessaroli, Andreini, Pellegri, & Frassinetti, 2013).

In similar neuroimaging studies, using familiar faces as stimuli, no difference in fusiform gyrus activity between children with autism and TD children was found (Pierce, Haist, Sedaghat, & Courchesne, 2004; Pierce & Redcay, 2008), suggesting that when controlling for factors such as facial familiarity and motivation (Pierce et al., 2004), attention (Hadjikhani et al., 2004), and gaze fixation (Dalton et al., 2005), the fusiform gyrus does appear to engage in individuals with ASD (Nomi & Uddin, 2015). While basic rapid face identification mechanisms appear to be functional in ASD, individuals with ASD failed to engage the subcortical brain regions involved in face detection and automatic emotional face processing, suggesting a core mechanism for impaired socio-emotional processing in ASD. Neural abnormalities in this system may contribute to early-emerging deficits in social orienting and attention, the putative precursors to abnormalities in social cognition and cortical face processing specialization (Kleinhans et al., 2011).

Agency and perspective-taking

Another physical manifestation of the self is the sense of agency, or ownership of one's actions (Gallagher, 2000). Behavioral work suggests that individuals with autism do not show deficits in action monitoring and attribution, despite significant impairments in mentalizing (David et al., 2008). David and colleagues have also demonstrated no impairments in visuospatial perspective-taking in adults with Asperger's syndrome (David et al., 2009). Williams and colleagues report that individuals with autism did not differ from typically developing individuals in finding it easier to monitor their own agency than to monitor the agency of the experimenter. Further, both groups showed a self-reference effect, in that they recalled their own actions better than those of the experimenter (D. Williams & Happe, 2009). These studies suggest that action monitoring and agency are relatively intact in individuals with ASD.

Most recently, Grainger and colleagues (2013) explored whether individuals with ASD experience difficulties with action monitoring. Two experimental tasks examined whether adults with ASD are able to monitor their own actions online, and whether they also show typical enactment effects in memory (enhanced memory for actions they have performed compared to actions they have observed being performed). Individuals with ASD and TD participants showed a similar pattern of performance on both tasks. When required to distinguish person-caused from computer-caused changes in phenomenology, both groups found it easier to monitor their own actions compared to those of an experimenter. Both groups also showed typical enactment effects, supporting earlier findings that action monitoring is unimpaired in ASD (Grainger, Williams, & Lind, 2013).

Intentional binding is an implicit way of measuring sense of agency. Intentional binding refers to the temporal attraction between a voluntary action and its outcome (Haggard, Clark, & Kalogeras, 2002) and is thought to result from predictive signals generated by the motor system. A recent study reports reduced intentional binding in ASD, which the authors suggest may be due to altered predictive mechanisms related to action planning and monitoring (Sperduti, Pieron, Leboyer, & Zalla, 2014). Whereas studies explicitly examining sense of agency in ASD have reported no deficits, this implicit measure of "pre-reflective" agency may reflect subtle deficits in self-monitoring in this population.

As we have discussed earlier, it has been suggested that the social symptoms of ASD could be caused in part by a dysfunctional MNS (Iacoboni & Dapretto, 2006). Furthermore, some of our functional imaging (Uddin et al., 2005) and transcranial magnetic stimulation (Uddin et al., 2006) work has shown that the right IPL, a brain area that is considered to be part of the human MNS, is involved in self-recognition and self–other discrimination tasks. If autism involves a dysfunctional MNS, and the MNS is necessary for self-awareness, then mirror neuron deficits could be one explanation for deficits in self-awareness seen in ASD (U. Frith & Happe, 1999). Because the recursive activity of a functioning MNS might enable the brain to integrate visual and motor sensations into a coherent body schema, the deficits in self-awareness often seen in ASD might be caused by the same mirror neuron dysfunction. Of note, however, other work examining the MNS in ASD has produced mixed results (Hamilton, 2013).

Root and colleagues (2014) studied CL, an autistic adolescent who is profoundly fascinated with his reflection, looking in mirrors at every opportunity. They demonstrated that CL's abnormal gait improved significantly when using a mirror for visual feedback. They also showed that both the fascination and the happiness that CL derived from looking at a computer-generated reflection diminished when a delay was introduced between the camera input and screen output. The authors believe that immediate, real-time visual feedback allows CL to integrate motor sensations with external visual ones into a coherent body schema that he cannot internally generate, perhaps due to a dysfunctional MNS (Root, Case, Burrus, & Ramachandran, 2015), as we have also previously proposed (Molnar-Szakacs & Uddin, 2012, 2013).

The majority of current research has found an intact sense of agency in individuals with autism using explicit judgments of agency (David et al., 2008). However, a recent study has revealed reduced intentional binding using implicit measures of agency (Sperduti et al., 2014). Taken together, these findings suggest that while there appears to be an intact explicit sense of agency, the diminished intentional binding in ASD participants might be due to altered predictive mechanisms, which are likely to be involved in action planning and monitoring. This explanation is in accordance with a large body of evidence documenting motor disturbances, as well as altered motor planning and action prediction, in individuals with ASD (Cattaneo et al., 2007; Martineau, Schmitz, Assaiante, Blanc, & Barthelemy, 2004; Nazarali, Glazebrook, & Elliott, 2009; Rinehart, Bradshaw, Brereton, & Tonge, 2001). In fact, a recent more general unifying theory put forth suggests that autism can be viewed as a disorder of prediction, and that several aspects of the autism phenotype may be manifestations of an underlying impairment in prediction abilities (Sinha et al., 2014). General sensorimotor impairments in autism have been documented in the domains of proprioception (Torres et al., 2013), gross and fine motor control (Bhat, Landa, & Galloway, 2011), and high-level motor planning (Gowen & Hamilton, 2013). How these deficits can contribute to specific aspects of physical self-related processing are currently under investigation. In particular, an "enactive account" (De Jaegher, 2013) posits that idiosyncratic ways in which individuals with ASD interact with the world can contribute to difficulties with self- and other-understanding.

To summarize, studies of the physical aspects of self-representation in individuals with ASD have revealed an intact ability for explicit face recognition, physical self–other distinction, and sense of agency. Further neuroimaging studies are required to explore this aspect of the disorder, as there is a dearth of empirical work on this topic. This need is further emphasized by findings that indicate some deficits in implicit aspects of physical self-recognition tasks, as well as tasks of agency that merit further exploration.

The psychological and evaluative self in autism

Personality traits

Self-related cognition of the evaluative type has been linked to a set of brain regions often termed "cortical midline structures" (Northoff & Bermpohl, 2004) or the "default mode network" (Gusnard, Akbudak, Shulman, & Raichle, 2001; Raichle *et al.*, 2001). Regions typically considered to belong to this system include the medial prefrontal cortex (MPFC), posterior cingulate cortex (PCC), IPL, and medial temporal lobes (MTL) (Greicius, Krasnow, Reiss, & Menon, 2003). While the MPFC and PCC are considered core "hubs" of the default mode network (DMN), some have suggested that the network can be fractionated into subcomponents. Recently, Salomon, Levy, and Malach (2013) have proposed that the inferior and posterior parietal aspects of the DMN can be further subdivided such that some show greater involvement in self-referential judgments than others (Salomon *et al.*, 2013). Andrews-Hanna and colleagues found that one subsystem including the dorsal MPFC, temporo-parietal junction, lateral temporal cortex, and temporal pole, is more engaged when individuals make self-referential judgments about their present situation or mental states, whereas a different subsystem comprised of the ventromedial prefrontal cortex (VMPFC), MTL, IPL, and retrosplenial cortex is more active during episodic judgments about the personal future (Andrews-Hanna, Reidler, Sepulcre, Poulin, & Buckner, 2010).

Additionally, the VMPFC shows activation during tasks requiring viewing of adjectives describing personality traits and judging whether or not they describe the self (Kelley *et al.*, 2002). Tasks involving self-knowledge generally activate the anterior region of the rostral medial frontal cortex, which is also an area engaged by mentalizing or ToM (Amodio & Frith, 2006). The observation that both self-related and social cognitive processes appear to overlap in this midline brain structure (Tamir & Mitchell, 2010) has lent credence to simulation theories positing that individuals may use their own minds to understand the minds of others (Gallese, 2003).

Lombardo and colleagues used a paradigm involving reflective mentalizing or physical judgments about the self and other to examine self-representation in adults with autism. They found that TD participants demonstrated greater activations in VMPFC for the self-judgments than for the other judgments. Individuals with autism, on the other hand, did not show differential responses during self and other judgments in this same region. In addition, they report reduced functional connectivity between the VMPFC and ventral premotor and somatosensory cortex in individuals with autism (Lombardo *et al.*, 2010). Furthermore, the magnitude of neural self–other distinction in VMPFC

was strongly related to the severity of early childhood social impairments in autism. Individuals whose VMPFC made the largest distinction between mentalizing about self and other were least socially impaired in early childhood, while those whose VMPFC made little to no distinction between mentalizing about self and other were the most socially impaired in early childhood. This study further points to functional abnormalities in the neural systems anchored in the MPFC that are associated with self-related evaluative processing.

In a study by Kennedy and colleagues, participants performed a task where they made true/false judgments for statements (describing either personality traits or observable external characteristics) about themselves or a close other person. Individuals with autism showed reduced activity in VMPFC across judgments involving both the self and other (Kennedy & Courchesne, 2008). In a recent study investigating self-appraisal across social and academic domains in ASD, Pfeifer and colleagues found hypoactivation of the VMPFC and insular cortex (IC) in children with the disorder. This study also found that stronger activity in the mid-cingulate cortex and IC during self-appraisals was associated with better social functioning in the ASD group (Pfeifer *et al.*, 2013). Taken together, these studies indicate a specificity in the deficit for neurally distinguishing self from other in ASD. Studies of social processing also point to medial prefrontal hypoactivity as a distinguishing feature of ASD. In an activation likelihood estimation meta-analysis of 24 neuroimaging studies examining social processing in ASD, it was also found that a region within the MPFC is hypoactive relative to TD adults (Di Martino *et al.*, 2009).

While these studies suggest that atypical engagement of the MPFC, and perhaps the larger DMN, is associated with altered self-related evaluative processing in ASD, growing literature supports the idea that in such a complex disorder, it is likely that atypical neural connectivity within and between large-scale brain networks, rather than focal deficits, underlie the symptoms (Belmonte *et al.*, 2004; Kana, Libero, & Moore, 2011; Kennedy & Adolphs, 2012; Minshew & Williams, 2007; Uddin & Menon, 2009). Several studies have found that functional connectivity of the DMN is reduced in adults and adolescents with the disorder (Assaf *et al.*, 2010; Cherkassky *et al.*, 2006; Kennedy *et al.*, 2006; Monk *et al.*, 2009; Weng *et al.*, 2010). However, contrary to what has been reported in adults and adolescents, childhood ASD may be characterized by greater instances of hyperconnectivity than hypoconnectivity (Supekar *et al.*, 2013; Uddin *et al.*, 2013). Most recently, Lynch and colleagues found that the PCC was hyperconnected with the medial and anterior temporal cortex in children with ASD, and this hyperconnectivity was linked with severity of social symptoms (Lynch *et al.*, 2013). This work lends further support to the notion that atypical patterns of DMN connectivity in ASD may lead to disrupted interactions at the neural level that could underlie social deficits in the disorder (Assaf *et al.*, 2010; Washington *et al.*, 2014).

We have recently proposed that simulation-based mechanisms of self- and other-understanding are supported by interactions of the human MNS with the DMN (Molnar-Szakacs & Uddin, 2012, 2013). These interactions produce the appropriate mappings to provide a coherent self-representation in the service of social-cognitive demands. Although the precise functional properties of the DMN are not yet established, a growing number of studies implicate this network in various aspects of self-related processing. For example, the DMN is implicated during self-related evaluations (Buckner & Carroll, 2007; Northoff *et al.*, 2006) and episodic and autobiographical memories (Sestieri, Corbetta, Romani, & Shulman, 2011; Spreng, Mar, & Kim, 2009).

Simulation-based representations serve to scaffold conceptual representations that allow us to understand the self in its social context. By virtue of their differential patterns of connectivity, subdivisions of the DMN can interact with the MNS. We proposed that two of the most important hubs for interaction between the DMN and MNS are the IC and the PCC, given their unique positions as "hubs" critical for information flow throughout the entire brain (Honey, Kotter, Breakspear, & Sporns, 2007; Menon & Uddin, 2010; Molnar-Szakacs & Uddin, 2013).

A recent meta-analysis of 87 self-related studies has lent further support to the view that high-level social cognitive processes such as mentalizing engage both the MPFC and circuitry involved in low-level embodied sensorimotor representations (Qin & Northoff, 2011). The role of somatosensory cortex in low-level shared representations of touch (Blakemore, Bristow, Bird, Frith, & Ward, 2005; Keysers *et al.*, 2004), self-experienced pain (Singer *et al.*, 2004), and action–perception mirroring (Gazzola *et al.*, 2006) is well established. Thus, the observation that the primary somatosensory cortex is also recruited for mentalizing about self and others suggests that low-level embodied simulative representations computed by

this region are also important for the processes underlying higher-level inference-based mentalizing when compared with reflecting on physical characteristics (Lombardo *et al.*, 2010). Taken together, these results provide strong evidence of the integration of function between the DMN and the MNS and suggest that disruptions to these inter-network interactions may underlie some of the self-related processing abnormalities in ASD (Uddin & Menon, 2009; Uddin *et al.*, 2014).

Alexithymia, or reduced ability to identify and describe one's emotions, often co-occurs with autism. Using functional neuroimaging, Silani and colleagues showed that high levels of alexithymia were associated with hypoactivation in the anterior insula in individuals with high-functioning autism (Silani *et al.*, 2008). Furthermore, there was a significant correlation between activity in the insular cortex not only with alexithymia scores, but also with scores on empathic concern and perspective-taking scales. In a more recent study, the same authors measured empathic brain responses in participants with ASD and neurotypical controls while they witnessed another person experiencing pain. The results were consistent with those of the original study, showing that the levels of alexithymia, but not a diagnosis of autism, were associated with the degree of empathic brain activation in anterior insula (Bird *et al.*, 2010). These results are important in showing that the empathy deficit widely attributed to ASD can be explained by the extent of alexithymic traits and does not necessarily constitute a universal social impairment in autism (Molnar-Szakacs & Heaton, 2012). These examples further highlight the ways in which self-representations (e.g., representations of one's own emotions) can relate to other-representations (e.g., empathy for another's pain) in ASD, and help us to better understand the precise nature of deficits in ASD.

Autobiographical memory and the temporally extended self

A critical aspect of self-related cognition is the ability to remember events from one's past. It has been suggested that individuals with autism experience difficulties with accessing specific autobiographical memories due to problems in using the self as an effective memory organizational system (Crane, Goddard, & Pring, 2009). In a study examining narratives of self-defining and everyday autobiographical memories in adults with ASD, it was shown that individuals with ASD generated fewer specific memories than TD controls. Individuals with ASD also extracted less meaning from their memories than controls, which the authors interpreted as a failure in using past experiences to update the self (Crane, Goddard, & Pring, 2010).

Bruck and colleagues report that children with ASD also have autobiographical memory recall that is marked by errors of omission, and that memory is particularly poor for early life events (Bruck, London, Landa, & Goodman, 2007). A recent case report examined the development of autobiographical memory in an 8-year-old boy with Asperger's syndrome. This child exhibited difficulties in strategic retrieval and ToM, as well as different patterns of performance with regards to autobiographical memory measured at three time points. The child showed (1) relative preservation of current year personal knowledge, but impairment for the previous and earlier years, and (2) impairment of episodic memory for the current and previous year, but performances similar to those of controls for the earlier years. The authors suggest that the abnormal functioning of social cognition in ASD, encompassing social, and personal points of view, has an impact on autobiographical memory (Bon *et al.*, 2012).

The most recent study on autobiographical memory in children with ASD has found that a deficit in specific memory retrieval in the ASD group was more characteristic of male participants. Females in both the TD and ASD groups generated more detailed and emotional memories than males. There was also evidence of enhanced recall of recent events in females with ASD as their recent memories were more detailed than their remote memories. Girls also demonstrated superior verbal fluency scores (Goddard *et al.*, 2014). Further research is required to study the developmental implications of these results on social behavior in children with ASD.

In neurotypical adults, autobiographical memory retrieval is associated with activation in the retrosplenial cortex and MPFC (Schacter & Addis, 2007), areas that are part of the DMN (Raichle *et al.*, 2001). A growing number of studies suggest the brain's default network becomes engaged when individuals recall their personal past or simulate their future (Buckner & Carroll, 2007; Molnar-Szakacs & Arzy, 2009). Recent reports of heterogeneity within the network raise the possibility that these autobiographical processes are comprised of multiple component processes, each supported by distinct functional–anatomic subsystems. Andrews-Hanna and colleagues hypothesized

that a medial temporal subsystem contributes to autobiographical memory and future thought by enabling individuals to retrieve prior information and bind this information into a mental scene, and conversely, a dorsal medial subsystem was proposed to support social-reflective aspects of autobiographical thought, allowing individuals to reflect on the mental states of one's self and others (i.e., "mentalizing"). They report that, across studies, laboratory-based episodic retrieval tasks were preferentially linked to the medial temporal subsystem, while mentalizing tasks were preferentially linked to the dorsal medial subsystem. In turn, autobiographical tasks engaged aspects of both subsystems. These results suggest the DMN is a heterogeneous brain system whose subsystems support distinct component processes of autobiographical thought (Andrews-Hanna, Saxe, & Yarkoni, 2014). Despite considerable evidence for impaired autobiographical memory in autism, no imaging studies of autobiographical memory in individuals with the disorder have yet been reported.

A recent set of reviews argue that individuals with ASD have reduced psychological self-knowledge resulting in a less elaborate self-concept. This is thought to contribute to impairments in autobiographical memory and a reduced self-reference effect. These deficits are thought to result in a diminished temporally extended self-concept in autism (Lind, 2010), specifically due to narrative memory deficits (Brezis, 2015).

Summary and conclusions

The studies summarized in this chapter suggest that while some aspects of physical and embodied self-representation are relatively intact in autism, there is still work to be done to understand the specific ways in which low-level sensorimotor processing abnormalities can lead to downstream difficulties in self-processing. Self-face recognition, agency, and perspective-taking studies in autism have not demonstrated explicit behavioral deficits in these abilities. Due to the small number of studies, however, we cannot rule out the possibility that there are implicit deficits that have not yet been revealed and may be hidden by effective compensatory strategies. Psychological and evaluative self-related cognition appears to be impaired to a greater extent in individuals with ASD. Despite a variety of methodological approaches and different operationalization of the "self," many studies on psychological aspects of the autistic self consistently point to a lack of differences between representations of self and other. Specifically, activity in the VMPFC, part of a larger default mode network which supports self-knowledge and autobiographical memory in typically developing adults, may be altered in the disorder. More generally, theory of mind impairments have been documented in autism over the past 25 years (Baron-Cohen, Leslie, & Frith, 1985), and the ability is also thought to rely on the MPFC (C. D. Frith & Frith, 1999).

In a meta-analysis of 24 studies examining social information processing in autism, Di Martino and colleagues (2009) found that the anterior cingulate cortex and IC were consistently reported as hypoactive in social information-processing tasks among individuals with ASD. The IC is essential to interoceptive self-referential processing and contributes to the phylogenetic and ontogenetic emergence of self-awareness (Bud Craig, 2009). Uddin and Menon (2009) have subsequently suggested that the anterior insula, most likely in conjunction with the anterior cingulate, serves as a hub mediating interactions between large scale brain networks that are "involved in externally oriented attention and internally oriented cognitive processes." It is likely that many of the same aberrant patterns of brain activity underlying impaired social cognitive abilities in autism may contribute to the deficits in self-related processing described here. In fact, it has been proposed that an early, chronic disturbance in the capacity for integrating self- and other-referenced information may have cascading effects on the development of self-awareness in autism (Mundy, Gwaltney, & Henderson, 2010).

Currently, there is a dearth of neuroimaging studies investigating self-recognition, agency, perspective-taking, autobiographical memory, and other forms of self-related cognition in autism, in stark contrast to the large body of literature examining social and interpersonal cognition in the disorder (Itier & Batty, 2009; Pelphrey, Adolphs, & Morris, 2004). As greater awareness of alterations in self-related cognition permeates throughout the field of autism research, and greater emphasis is placed on understanding these alterations as they relate to social cognition in ASD, we can expect increasingly sophisticated insights into the neural basis of the self in the disorder.

Directions for future research include neuroimaging studies designed to more closely examine autobiographical memory and self-knowledge deficits in ASD, which could be related to integrity of the default mode network. Bringing together behavioral approaches to studying self-related cognition with imaging methods will ultimately lead to a more complete understanding of the nature of the self and self-processing in ASD. Future research should consider that: (i) taking a systems-based approach to the study of brain disorders such as ASD can be informative beyond traditional localizationist approaches, and (ii) examining relatively "simple" self-related processing deficits in ASD can provide a more comprehensive framework for understanding the "complex" social, cognitive, and affective symptomatology of the disorder.

Acknowledgments
This work was supported by K01MH092288 from the National Institute of Mental Health (LQU). The content is solely the responsibility of the author and does not necessarily represent the official views of the NIMH or the NIH.

References
Amodio, D. M., & Frith, C. D. (2006). Meeting of minds: The medial frontal cortex and social cognition. *Nature Reviews Neuroscience*, 7(4), 268–277.

Amsterdam, B. (1972). Mirror self-image reactions before age two. *Developmental Psychobiology*, 5(4), 297–305.

Andrews-Hanna, J. R., Reidler, J. S., Sepulcre, J., Poulin, R., & Buckner, R. L. (2010). Functional–anatomic fractionation of the brain's default network. *Neuron*, 65(4), 550–562.

Andrews-Hanna, J. R., Saxe, R., & Yarkoni, T. (2014). Contributions of episodic retrieval and mentalizing to autobiographical thought: Evidence from functional neuroimaging, resting-state connectivity, and fMRI meta-analyses. *Neuroimage*, 91, 324–335.

APA. (2013). *Diagnostic and Statistical Manual of Mental Disorders* (5th ed.). Arlington, VA: American Psychiatric Publishing.

Arbib, M. A. (2005). From monkey-like action recognition to human language: An evolutionary framework for neurolinguistics. *The Behavioral and Brain Sciences*, 28(2), 105–124; discussion 125–167.

Assaf, M., Jagannathan, K., Calhoun, V. D., *et al.* (2010). Abnormal functional connectivity of default mode sub-networks in autism spectrum disorder patients. *Neuroimage*, 53(1), 247–256.

Baltaxe, C. A., & Simmons, J. Q. (1977). Bedtime soliloquies and linguistic competence in autism. *Journal of Speech and Hearing Disorders*, 42(3), 376–393.

Baron-Cohen, S., Leslie, A. M., & Frith, U. (1985). Does the autistic child have a "theory of mind"? *Cognition*, 21(1), 37–46.

Belmonte, M. K., Allen, G., Beckel-Mitchener, A., *et al.* (2004). Autism and abnormal development of brain connectivity. *Journal of Neuroscience*, 24(42), 9228–9231.

Bhat, A. N., Landa, R. J., & Galloway, J. C. (2011). Current perspectives on motor functioning in infants, children, and adults with autism spectrum disorders. *Physical Therapies*, 91(7), 1116–1129.

Bird, G., Silani, G., Brindley, R., *et al.* (2010). Empathic brain responses in insula are modulated by levels of alexithymia but not autism. *Brain*, 133(Pt 5), 1515–1525.

Blakemore, S. J., Bristow, D., Bird, G., Frith, C., & Ward, J. (2005). Somatosensory activations during the observation of touch and a case of vision–touch synaesthesia. *Brain*, 128(Pt 7), 1571–1583.

Bon, L., Baleyte, J. M., Piolino, P., *et al.* (2012). Growing up with Asperger's Syndrome: Developmental trajectory of autobiographical memory. *Frontiers in Psychology*, 3, 605.

Brezis, R. S. (2015). Memory integration in the autobiographical narratives of individuals with autism. *Frontiers in Human Neuroscience*, 9, 76

Bruck, M., London, K., Landa, R., & Goodman, J. (2007). Autobiographical memory and suggestibility in children with autism spectrum disorder. *Developmental Psychopathology*, 19(1), 73–95.

Buccino, G., Vogt, S., Ritzl, A., *et al.* (2004). Neural circuits underlying imitation learning of hand actions: An event-related fMRI study. *Neuron*, 42(2), 323–334.

Buckner, R. L., & Carroll, D. C. (2007). Self-projection and the brain. *Trends in Cognitive Science*, 11(2), 49–57.

Bud Craig, A. D. (2009). How do you feel – now? The anterior insula and human awareness. *Nature Reviews Neuroscience*, 10(1), 59–70.

Carr, L., Iacoboni, M., Dubeau, M. C., Mazziotta, J. C., & Lenzi, G. L. (2003). Neural mechanisms of empathy in humans: A relay from neural systems for imitation to limbic areas. *Proceedings of the National Academy of Sciences of the USA*, 100(9), 5497–5502.

Cattaneo, L., Fabbri-Destro, M., Boria, S., *et al.* (2007). Impairment of actions chains in autism and its possible role in intention understanding. *Proceedings of the National Academy of Sciences of the USA*, 104(45), 17825–17830.

Charman, T., Swettenham, J., Baron-Cohen, S., *et al.* (1997). Infants with autism: An investigation of empathy, pretend play, joint attention, and imitation. *Developmental Psychology*, 33(5), 781–789.

Cherkassky, V. L., Kana, R. K., Keller, T. A., & Just, M. A. (2006). Functional connectivity in a baseline resting-state network in autism. *Neuroreport*, 17(16), 1687–1690.

Crane, L., Goddard, L., & Pring, L. (2009). Specific and general autobiographical knowledge in adults with autism spectrum disorders: the role of personal goals. *Memory*, 17(5), 557–576.

Crane, L., Goddard, L., & Pring, L. (2010). Brief report: Self-defining and everyday autobiographical memories in adults with autism spectrum disorders. *Journal of Autism and Developmental Disorders*, 40(3), 383–391.

Cygan, H. B., Tacikowski, P., Ostaszewski, P., Chojnicka, I., & Nowicka, A. (2014). Neural correlates of own name and own face detection in autism spectrum disorder. *PLoS ONE*, 9(1), e86020.

Dalton, K. M., Nacewicz, B. M., Johnstone, T., *et al.* (2005). Gaze fixation and the neural circuitry of face processing in autism. *Nature Neuroscience*, 8(4), 519–526.

David, N., Aumann, C., Bewernick, B. H., *et al.* (2009). Investigation of mentalizing and visuospatial perspective taking for self and other in Asperger syndrome. *Journal of Autism and Developmental Disorders*, 40(3), 290–299.

David, N., Gawronski, A., Santos, N. S., *et al.* (2008). Dissociation between key processes of social cognition in autism: Impaired mentalizing but intact sense of agency. *Journal of Autism and Developmental Disorders*, 38(4), 593–605.

Dawson, G., & McKissick, F. C. (1984). Self-recognition in autistic children. *Journal of Autism and Developmental Disorders*, 14(4), 383–394.

Dawson, G., Webb, S. J., Carver, L., Panagiotides, H., & McPartland, J. (2004). Young children with autism show atypical brain responses to fearful versus neutral facial expressions of emotion. *Developmental Science*, 7(3), 340–359.

De Jaegher, H. (2013). Embodiment and sense-making in autism. *Frontiers in Integrated Neuroscience*, 7, 15.

Devue, C., & Bredart, S. (2011). The neural correlates of visual self-recognition. *Conscious Cognition*, 20(1), 40–51.

Di Martino, A., Ross, K., Uddin, L. Q., *et al.* (2009). Functional brain correlates of social and nonsocial processes in autism spectrum disorders: An activation likelihood estimation meta-analysis. *Biological Psychiatry*, 65(1), 63–74.

Frith, C. D., & Frith, U. (1999). Interacting minds – A biological basis. *Science*, 286(5445), 1692–1695.

Frith, U., & de Vignemont, F. (2005). Egocentrism, allocentrism, and Asperger syndrome. *Conscious Cognition*, 14(4), 719–738.

Frith, U., & Happe, F. (1999). Theory of mind and self-consciousness: What is it like to be autistic? *Mind & Language*, 14(1), 82–89.

Gallagher, S. (2000). Philosophical conceptions of the self: Implications for cognitive science. *Trends in Cognitive Sciences*, 4(1), 14–21.

Gallese, V. (2003). The roots of empathy: The shared manifold hypothesis and the neural basis of intersubjectivity. *Psychopathology*, 36(4), 171–180.

Gallese, V., & Goldman, A. (1998). Mirror neurons and the simulation theory of mind-reading. *Trends in Cognitive Science*, 2(12), 493–501.

Gallese, V., Keysers, C., & Rizzolatti, G. (2004). A unifying view of the basis of social cognition. *Trends in Cognitive Science*, 8(9), 396–403.

Gallup, G. G. (1970). Chimpanzees: Self-recognition. *Science*, 167, 86–87.

Gallup, G. G., Jr. (1977). Self-recognition in primates: A comparative approach to the bidirectional properties of consciousness. *American Psychologist*, 32(5), 329–338.

Gazzola, V., Aziz-Zadeh, L., & Keysers, C. (2006). Empathy and the somatotopic auditory mirror system in humans. *Current Biology*, 16(18), 1824–1829.

Gessaroli, E., Andreini, V., Pellegri, E., & Frassinetti, F. (2013). Self-face and self-body recognition in autism. *Research in Autism Spectrum Disorders*, 7, 793–800.

Gillihan, S. J., & Farah, M. J. (2005). Is self special? A critical review of evidence from experimental psychology and cognitive neuroscience. *Psychology Bulletin*, 131(1), 76–97.

Goddard, L., Dritschel, B., Robinson, S., & Howlin, P. (2014). Development of autobiographical memory in children with autism spectrum disorders: Deficits, gains, and predictors of performance. *Development and Psychopathology*, 26(1), 215–228.

Gowen, E., & Hamilton, A. (2013). Motor abilities in autism: A review using a computational context. *Journal of Autism and Developmental Disorders*, 43(2), 323–344.

Grainger, C., Williams, D. M., & Lind, S. E. (2013). Online action monitoring and memory for self-performed actions in autism spectrum disorder. *Journal of Autism and Developmental Disorders*, 44(5), 1193–1206.

Greicius, M. D., Krasnow, B., Reiss, A. L., & Menon, V. (2003). Functional connectivity in the resting brain: A network analysis of the default mode hypothesis. *Proceedings of the National Academy of Sciences of the USA*, 100(1), 253–258.

Gunji, A., Inagaki, M., Inoue, Y., Takeshima, Y., & Kaga, M. (2009). Event-related potentials of self-face recognition in children with pervasive developmental disorders. *Brain Development*, 31(2), 139–147.

Gusnard, D. A., Akbudak, E., Shulman, G. L., & Raichle, M. E. (2001). Medial prefrontal cortex and self-referential mental activity: Relation to a default mode of brain function. *Proceedings of the National Academy of Sciences of the USA*, 98(7), 4259–4264.

Hadjikhani, N., Joseph, R. M., Snyder, J., et al. (2004). Activation of the fusiform gyrus when individuals with autism spectrum disorder view faces. *Neuroimage*, 22(3), 1141–1150.

Hadjikhani, N., Joseph, R. M., Snyder, J., & Tager-Flusberg, H. (2007). Abnormal activation of the social brain during face perception in autism. *Human Brain Mapping*, 28(5), 441–449.

Haggard, P., Clark, S., & Kalogeras, J. (2002). Voluntary action and conscious awareness. *Nature Neuroscience*, 5(4), 382–385.

Hamilton, A. F. (2013). Reflecting on the mirror neuron system in autism: A systematic review of current theories. *Developmental and Cognitive Neuroscience*, 3, 91–105.

Honey, C. J., Kotter, R., Breakspear, M., & Sporns, O. (2007). Network structure of cerebral cortex shapes functional connectivity on multiple time scales. *Proceedings of the National Academy of Sciences of the USA*, 104(24), 10240–10245.

Iacoboni, M., & Dapretto, M. (2006). The mirror neuron system and the consequences of its dysfunction. *Nature Reviews in Neuroscience*, 7(12), 942–951.

Iacoboni, M., & Mazziotta, J. C. (2007). Mirror neuron system: Basic findings and clinical applications. *Annals of Neurology*, 62(3), 213–218.

Iacoboni, M., Molnar-Szakacs, I., Gallese, V., et al. (2005). Grasping the intentions of others with one's own mirror neuron system. *PLoS Biology*, 3(3), e79.

Iacoboni, M., Woods, R. P., Brass, M., et al. (1999). Cortical mechanisms of human imitation. *Science*, 286(5449), 2526–2528.

Itier, R. J., & Batty, M. (2009). Neural bases of eye and gaze processing: The core of social cognition. *Neuroscience and Biobehavioral Reviews*, 33(6), 843–863.

James, W. (1983). *The Principles of Psychology*. Cambridge, MA: Harvard University Press.

Jeannerod, M. (2003). The mechanism of self-recognition in humans. *Behavior and Brain Research*, 142(1–2), 1–15.

Jemel, B., Mottron, L., & Dawson, M. (2006). Impaired face processing in autism: Fact or artifact? *Journal of Autism and Developmental Disorders*, 36(1), 91–106.

Kana, R. K., Libero, L. E., & Moore, M. S. (2011). Disrupted cortical connectivity theory as an explanatory model for autism spectrum disorders. *Physics of Life Reviews*, 8(4), 410–437.

Kanner, L. (1943). Autistic disturbances of affective contact. *Nervous Child*, 2, 217–250.

Kanwisher, N., McDermott, J., & Chun, M. M. (1997). The fusiform face area: A module in human extrastriate cortex specialized for face perception. *Journal of Neuroscience*, 17(11), 4302–4311.

Kelley, W. M., Macrae, C. N., Wyland, C. L., *et al.* (2002). Finding the self? An event-related fMRI study. *Journal of Cognitive Neuroscience*, 14(5), 785–794.

Kennedy, D. P., & Adolphs, R. (2012). The social brain in psychiatric and neurological disorders. *Trends in Cognitive Science*, 16(11), 559–572.

Kennedy, D. P., & Courchesne, E. (2008). Functional abnormalities of the default network during self- and other-reflection in autism. *Social Cognition and Affective Neuroscience*, 3(2), 177–190.

Kennedy, D. P., Redcay, E., & Courchesne, E. (2006). Failing to deactivate: Resting functional abnormalities in autism. *Proceedings of the National Academy of Sciences*, 103(21), 8275–8280.

Keysers, C., Wicker, B., Gazzola, V., *et al.* (2004). A touching sight: SII/PV activation during the observation and experience of touch. *Neuron*, 42(2), 335–346.

Kita, Y., Gunji, A., Inoue, Y., *et al.* (2011). Self-face recognition in children with autism spectrum disorders: A near-infrared spectroscopy study. *Brain and Development*, 33(6), 494–503.

Kleinhans, N. M., Richards, T., Johnson, L. C., *et al.* (2011). fMRI evidence of neural abnormalities in the subcortical face processing system in ASD. *Neuroimage*, 54(1), 697–704.

Koski, L., Iacoboni, M., Dubeau, M. C., Woods, R. P., & Mazziotta, J. C. (2003). Modulation of cortical activity during different imitative behaviors. *Journal of Neurophysiology*, 89(1), 460–471.

Leslie, K. R., Johnson-Frey, S. H., & Grafton, S. T. (2004). Functional imaging of face and hand imitation: Towards a motor theory of empathy. *Neuroimage*, 21(2), 601–607.

Lethmate, J., & Ducker, G. (1973). [Studies on self-recognition in a mirror in orang-utans, chimpanzees, gibbons and various other monkey species]. *Zeitschrift für Tierpsychologie*, 33(3), 248–269.

Lieberman, M. D. (2007). Social cognitive neuroscience: A review of core processes. *Annual Review of Psychology*, 58, 259–289.

Lind, S. E. (2010). Memory and the self in autism: A review and theoretical framework. *Autism*, 14(5), 430–456.

Lind, S. E., & Bowler, D. M. (2009). Delayed self-recognition in children with autism spectrum disorder. *Journal of Autism and Developmental Disorders*, 39(4), 643–650.

Lombardo, M. V., Barnes, J. L., Wheelwright, S. J., & Baron-Cohen, S. (2007). Self-referential cognition and empathy in autism. *PLoS ONE*, 2(9), e883.

Lombardo, M. V., Chakrabarti, B., Bullmore, E. T., *et al.* (2010). Atypical neural self-representation in autism. *Brain*, 133(Pt 2), 611–624.

Lord, C., Risi, S., Lambrecht, L., *et al.* (2000). The autism diagnostic observation schedule-generic: A standard measure of social and communication deficits associated with the spectrum of autism. *Journal of Autism and Developmental Disorders*, 30(3), 205–223.

Lord, C., Rutter, M., & Le Couteur, A. (1994). Autism Diagnostic Interview – Revised: A revised version of a diagnostic interview for caregivers of individuals with possible pervasive developmental disorders. *Journal of Autism and Developmental Disorders*, 24(5), 659–685.

Lynch, C. J., Uddin, L. Q., Supekar, K., *et al.* (2013). Default mode network in childhood autism: Posteromedial cortex heterogeneity and relationship with social deficits. *Biological Psychiatry*, 74(3), 212–219.

Martineau, J., Schmitz, C., Assaiante, C., Blanc, R., & Barthelemy, C. (2004). Impairment of a cortical event-related desynchronisation during a bimanual load-lifting task in children with autistic disorder. *Neuroscience Letters*, 367(3), 298–303.

Menon, V., & Uddin, L. Q. (2010). Saliency, switching, attention and control: A network model of insula function. *Brain Structure and Function*, 214(5–6), 655–667.

Minshew, N. J., & Williams, D. L. (2007). The new neurobiology of autism: Cortex, connectivity, and neuronal organization. *Archives of Neurology*, 64(7), 945–950.

Molnar-Szakacs, I., & Arzy, S. (2009). Searching for an integrated self-representation. *Communications in Integrated Biology*, 2(4), 365–367.

Molnar-Szakacs, I., & Heaton, P. (2012). Music: A unique window into the world of autism. *Annals of the New York Academy of Sciences*, 1252, 318–324.

Molnar-Szakacs, I., Iacoboni, M., Koski, L., & Mazziotta, J. C. (2005). Functional segregation within pars opercularis of the inferior frontal gyrus: Evidence from fMRI studies of imitation and action observation. *Cerebral Cortex*, 15(7), 986–994.

Molnar-Szakacs, I., & Overy, K. (2006). Music and mirror neurons: From motion to 'e'motion. *Social Cognitive Affective Neuroscience*, 1(3), 235–241.

Molnar-Szakacs, I., & Uddin, L. Q. (2012). The emergent self: How distributed neural networks support self-representation. In D. D. Franks & J. H. Turner (Eds.), *Handbook of Neurosociology*: New York, NY: Springer.

Molnar-Szakacs, I., & Uddin, L. Q. (2013). Self-processing and the default mode network: Interactions with the mirror neuron system. *Frontiers in Human Neuroscience*, 7, 571.

Monk, C. S., Peltier, S. J., Wiggins, J. L., *et al.* (2009). Abnormalities of intrinsic functional connectivity in autism spectrum disorders. *Neuroimage*, 47(2), 764–772.

Mundy, P., Gwaltney, M., & Henderson, H. (2010). Self-referenced processing, neurodevelopment and joint attention in autism. *Autism*, 14(5), 408–429.

Nazarali, N., Glazebrook, C. M., & Elliott, D. (2009). Movement planning and reprogramming in individuals with autism. *Journal of Autism and Developmental Disorders*, 39(10), 1401–1411.

Nomi, J. S., & Uddin, L. Q. (2015). Face processing in autism spectrum disorders: From brain regions to brain networks. *Neuropsychologia*, 71, 201–216.

Northoff, G., & Bermpohl, F. (2004). Cortical midline structures and the self. *Trends in Cognitive Science*, 8(3), 102–107.

Northoff, G., Heinzel, A., de Greck, M., *et al.* (2006). Self-referential processing in our brain – A meta-analysis of imaging studies on the self. *Neuroimage*, 31(1), 440–457.

Oberman, L. M., & Ramachandran, V. S. (2007). The simulating social mind: The role of the mirror neuron system and simulation in the social and communicative deficits of autism spectrum disorders. *Psychology Bulletin*, 133(2), 310–327.

Pelphrey, K., Adolphs, R., & Morris, J. P. (2004). Neuroanatomical substrates of social cognition dysfunction in autism. *Mental Retardation and Developmental Disabilities Research Review*, 10(4), 259–271.

Pfeifer, J. H., Merchant, J. S., Colich, N. L., *et al.* (2013). Neural and behavioral responses during self-evaluative processes differ in youth with and without autism. *Journal of Autism and Developmental Disorders*, 43(2), 272–285.

Pierce, K., Haist, F., Sedaghat, F., & Courchesne, E. (2004). The brain response to personally familiar faces in autism: Findings of fusiform activity and beyond. *Brain*, 127(Pt 12), 2703–2716.

Pierce, K., Muller, R. A., Ambrose, J., Allen, G., & Courchesne, E. (2001). Face processing occurs outside the fusiform 'face area' in autism: Evidence from functional MRI. *Brain*, 124(Pt 10), 2059–2073.

Pierce, K., & Redcay, E. (2008). Fusiform function in children with an autism spectrum disorder is a matter of "who". *Biological Psychiatry*, 64(7), 552–560.

Plotnik, J. M., de Waal, F. B., & Reiss, D. (2006). Self-recognition in an Asian elephant. *Proceedings of the National Academy of Science of the USA*, 103(45), 17053–17057.

Povinelli, D. J., & Gallup, G. G., Jr. (1997). Chimpanzees recognize themselves in mirrors. *Animal Behavior*, 53, 1083–1088.

Qin, P., & Northoff, G. (2011). How is our self related to midline regions and the default-mode network? *Neuroimage*, 57(3), 1221–1233.

Raichle, M. E., MacLeod, A. M., Snyder, A. Z., *et al.* (2001). A default mode of brain function. *Proceedings of the National Academy of Science of the USA*, 98(2), 676–682.

Reiss, D., & Marino, L. (2001). Mirror self-recognition in the bottlenose dolphin: A case of cognitive convergence. *Proceedings of the National Academy of Science of the USA*, 98(10), 5937–5942.

Rinehart, N. J., Bradshaw, J. L., Brereton, A. V., & Tonge, B. J. (2001). Movement preparation in high-functioning autism and Asperger disorder: A serial choice reaction time task involving motor reprogramming. *Journal of Autism and Developmental Disorders*, 31(1), 79–88.

Rizzolatti, G., & Arbib, M. A. (1998). Language within our grasp. *Trends in Neuroscience*, 21(5), 188–194.

Rizzolatti, G., & Craighero, L. (2004). The mirror-neuron system. *Annual Review of Neuroscience*, 27, 169–192.

Rizzolatti, G., & Sinigaglia, C. (2010). The functional role of the parieto-frontal mirror circuit: Interpretations and misinterpretations. *Nature Reviews Neuroscience*, 11(4), 264–274.

Root, N. B., Case, L. K., Burrus, C. J., & Ramachandran, V. S. (2015). External self-representations improve self-awareness in a child with autism. *Neurocase*, 21(2), 206–210.

Salomon, R., Levy, D. R., & Malach, R. (2014). Deconstructing the default: Cortical subdivision of the default mode/intrinsic system during self-related processing. *Human Brain Mapping*, 35(4), 1491–1502.

Schacter, D. L., & Addis, D. R. (2007). The cognitive neuroscience of constructive memory: Remembering the past and imagining the future. *Philosophical Transactions of the Royal Society of London, Series B Biological Science*, 362(1481), 773–786.

Schultz, R. T., Gauthier, I., Klin, A., *et al.* (2000). Abnormal ventral temporal cortical activity during face discrimination among individuals with autism and Asperger syndrome. *Archives of General Psychiatry*, 57(4), 331–340.

Sestieri, C., Corbetta, M., Romani, G. L., & Shulman, G. L. (2011). Episodic memory retrieval, parietal cortex, and the default mode network: Functional and topographic analyses. *Journal of Neuroscience*, 31(12), 4407–4420.

Silani, G., Bird, G., Brindley, R., *et al.* (2008). Levels of emotional awareness and autism: An fMRI study. *Social Neuroscience*, 3(2), 97–112.

Singer, T., Seymour, B., O'Doherty, J., *et al.* (2004). Empathy for pain involves the affective but not sensory components of pain. *Science*, 303(5661), 1157–1162.

Sinha, P., Kjelgaard, M. M., Gandhi, T. K., *et al.* (2014). Autism as a disorder of prediction. *Proceedings of the National Academy of Science of the USA,* 111(42), 15220–15225.

Sperduti, M., Pieron, M., Leboyer, M., & Zalla, T. (2014). Altered pre-reflective sense of agency in autism spectrum disorders as revealed by reduced intentional binding. *Journal of Autism and Developmental Disorders*, 44(2), 343–352.

Spiker, D., & Ricks, M. (1984). Visual self-recognition in autistic children: Developmental relationships. *Child Development*, 55(1), 214–225.

Spreng, R. N., Mar, R. A., & Kim, A. S. (2009). The common neural basis of autobiographical memory, prospection, navigation, theory of mind, and the default mode: A quantitative meta-analysis. *Journal of Cognitive Neuroscience*, 21(3), 489–510.

Supekar, K., Uddin, L. Q., Khouzam, A., *et al.* (2013). Brain hyperconnectivity in children with autism and its links to social deficits. *Cell Reports*, 5(3), 738–747.

Tamir, D. I., & Mitchell, J. P. (2010). Neural correlates of anchoring-and-adjustment during mentalizing. *Proceedings of the National Academy of Science of the USA*, 107(24), 10827–10832.

Torres, E. B., Brincker, M., Isenhower, R. W., *et al.* (2013). Autism: The micro-movement perspective. *Frontiers in Integrated Neuroscience*, 7, 32.

Uddin, L. Q. (2011). The self in autism: An emerging view from neuroimaging. *Neurocase*, 17(3), 201–208.

Uddin, L. Q., Davies, M. S., Scott, A. A., *et al.* (2008). Neural basis of self and other representation in autism: An FMRI study of self-face recognition. *PLoS ONE*, 3(10), e3526.

Uddin, L. Q., Iacoboni, M., Lange, C., & Keenan, J. P. (2007). The self and social cognition: The role of cortical midline structures and mirror neurons. *Trends in Cognitive Science,* 11(4), 153–157.

Uddin, L. Q., Kaplan, J. T., Molnar-Szakacs, I., Zaidel, E., & Iacoboni, M. (2005). Self-face recognition activates a frontoparietal "mirror" network in the right hemisphere: An event-related fMRI study. *Neuroimage*, 25(3), 926–935.

Uddin, L. Q., & Menon, V. (2009). The anterior insula in autism: Under-connected and under-examined. *Neuroscience and Biobehavioral Review*, 33(8), 1198–1203.

Uddin, L. Q., Molnar-Szakacs, I., Zaidel, E., & Iacoboni, M. (2006). rTMS to the right inferior parietal lobule disrupts self-other discrimination. *Social Cognitive and Affective Neuroscience*, 1(1), 65–71.

Uddin, L. Q., Supekar, K., Lynch, C. J., *et al.* (2014). Brain state differentiation and behavioral inflexibility in autism. *Cerebral Cortex*.

Uddin, L. Q., Supekar, K., Lynch, C. J., *et al.* (2013). Salience network-based classification and prediction of symptom severity in children with autism. *JAMA Psychiatry*, 70(8), 869–879.

Washington, S. D., Gordon, E. M., Brar, J., *et al.* (2013). Dysmaturation of the default mode network in autism. *Human Brain Mapping*, 35(4), 1284–1296.

Weng, S. J., Wiggins, J. L., Peltier, S. J., *et al.* (2010). Alterations of resting state functional connectivity in the default network in adolescents with autism spectrum disorders. *Brain Research*, 1313, 202–214.

Williams, D., & Happe, F. (2009). Pre-conceptual aspects of self-awareness in autism spectrum disorder: The case of action-monitoring. *Journal of Autism and Developmental Disorders*, 39(2), 251–259.

Williams, J. H., Whiten, A., Suddendorf, T., & Perrett, D. I. (2001). Imitation, mirror neurons and autism. *Neuroscience and Biobehavioral Reviews*, 25(4), 287–295.

Chapter

16

Basic self disturbance in the schizophrenia spectrum: a review and future directions

Barnaby Nelson, Louis A. Sass, and Josef Parnas

Many classic texts about schizophrenia proposed that forms of self-disturbance are at the core of the disorder (Parnas, 2011; Sass, 2001). This formulation faded somewhat with the attempt in psychiatric diagnostic manuals to improve diagnostic reliability and to operationalize psychiatric concepts (Andreasen, 2007; Parnas, 2011). However, over the last decade or so, there seems to have been something of a resurgence of interest in the concept of "self" in schizophrenia and related disorders (Maj, 2012; Nelson, 2013; Park & Nasrallah, 2014; Parnas, Sass, & Zahavi, 2013). Lysaker and Lysaker (2010) recently delineated six accounts of disturbance of self-experience in schizophrenia: those presented in early psychiatry, existential psychiatry, psychoanalysis, phenomenology, psychosocial rehabilitation, and dialogical psychology. In this chapter we will focus on self-disturbance in schizophrenia as formulated in phenomenological psychiatry. We review the phenomenological model of disturbance of the minimal or basic self in schizophrenia spectrum disorders, summarize the empirical findings relating to this model, discuss the possible neurocognitive correlates and developmental pathways to basic self-disturbance, briefly mention implications for therapy, and suggest pathways for future research.

The phenomenological model of basic self-disturbance in schizophrenia

Although there is much debate in philosophy and cognitive science about the notion of the "self" (Gallagher, 2011; Gallagher & Zahavi, 2012), two levels of the experiential self are widely accepted. These include the following.

1. "Minimal" self, also referred to as "basic" or "core" self or as "ipseity" (referred to in this chapter as "basic self"). This is a *pre-reflective, tacit* level of selfhood. It refers to the implicit first-person quality of consciousness, i.e., the implicit awareness that all experience articulates itself in first person perspective as "*my*" experience. In other words, all conscious acts are intrinsically self-conscious (Janzen, 2008), in that they imply a perceiving or experiencing subject. This feature of consciousness is sometimes designated as "self-affection" or as "self-presence." The basic self constitutes the foundational or ground level of selfhood on which other levels of selfhood are built (Janzen, 2008; Parnas, 2003; Zahavi, 2005).

2. "Narrative" or social self. This somewhat heterogeneous category refers to characteristics such as social identity, personality, habits, style, personal history, and so on. Psychological concepts such as "self-esteem," "self concept," or "self-image" refer to this level of selfhood. This level is widely understood to *presuppose* the sense of existing as a subject of experience ("basic self"), and often involves reflective, meta-cognitive processes, in which one's self is largely an *object* of awareness (Damasio, 2000; Goldman, 2006; Zahavi, 2005). For example, when asked to reflect on what sort of a person you are, the narrative or social self is being elicited.

Phenomenologically oriented researchers propose that a disturbance of the basic sense of self is at the clinical core of the schizophrenia spectrum and that it is therefore a phenotypic trait marker of these conditions (Nelson, Yung, Bechdolf, & McGorry, 2008; Parnas,

The Self in Understanding and Treating Psychological Disorders, ed. Michael Kyrios, Richard Moulding, Guy Doron, Sunil S. Bhar, Maja Nedeljkovic, and Mario Mikulincer. Published by Cambridge University Press. © Cambridge University Press, 2016.

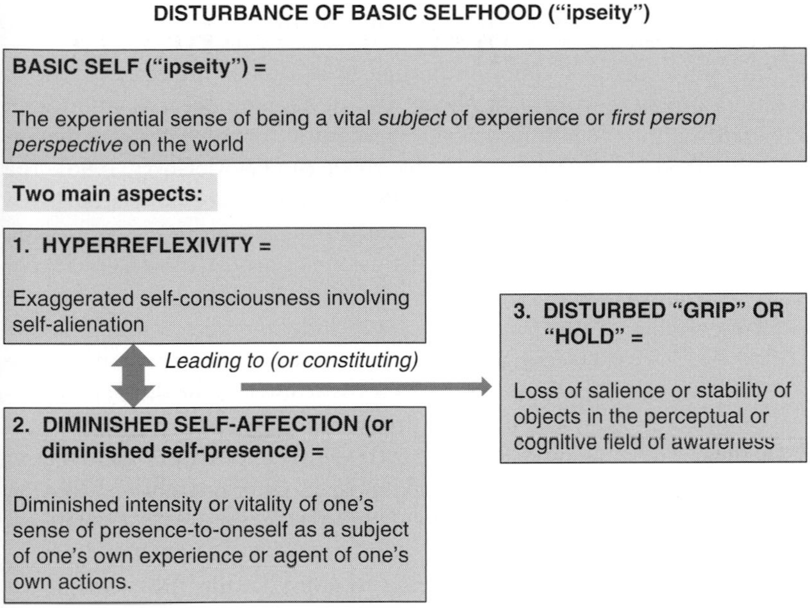

DISTURBANCE OF BASIC SELFHOOD ("ipseity")

Figure 16.1 Basic self-disturbance in schizophrenia.

BASIC SELF ("ipseity") =

The experiential sense of being a vital *subject* of experience or *first person perspective* on the world

Two main aspects:

1. HYPERREFLEXIVITY =

Exaggerated self-consciousness involving self-alienation

Leading to (or constituting)

2. DIMINISHED SELF-AFFECTION (or diminished self-presence) =

Diminished intensity or vitality of one's sense of presence-to-oneself as a subject of one's own experience or agent of one's own actions.

3. DISTURBED "GRIP" OR "HOLD" =

Loss of salience or stability of objects in the perceptual or cognitive field of awareness

2003, 2012; Parnas, Handest, Jansson, & Saebye, 2005; Sass, 1992; Sass & Parnas, 2003). This notion was implied in many early accounts of schizophrenia and expressed in different forms by phenomenological psychiatrists (see Parnas, 2011; Parnas & Henriksen, 2014; Sass, 2014 for reviews). It has been developed and extended over recent years by Sass and Parnas in the form of the "ipseity-disturbance model" (IDM, see Figure 16.1; Nelson, Parnas, & Sass, 2014; Sass & Parnas, 2003, 2007), which has emerged from a combination of clinical exploration, empirical research, and philosophical considerations (Møller & Husby, 2000; Parnas, 2000, 2003; Parnas, Handest, *et al.*, 2005; Parnas, Jansson, Sass, & Handest, 1998; Parnas, Møller, *et al.*, 2005; Sass & Parnas, 2003, 2007; Sass, Parnas, & Zahavi, 2011).

Various anomalies of subjective experience have been described in schizophrenia spectrum conditions which collectively point towards an instability or disturbance of basic selfhood, captured in the IDM. Although intimately interrelated, these anomalies have been organized into the categories of disturbed stream of consciousness, sense of presence, corporeality, self-demarcation, and existential reorientation (Parnas, 2003; Parnas, Møller, *et al.*, 2005). They have been comprehensively catalogued in the Examination of Anomalous Self-Experience (EASE) instrument (Parnas, Møller, *et al.*, 2005), which is a semi-structured interview designed to elicit and

measure aspects of basic self-disturbance. Brief descriptions of the anomalous subjective experiences are provided below.

Categories of anomalous self experience in schizophrenia

Stream of consciousness

A "gap" emerges in experience between the self and mental or cognitive content. The implicit sense of "mineness" of mental content is disrupted, as if thoughts were taking on an almost autonomous and anonymous identity and were no longer a lived aspect of subjectivity. A person may describe thoughts as having a physical, object-like, or acoustic quality, or as being disturbed in their normal flow, such as being pressured or appearing to be blocked. These experiences may evolve into frank psychotic symptoms, such as thought insertion, thought withdrawal, and thought broadcasting.

Presence

Normal human experience consists of being absorbed in activity among a world of (animate and inanimate) objects. As described above, this absorption provides us with a sense of "inhabiting" our self in a pre-reflective, tacit, or automatic fashion. This is referred to as *self-presence* or *self-affection*. As described above, our experiences appear to us in a first-person mode of presentation – that is, we automatically or pre-reflectively experience them as *our* experience. This sense of "mineness" constitutes a basic form of self-awareness. Disturbed presence is often evident in the schizophrenia spectrum, with a characteristic sense that the self no longer "saturates experience" (Parnas & Handest, 2003, p. 125) but instead stands alienated from itself. Patients may describe various forms of depersonalization or derealization, a sense of inner void, and a reduced ability to be affected or influenced by events or other people.

Corporeality

A disjunction between one's subjectivity and bodily experience is often present in schizophrenia spectrum conditions, particularly during the pre-onset or prodromal phase. This is represented in many of the bodily basic symptoms, such as cenesthesias and impaired bodily sensations (Klosterkötter, Hellmich, Steinmeyer, & Schultze-Lutter, 2001). The transformation in the experience of the "lived body" (Merleau-Ponty, 1964) is characterized by an experiential gap or distance emerging between the sense of self and bodily experience. That is, rather than automatically "inhabiting" one's body and experiencing it as a "background" feature, as in normal experience, aspects of physical experience can come to seem object- or thing-like in schizophrenia spectrum conditions. For example, parts of the body can appear to the person to have changed in some way (e.g., "my hand is thinner, longer") or to appear strange, alien or lifeless (to use an example from the EASE: "It is as if his body was alien. He knows that it is his body, but it feels 'as if it did not hang together', it feels 'as if his head was just fixed to the body.'")

Self-demarcation

A diminution or permeability of self–other/self–world boundaries ("transitivism") is often apparent in schizophrenia spectrum conditions. This can be represented in a variety of subtle phenomena. Examples include confusion of boundaries between self and others (e.g., losing sense of whether thoughts, feelings, etc., originated in oneself or another person or whether a reflected image is of oneself or another person), a sense of passivity in relation to the world and others (being "at the mercy of the world," lacking agency), or experiencing the physical presence and contact of others as threatening to one's existence in some way.

Existential reorientation

A common finding in studies of the early psychotic phase has been of a developing preoccupation with philosophical, supernatural, and metaphysical themes (Møller & Husby, 2000; Yung & McGorry, 1996). The rupture in "normal" self-experience motivates such a preoccupation. The person is attempting to explain, justify, or perhaps just to explore their anomalous experience. Feelings of centrality or solipsism may come to the fore. Examples include: the person may describe fleeting feelings that the only things existing in the world are those that are in his visual field, and that people and objects that he cannot see do not exist. The person may also be extremely occupied by thoughts about living up to impossible ideals of thought or behavior, and may search world religions for ultimate metaphysical answers.

It is important to note that the IDM view of the schizophrenia spectrum posits a Gestalt or structural shift in self-world experience (Parnas, 2012; Parnas & Sass, 2011; Sass & Parnas, 2003). Accordingly, the notion of "core" disturbance is often invoked (Parnas, 2012). This is consistent with psychotic symptomatology not being restricted to any particular modality of consciousness (i.e., it can appear as a disruption of cognitive functioning or sensory perception, etc.), and indeed can manifest as disturbance of different senses (e.g., auditory versus visual hallucinations, etc.), as well as being consistent with the variable expression of its single features (i.e., why one symptom might recede and another become more prominent; Parnas, 2011; Sass & Parnas, 2007). An instability in basic selfhood can have a reverberating effect through the different modalities of conscious experience (Sass & Parnas, 2003). In this sense, the basic self might be thought of as the center of experiential gravity, so that when this central organizing dynamic is disturbed, the various modalities of consciousness are thrown off-kilter, resulting in the aberrations of experience in psychotic symptoms. This formulation stands in contrast to the "single symptom" approach often advocated in the cognitive-behavioral tradition (Bentall, 2003; Spaulding, Sullivan, & Poland, 2003), sometimes referred to as an atomistic or "zoom in" approach (Murphy, 2013; Skodlar, Henriksen, Sass, Nelson, & Parnas, 2013).

The IDM describes instability of the basic self as consisting of two complementary aspects: hyperreflexivity and diminished self-affection (or self-presence; Sass, 1992; Sass & Parnas, 2003). Hyperreflexivity is a form of exaggerated self-consciousness and heightened awareness of aspects of one's experience. This style of awareness objectifies aspects of oneself that are normally tacit (e.g., awareness of the act of breathing or sensations while walking), thereby forcing them to be experienced as if they were external objects. Hyperreflexivity is a concept that includes hyperreflectivity (or "*reflective* hyperreflexivity," an exaggerated intellectual or reflective process) but is not limited to this: it also refers to acts of awareness that are not intellectual in nature, and that may occur involuntarily, as in the case of kinaesthetic experiences "popping" into awareness; these latter, which are probably more basic in a pathogenic sense, are termed "*operative* hyperreflexivity" (Sass & Parnas, 2007).

Diminished self-affection or self-presence refers to a weakened sense of existing as a *vital subject* of awareness, a diminished "saturation" of experience with implicit self-awareness. Hyperreflexivity and diminished self-affection are considered to be complementary, mutually implicating aspects of self-disturbance: "Whereas the notion of hyper-reflexivity emphasizes the way in which something normally tacit becomes focal and explicit, the notion of diminished self-affection emphasises a complementary aspect of this very same process – the fact that what once *was* tacit is no longer being inhabited as a medium of taken-for-granted selfhood" (Sass & Parnas, 2003, p. 430). The complementary distortions of hyperreflexivity and diminished self-affection are necessarily accompanied by certain alterations of a person's "grip" or "hold" on the conceptual or perceptual field of awareness. This refers to the sharpness or stability with which figures or meanings emerge against a background context. For example, there may be an unusual salience of particular features of the perceptual world (e.g., a striking prominence of the visual image of the chair in front of me) or of particular thoughts (e.g., a preoccupation with the meaning of a blue umbrella). This can often lead to the sense of perplexity commonly seen in schizophrenia. An important feature of basic self-experience is what Heidegger captured in the concept of "mattering," i.e., the self as a point of orientation directed by needs, desires, and purposes and the resulting pattern of meanings that make for a coherent and significant world (Nelson & Sass, 2009). A diminished vitality of subjectivity (diminished self-affection or self-presence) implies a weakening of these needs, desires and purposes, and therefore of the structuring and organizing influence they have on

the cognitive and perceptual domains (i.e., disturbed "grip" or "hold").

Finally, as has been more or less implicit in the description above, it is important to note that being self-present and present in the world of others and objects (the self-world *structure*) exist as two sides of the same coin (Henriksen & Parnas, 2014). Accordingly, basic self-disturbance involves diminished attunement to others and immersion in the world, inadequate spontaneous grasp of self-evident meanings (perplexity, diminished "common sense"), and hyperreflectivity.

Empirical studies

The IDM of schizophrenia has gained substantial empirical support. Two in-depth qualitative studies revealed alterations of basic self-experience to be a central feature of the prodromal phase of schizophrenia spectrum disorders (Møller & Husby, 2000; Parnas *et al.*, 1998). In subsequent studies, a Danish research group found that basic self-disturbance: (1) is specific to schizophrenia spectrum conditions compared to remitted psychotic bipolar patients and a mixed group of first-admitted patients, (2) is characteristic of pre-schizophrenic prodromes, and (3) frequently occurs in hospitalized schizotypal conditions (Handest, 2003; Handest & Parnas, 2005; Nordgaard & Parnas, 2014; Parnas, 2003; Parnas, Handest, Saebye, & Jansson, 2003). Also, they found that: (4) self-disturbance correlated positively with the duration of pre-onset social dysfunction and aggregated significantly in patients with a positive family history of schizophrenia, and (5) self-disturbance correlated both with negative and positive psychotic symptom scales in schizophrenia patients. Five-year follow-up data of 155 first-admission cases indicated that basic self-disturbance (but not PANSS-scored positive and negative symptoms) was a strong predictor of a future schizophrenia spectrum diagnosis in those who presented with non-psychotic conditions (Parnas, Raballo, Handest, Vollmer-Larsen, & Saebye, 2011).

Genetic linkage data has indicated a similar pattern of findings. Raballo and Parnas (2011) analyzed data from 218 unaffected members of 6 extended families of schizophrenia patients (i.e., individuals at high genetic risk). Basic self-disturbance was incrementally present in groupings of family members with no mental illness, no mental illness but with schizotypal traits, personality disorders other than schizotypal personality disorder (the majority of whom had comorbid schizotypal traits), and schizotypal personality disorder, independent of sociodemographics, negative symptoms, and formal thought disorder. Similar findings were evident when this data set was analysed according to schizophrenia spectrum conditions, with basic self-disturbance being characteristic of schizophrenia spectrum conditions and levels of basic self-disturbance increasing with diagnostic severity (no mental illness, mental illness not in the schizophrenia spectrum, schizotypal personality disorder, schizophrenia; Raballo, Saebye, & Parnas, 2011).

A somewhat different approach was adopted in two quasi-empirical studies that compared self-disturbances in schizophrenia (as defined in the EASE; Sass, Pienkos, Nelson, & Medford, 2013) with self-anomalies found in two non-schizophrenic conditions: depersonalization disorder (which involves loss of self-presence) and intense introspection (which involves reflective or largely volitional forms of hyper-reflexivity; Sass, Pienkos, & Nelson, 2013). Whereas some EASE items did appear to be fairly common in these latter conditions, the most severe indications of a fundamental disturbance of ipseity seemed to occur only in the schizophrenia spectrum.

Other work provides further evidence that basic self-disturbance is a central feature of the pre-onset phase of psychotic disorders, particularly of schizophrenia spectrum disorders. In a follow-back study using objective data, Hartmann et al. (1984) found that fluidity of self-demarcation, lack of a coherent narrative–historical self-identity, and other self-disturbances were prominent features of pre-schizophrenic states at school age. "Basic symptoms," some of which reflect basic self-disturbance (e.g., varieties of depersonalization, disturbances of the stream of consciousness, distorted bodily experiences), have consistently been identified early in the pre-onset phase (Klosterkötter et al., 2001). Davidsen (2009) found that, although there was a difference in the kind and number of single features, disorders of self-experience were evident in all subjects in a clinical high-risk sample ($N = 11$), i.e., those with sub-threshold positive psychotic symptoms. In another clinical high-risk study, Nelson, Thompson, & Yung (2012) found that basic self-disturbance, assessed using the EASE, predicted onset of fully fledged psychotic disorder over a 1.5-year follow-up period. Although statistical power was limited, the data indicated that basic self-disturbance was particularly predictive of schizophrenia spectrum disorders. Recent work has also indicated that basic self-disturbance

correlates with suicidality (more strongly than positive symptoms; Haug, Melle, et al., 2012; Skodlar & Parnas, 2010; Skodlar, Tomori, & Parnas, 2008), lack of insight (Henriksen & Parnas, 2014; Parnas & Henriksen, 2013), and social dysfunction (Haug et al., 2014) in schizophrenia spectrum disorders.

In sum, empirical findings indicate that basic self-disturbance distinguishes schizophrenia spectrum conditions from other psychoses (Nelson, Thompson, & Yung, 2013; Parnas et al., 2003), characterizes the schizophrenia prodrome in retrospective studies (Møller & Husby, 2000; Parnas & Handest, 2003; Parnas, Handest, et al., 2005; Parnas et al., 1998), is present in non-psychotic family members of schizophrenia spectrum patients (Raballo & Parnas, 2011; Raballo, Saebye, & Parnas, 2011), predicts onset of schizophrenia spectrum disorders in those who present with non-psychotic conditions (Parnas et al., 2011), is prominent in "ultra high-risk" (UHR) patients (Davidsen, 2009; Nelson et al., 2012), and predicts future onset of psychotic disorder in UHR patients, particularly schizophrenia spectrum cases (Nelson et al., 2012). These findings are strong indicators that the construct may be considered a phenotypic trait marker of schizophrenic vulnerability and may therefore be useful in early identification and diagnosis.

Neurocognitive correlates

Recent work has started to address the neurocognitive and neurobiological processes related to basic self-disturbance. A study by a Norwegian group (Haug, Oie, et al., 2012) examined basic self-disturbance (using the EASE instrument) and neurocognitive variables in a group of patients in the early phase of schizophrenia. The neurocognitive variables included measures of psychomotor speed, working memory, and executive and memory functions. Few associations were found between basic self-disturbance and neurocognitive impairment, with impaired verbal memory emerging as the single correlate. We have recently argued that the lack of association between neurocognitive measures and basic self-disturbance in this study may have been due to the fact that the particular neurocognitive measures used were standard, reasonably broad measures (Nelson, Whitford, Lavoie, & Sass, 2014a, 2014b). It may be that the neurocognitive disturbances underpinning basic self-disturbance are more specific and subtle, requiring different tests. The "traditional" neurocognitive measures used in psychosis research were, after all, devised for assessing acquired brain injury and intellectual disability (Keefe, Kraus, & Krishnan, 2011) and therefore may not be sufficiently sensitive to detect specific deficits in schizophrenia. We proposed that two streams of neurocognitive research in psychosis show particular affinity with the IDM. Broadly speaking, they consist of (1) source monitoring deficits, and (2) aberrant salience. These will be addressed briefly in turn.

Various neurocognitive models of schizophrenia are based on the idea that psychotic symptoms emerge from a difficulty distinguishing between the origins of endogenous (i.e., internally or self-generated) and exogenous (i.e., externally or other-generated) stimuli. These "source monitoring" deficits, as they are known, are believed to arise from failures in the neural mechanisms involved in distinguishing endogenous from exogenous stimuli, namely corollary discharges (i.e., a copy of a motor command that is directed to sensory brain areas to inform them of an impending movement). Although the models differ in detail, a common tenet is that positive psychotic symptoms result from the *predictions* we make and the extent to which these predictions are fulfilled. This has been dubbed the comparator model (Frith, 2012) as the predicted outcomes are *compared* with the actual outcomes. A key difference between self- and other-generated stimuli is that the former are predictable and controllable whereas the latter are not. When stimuli are predictable (i.e., self-generated) they are "dampened" in perception. When these self-generated stimuli are not effectively "dampened," they might be experienced as if they were external in origin (Feinberg, 1978). A range of studies have yielded data consistent with the view that in schizophrenia there is some form of disconnection between a (self-generated) motor act and the sensory consequences of that act (see Nelson, Whitford, *et al.*, 2014b for review). We have argued that various aspects of the IDM, particularly diminished ownership of experience, self–other boundary confusion, and hyperreflexivity, are congruent with the types of disturbances one would expect from source monitoring deficits (see Nelson, Whitford, *et al.*, 2014b for full discussion).

A considerable amount of research indicates the presence of attention and memory disturbances in schizophrenia. A major theme in these findings is the failed suppression of attention to irrelevant or familiar information or stimuli in the environment, leading to aberrant salience of objects and associations (Hemsley, 2005a, 2005b; Kapur, Mizrahi, & Li, 2005) – or, to reverse the terminology, excessive

attention to information that is irrelevant or highly familiar. A number of neurocognitive models and experimental paradigms have yielded findings consistent with this view, including Keefe and colleagues' memory-prediction model of cortical function (Keefe & Kraus, 2009; Keefe *et al.*, 2011; Kraus, Keefe, & Krishnan, 2009); the salience dysregulation model based on dopamine system abnormalities (Gray, Feldon, Rawlins, Hemsley, & Smith, 1991; Hemsley, 1992; Kapur, 2003); mismatch negativity reduction findings (Todd, Michie, Schall, Ward, & Catts, 2012); the latent inhibition theory (Gray, 1998; Gray, Hemsley, & Gray, 1992; Lubow & Gewirtz, 1995); and Corlett's model of ketamine as a pharmacological model of psychosis (Corlett *et al.*, 2006; Corlett, Honey, & Fletcher, 2007). We have argued that this line of neurocognitive research, broadly referred to as "aberrant salience" research, is congruent with important aspects of the IDM, including hyperreflexivity, disturbed "grip" or "hold" on the perceptual and conceptual field, and disturbances of intuitive social understanding ("common sense"; Nelson, Whitford, *et al.*, 2014a).

Developmental pathways

Little is known about the etiological pathways leading to disturbance or instability in the basic sense of self. This is perhaps not surprising given that the development or formation of the normal or non-pathological experience of the basic self is not well understood (Gallagher, 2011). However, there are some promising avenues of enquiry that should be the focus of future research. If the neurocognitive constructs (aberrant salience and source monitoring deficits) described above do indeed prove to have a role in basic self-disturbance, then tracing the development of these disturbances may inform our understanding of basic self-disturbance. Another area of research from developmental psychology, "intermodal integration," otherwise referred to as "multisensory integration" (Gamma *et al.*, 2014; Parnas, Bovet, & Innocenti, 1996; Postmes *et al.*, 2014), may also be of relevance. Intermodal integration refers to the integration of perceptual experience across modalities (vision, touch, hearing, proprioception), as well as the integration or linking of perception with motility. Intermodal integration occurs from birth onwards and much research in developmental psychology indicates that it is critical to the development of self/non-self discrimination and, by implication, a basic sense of self (Bahrick & Watson,

1985; Damasio, 2012; Parnas *et al.*, 1996; Rochat, 2001; Rochat & Striano, 2002).

If early intermodal integration contributes to the development of the basic sense of self (and associated components of self–other differentiation, motor awareness, and social cognition), then some form of disruption of this process may contribute to basic self-disturbance, and therefore to vulnerability to schizophrenia spectrum disorders. Testing this etiological model obviously requires challenging longitudinal work. However, some consistent data have already emerged. Gamma and colleagues (2014) report data from the New England Family Study, which consisted of over 17,000 pregnant women recruited between 1959 and 1966. They ascertained a "high-risk" sample of infants of parents with schizophrenia (*n* = 58) and compared data from this sample with infants of parents with affective psychoses (*n* =128) and healthy controls (*n* = 174). Infants were assessed with a range of measures at eight months of age. Early intermodal integration measures were grouped into three domains characterizing different aspects of infant development: sense of one's own body, object awareness, and social interactions. Results indicated that body and object-related early intermodal integration abnormalities were significantly increased for infants of parents with schizophrenia compared with control infants. These abnormalities were not detected in infants of parents with affective psychoses. However, early intermodal integration abnormalities in relation to social interactions were significantly increased both in infants of parents with schizophrenia and affective psychoses. These data support the notion of dysfunction in intermodal integration as a risk marker for vulnerability to schizophrenia. Similar intermodal integration deficits have been observed in infants at risk of autism (Guiraud *et al.*, 2012). Future work needs to investigate how this early dysfunction evolves over the developmental trajectory, how it relates to other neurodevelopmental dysfunctions in young people at risk for psychosis, and if it predicts the anomalies of subjective experience associated with basic self-disturbance and onset of psychotic symptoms. Genetic high-risk and clinical high-risk populations provide ideal groups in which to investigate these questions.

Treatment

No treatment studies addressing basic self-disturbance have been published to date. However, several theoretical papers and a case study addressing the implications of the basic self-disturbance model for psychotherapy with schizophrenia patients have been published (Nelson & Sass, 2009; Nelson, Sass, & Skodlar, 2009; Skodlar *et al.*, 2013). These papers have highlighted the possible limitations of the cognitive-behavioral therapy (CBT) approach, particularly "second-wave" CBT, for this patient group, and they suggested avenues that may be more productive given their superior "fit" with the vulnerabilities associated with basic self-disturbance. Specifically, it has been proposed that CBT's emphasis on cognitive challenging, testing assumptions, and analyzing the content of thoughts may at times in fact *encourage* a central pathological process associated with basic self-disturbance, namely hyperreflexive awareness. CBT may therefore even be counterproductive in this patient population.

There is often an atomization and reification of mental phenomena at play in cognitive-behavioral approaches (Skodlar *et al.*, 2013), in their attempt to "… identify which kinds of cognitive abnormalities are implicated in which symptoms, and to thereby construct a kind of 'cognitive table' of psychopathological states analogous to the periodic table in chemistry." This single-symptom approach can prevent a more nuanced understanding of the disturbances of subjective experience at play in schizophrenia spectrum disorders that takes into account the structural alterations described above. An example of this is CBT's approach to the so-called negative symptoms. Rather than considering the subjective experiences associated with negative symptoms (e.g., disturbed sense of presence and correlated problems with immersion in the intersubjective world, as described above), CBT has tended to automatically import the orientation and techniques used in the treatment of depression (identifying and challenging "negative" beliefs and anticipations). In a similar fashion, delusions have tended to be targeted by challenging and attempting to re-frame these "false beliefs" (i.e., an attempt to prove the empirical falsity of the belief) rather than recognizing the delusional content as a metaphorical extension of a profoundly altered subjectivity and self–world relationship.

The phenomenological perspective emphasizes affective, experiential and behavioral processes above "cognitive appraisals." Hence the role of the therapeutic relationship is critical. A central objective is to cultivate an intersubjective space where patients can evolve a more robust sense of pre-reflective first-person perspective. A focus on the "here-and-now" of the therapeutic relationship might be useful in this regard

(Stanghellini & Lysaker, 2007). The phenomenological approach's sensitivity to structural shifts in experience may strengthen empathic attunement with the patient. Given the alienation from constitutive features of selfhood, strategies that encourage a form of immediate engagement, immersion or absorption in present activity may be of value. Such strategies may include certain elements of so-called "third-wave" CBT, such as mindfulness and acceptance and commitment therapy (ACT), creative "flow," or physical activities. As such, we suggest that a systematic trial of psychotherapy for schizophrenia spectrum patients informed by the IDM is warranted.

Conclusions

The concept of basic self-disturbance in schizophrenia posits a characteristic Gestalt of expressive and subjective features marked by an unstable first-person perspective, diminished sense of presence, and loss of vital contact with reality. Importantly, basic self-disturbance is characterized by a *structural shift* in experience; the *form* of experience seems to be altered, rather than the particular contents of experience or disturbance of particular modalities. The model provides a unifying comprehensibility to various symptoms of schizophrenia (the so-called positive, negative, and disorganization symptoms), akin to a psychological formulation, which stands in contrast to Jaspers' (1963) assertion regarding the essential "un-understandability" of psychotic symptoms. Empirical research indicates that this form of disturbance is specific to the schizophrenia spectrum, in contrast to the "unitary psychosis" view (Berrios, 1995; Kendell, 1991), which lumps all psychoses into a single category. It is a trait disturbance that antedates the onset of psychotic symptoms, is present after remission of symptoms, and is present in unaffected family members of patients. The concept may therefore be of value in etiological and pathogenetic research, as well as in diagnostic clarification and early identification. It may serve a useful unifying or integrative function across "levels" of inquiry in schizophrenia research, including psychopathological/clinical, neurocognitive, and neurobiological domains. There are a number of important avenues for future research, as highlighted above. The developmental pathways to basic self-disturbance need to be clarified and psychotherapeutic approaches built around the basic self-disturbance concept should be developed and trialled.

References

Andreasen, N. C. (2007). DSM and the death of phenomenology in America: An example of unintended consequences. *Schizophrenia Bulletin*, 33(1), 108–112.

Bahrick, L. E., & Watson, J. S. (1985). Detection of intermodal proprioceptive-visual contingency as a potential basis of self-perception in infancy. *Developmental Psychology*, 21, 963–973.

Bentall, R. (2003). *Madness Explained*. London: Allen Lane.

Berrios, C. E. (1995). Conceptual problems in diagnosing schizophrenic disorders. In J. A. D. Boer, H. G. M. Westenberg, & H. M. v. Praag (Eds.), *Advances in the Neurobiology of Schizophrenia* (pp. 7–25). Chichester: Wiley.

Corlett, P. R., Honey, G. D., Aitken, M. R., *et al.* (2006). Frontal responses during learning predict vulnerability to the psychotogenic effects of ketamine: Linking cognition, brain activity, and psychosis. *Archives of General Psychiatry*, 63(6), 611–621.

Corlett, P. R., Honey, G. D., & Fletcher, P. C. (2007). From prediction error to psychosis: Ketamine as a pharmacological model of delusions. *Journal of Psychopharmacology*, 21(3), 238–252.

Damasio, A. (2000). *The Feeling of What Happens: Body, Emotion and the Making of Consciousness*. London: Vintage.

Damasio, A. R. (2012). *Self Comes to Mind: Constructing the Conscious Brain*. New York, NY: Vintage Books.

Davidsen, K. A. (2009). Anomalous self-experience in adolescents at risk of psychosis. Clinical and conceptual elucidation. *Psychopathology*, 42(6), 361–369.

Feinberg, I. (1978). Efference copy and corollary discharge: Implications for thinking and its disorders. *Schizophrenia Bulletin*, 4(4), 636–640.

Frith, C. (2012). Explaining delusions of control: The comparator model 20 years on. *Consciousness and Cognition*, 21(1), 52–54.

Gallagher, S. (Ed.). (2011). *The Oxford Handbook of the Self*. Oxford: Oxford University Press.

Gallagher, S., & Zahavi, D. (2012). *The Phenomenological Mind* (2nd ed.). New York, NY: Routledge.

Gamma, F., Goldstein, J. M., Seidman, L. J., *et al.* (2014). Early intermodal integration in offspring of parents with psychosis. *Schizophrenia Bulletin*, 40(5), 992–1000.

Goldman, A. I. (2006). *Simulating Minds: The Philosophy, Psychology, and Neuroscience of Mindreading*. Oxford: Oxford University Press.

Gray, J. A. (1998). Integrating schizophrenia. *Schizophrenia Bulletin*, 24(2), 249–266.

Gray, J. A., Feldon, J., Rawlins, J. N. P., Hemsley, D. R., & Smith, A. D. (1991). The neuropsychology of schizophrenia. *Behavioral and Brain Sciences*, 14(1), 1–20.

Gray, N. S., Hemsley, D. R., & Gray, J. A. (1992). Abolition of latent inhibition in acute, but not chronic, schizophrenics. *Neurology, Psychiatry, and Brain Research*, 1, 83–89.

Guiraud, J. A., Tomalski, P., Kushnerenko, E., *et al.* (2012). Atypical audiovisual speech integration in infants at risk for autism. *PloS ONE*, 7(5), e36428.

Handest, P. (2003). *The prodomes of schizophrenia*. Doctoral thesis, University of Copenhagen, Copenhagen.

Handest, P., & Parnas, J. (2005). Clinical characteristics of first-admitted patients with ICD-10 schizotypal disorder. *British Journal of Psychiatry – Supplementum*, 48, s49–54.

Hartmann, E., Milofsky, E., Vaillant, G., *et al.* (1984). Vulnerability to schizophrenia. Prediction of adult schizophrenia using childhood information. *Archives of General Psychiatry*, 41(11), 1050–1056.

Haug, E., Melle, I., Andreassen, O. A., *et al.* (2012). The association between anomalous self-experience and suicidality in first-episode schizophrenia seems mediated by depression. *Comprehensive Psychiatry*, 53(5), 456–460.

Haug, E., Oie, M., Andreassen, O. A., *et al.* (2014). Anomalous self-experiences contribute independently to social dysfunction in the early phases of schizophrenia and psychotic bipolar disorder. *Comprehensive Psychiatry*, 55(3), 475–482.

Haug, E., Oie, M., Melle, I., *et al.* (2012). The association between self-disorders and neurocognitive dysfunction in schizophrenia. *Schizophrenia Research*, 135(1–3), 79–83.

Hemsley, D. R. (1992). Cognitive abnormalities and schizophrenic symptoms. *Psychological Medicine*, 22(4), 839–842.

Hemsley, D. R. (2005a). The development of a cognitive model of schizophrenia: Placing it in context. *Neuroscience & Biobehavioral Reviews*, 29(6), 977–988.

Hemsley, D. R. (2005b). The schizophrenic experience: Taken out of context? *Schizophrenia Bulletin*, 31(1), 43–53.

Henriksen, M. G., & Parnas, J. (2014). Self-disorders and schizophrenia: A phenomenological reappraisal of poor insight and noncompliance. *Schizophrenia Bulletin*, 40(3), 542–547.

Janzen, G. (2008). *The Reflexive Nature of Consciousness*. Amsterdam: John Benjamins.

Jaspers, K. (1963). *General Psychopathology* (J. Hoenig & M. W. Hamilton, Trans.). Chicago, IL: University of Chicago Press.

Kapur, S. (2003). Psychosis as a state of aberrant salience: A framework linking biology, phenomenology, and pharmacology in schizophrenia. *American Journal of Psychiatry*, 160(1), 13–23.

Kapur, S., Mizrahi, R., & Li, M. (2005). From dopamine to salience to psychosis – Linking biology, pharmacology and phenomenology of psychosis. *Schizophrenia Research*, 79(1), 59–68.

Keefe, R. S., & Kraus, M. S. (2009). Measuring memory-prediction errors and their consequences in youth at risk for schizophrenia. *Annals of the Academy of Medicine, Singapore*, 38(5), 414–416.

Keefe, R. S., Kraus, M. S., & Krishnan, R. R. (2011). Failures in learning-dependent predictive perception as the key cognitive vulnerability to psychosis in schizophrenia. *Neuropsychopharmacology*, 36(1), 367–368.

Kendell, R. E. (1991). The major functional psychoses: Are they independent entities or part of a continuum? Philosophical and conceptual issues underlying the debate. In A. Kerr & H. McClelland (Eds.), *Concepts of Mental Disorder: A Continuing Debate* (pp. 1–16). London: Gaskell.

Klosterkötter, J., Hellmich, M., Steinmeyer, E. M., & Schultze-Lutter, F. (2001). Diagnosing schizophrenia in the initial prodromal phase. *Archives of General Psychiatry*, 58, 158–164.

Kraus, M. S., Keefe, R. S., & Krishnan, R. K. (2009). Memory-prediction errors and their consequences in schizophrenia. *Neuropsychology Review*, 19(3), 336–352.

Lubow, R. E., & Gewirtz, J. C. (1995). Latent inhibition in humans: Data, theory, and implications for schizophrenia. *Psychological Bulletin*, 117(1), 87–103.

Lysaker, P. H., & Lysaker, J. T. (2010). Schizophrenia and alterations in self-experience: A comparison of 6 perspectives. *Schizophrenia Bulletin*, 36(2), 331–340.

Maj, M. (2012). The self and schizophrenia: Some open issues. *World Psychiatry*, 11(2), 65–66.

Merleau-Ponty, M. (1964). *The Primacy of Perception*. Evanston, IL: Northwestern University Press.

Møller, P., & Husby, R. (2000). The initial prodrome in schizophrenia: Searching for naturalistic core dimensions of experience and behavior. *Schizophrenia Bulletin*, 26(1), 217–232.

Murphy, D. (2013). Philosophy of psychiatry. *The Stanford Encyclopedia of Philosophy*. from <http://plato.stanford.edu/archives/fall2013/entries/psychiatry/%3E

Nelson, B. (2013). Varieties of self-disturbance: A prism through which to view mental disorder. *Early Intervention in Psychiatry*, 7, 231–234.

Nelson, B., Parnas, J., & Sass, L. A. (2014). Disturbance of minimal self (ipseity) in schizophrenia: Clarification and current status. *Schizophrenia Bulletin*, 40(3), 479–482.

Nelson, B., & Sass, L. A. (2009). Medusa's stare: A case study of working with self-disturbance in the early phase of schizophrenia. *Clinical Case Studies*, 8(6), 489–504.

Nelson, B., Sass, L. A., & Skodlar, B. (2009). The phenomenological model of psychotic vulnerability and its possible implications for psychological interventions in the ultra-high risk ('prodromal') population. *Psychopathology*, 42, 283–292.

Nelson, B., Thompson, A., & Yung, A. R. (2012). Basic self-disturbance predicts psychosis onset in the ultra high risk for psychosis "prodromal" population. *Schizophrenia Bulletin*, 38(6), 1277–1287.

Nelson, B., Thompson, A., & Yung, A. R. (2013). Not all first-episode psychosis is the same: Preliminary evidence of greater basic self-disturbance in schizophrenia spectrum cases. *Early Intervention in Psychiatry*, 7(2), 200–204.

Nelson, B., Whitford, T. J., Lavoie, S., & Sass, L. A. (2014a). What are the neurocognitive correlates of basic self-disturbance in schizophrenia? Integrating phenomenology and neurocognition: Part 2 (Aberrant salience). *Schizophrenia Research*, 152(1), 20–27.

Nelson, B., Whitford, T. J., Lavoie, S., & Sass, L. A. (2014b). What are the neurocognitive correlates of basic self-disturbance in schizophrenia? Integrating phenomenology and neurocognition. Part 1 (Source monitoring deficits). *Schizophrenia Research*, 152(1), 12–19.

Nelson, B., Yung, A. R., Bechdolf, A., & McGorry, P. D. (2008). The phenomenological critique and self-disturbance: Implications for ultra-high risk ("prodrome") research. *Schizophrenia Bulletin*, 34(2), 381–392.

Nordgaard, J., & Parnas, J. (2014). Self-disorders and the schizophrenia spectrum: A study of 100 first hospital admissions. *Schizophrenia Bulletin*, 40(6), 1300–1307.

Park, S., & Nasrallah, H. A. (2014). The varieties of anomalous self experiences in schizophrenia: Splitting of the mind at a crossroad. *Schizophrenia Research*, 152(1), 1–4.

Parnas, J. (2000). The self and intentionality in the pre-psychotic stages of schizophrenia: A phenomenological study. In D. Zahavi (Ed.), *Exploring the Self: Philosophical and Psychopathological Perspectives on Self-experience* (pp. 115–148). Amsterdam: John Benjamins.

Parnas, J. (2003). Self and schizophrenia: A phenomenological perspective. In T. Kircher & A. David (Eds.), *The Self in Neuroscience and Psychiatry* (pp. 127–141). Cambridge: Cambridge University Press.

Parnas, J. (2011). A disappearing heritage: The clinical core of schizophrenia. *Schizophrenia Bulletin*, 37(6), 1121–1130.

Parnas, J. (2012). The core Gestalt of schizophrenia. *World Psychiatry*, 11(2), 67–69.

Parnas, J., Bovet, P., & Innocenti, G. M. (1996). Schizophrenic trait features, binding, and cortico-cortical connectivity: A neurodevelopmental pathogenetic hypothesis. *Neurology, Psychiatry and Brain Research*, 4, 185–196.

Parnas, J., & Handest, P. (2003). Phenomenology of anomalous self-experience in early schizophrenia. *Comprehensive Psychiatry*, 44(2), 121–134.

Parnas, J., Handest, P., Jansson, L., & Saebye, D. (2005). Anomalous subjective experience among first-admitted schizophrenia spectrum patients: Empirical investigation. *Psychopathology*, 38(5), 259–267.

Parnas, J., Handest, P., Saebye, D., & Jansson, L. (2003). Anomalies of subjective experience in schizophrenia and psychotic bipolar illness. *Acta Psychiatrica Scandinavica*, 108(2), 126–133.

Parnas, J., & Henriksen, M. G. (2013). Subjectivity and schizophrenia: Another look at incomprehensibility and treatment nonadherence. *Psychopathology*, 46(5), 320–329.

Parnas, J., & Henriksen, M. G. (2014). Disordered self in the schizophrenia spectrum: A clinical and research perspective. *Harvard Review of Psychiatry*, 22(5), 251–265.

Parnas, J., Jansson, L., Sass, L. A., & Handest, P. (1998). Self-experience in the prodromal phases of schizophrenia: A pilot study of first-admissions. *Neurology, Psychiatry and Brain Research*, 6(2), 97–106.

Parnas, J., Møller, P., Kircher, T., *et al.* (2005). EASE: Examination of Anomalous Self-Experience. *Psychopathology*, 38(5), 236–258.

Parnas, J., Raballo, A., Handest, P., *et al.* (2011). Self-experience in the early phases of schizophrenia: 5-year follow-up of the Copenhagen Prodromal Study. *World Psychiatry*, 10(3), 200–204.

Parnas, J., & Sass, L. A. (2011). The structure of self-consciousness in schizophrenia. In S. Gallagher (Ed.), *The Oxford Handbook of the Self* (pp. 521–546). Oxford: Oxford University Press.

Parnas, J., Sass, L. A., & Zahavi, D. (2013). Rediscovering psychopathology: The epistemology and phenomenology of the psychiatric object. *Schizophrenia Bulletin*, 39(2), 270–277.

Postmes, L., Sno, H. N., Goedhart, S., *et al.* (2014). Schizophrenia as a self-disorder due to perceptual incoherence. *Schizophrenia Research*, 152(1), 41–50.

Raballo, A., & Parnas, J. (2011). The silent side of the spectrum: Schizotypy and the schizotaxic self. *Schizophrenia Bulletin*, 37(5), 1017–1026.

Raballo, A., Saebye, D., & Parnas, J. (2011). Looking at the schizophrenia spectrum through the prism of self-disorders: An empirical study. *Schizophrenia Bulletin*, 37(2), 344–351.

Rochat, P. (2001). *The Infant's World*. Cambridge, MA: Harvard University Press.

Rochat, P., & Striano, T. (2002). Who's in the mirror? Self-other discrimination in specular images by four- and nine-month-old infants. *Child Development*, 73(1), 35–46.

Sass, L. A. (1992). *Madness and Modernism: Insanity in the Light of Modern Art, Literature, and Thought*. Cambridge, MA: Harvard University Press.

Sass, L. A. (2001). Self and world in schizophrenia: Three classic approaches. *Philosophy, Psychiatry & Psychology*, 8(4), 251–270.

Sass, L. A. (2014). Self-disturbance and schizophrenia: Structure, specificity, pathogenesis (current issues, new directions). *Schizophrenia Research,* 152(1), 5–11.

Sass, L. A., & Parnas, J. (2003). Schizophrenia, consciousness, and the self. *Schizophrenia Bulletin*, 29(3), 427–444.

Sass, L. A., & Parnas, J. (2007). Explaining schizophrenia: The relevance of phenomenology. In M. C. Chung, K. W. M. Fulford, & G. Graham (Eds.), *Reconceiving Schizophrenia* (pp. 63–96). New York, NY: Oxford University Press.

Sass, L. A., Parnas, J., & Zahavi, D. (2011). Phenomenological psychopathology and schizophrenia: Contemporary approaches and misunderstandings. *Philosophy, Psychiatry & Psychology*, 18(1), 1–23.

Sass, L. A., Pienkos, E., & Nelson, B. (2013). Introspection and schizophrenia: A comparative investigation of anomalous self experiences. *Consciousness and Cognition*, 22(3), 853–867.

Sass, L. A., Pienkos, E., Nelson, B., & Medford, N. (2013). Anomalous self-experience in depersonalization and schizophrenia: A comparative investigation. *Consciousness and Cognition*, 22, 430–441.

Skodlar, B., Henriksen, M. G., Sass, L. A., Nelson, B., & Parnas, J. (2013). Cognitive-behavioral therapy for schizophrenia: A critical evaluation of its theoretical framework from a clinical–phenomenological perspective. *Psychopathology*, 46(4), 249–265.

Skodlar, B., & Parnas, J. (2010). Self-disorder and subjective dimensions of suicidality in schizophrenia. *Comprehensive Psychiatry*, 51(4), 363–366.

Skodlar, B., Tomori, M., & Parnas, J. (2008). Subjective experience and suicidal ideation in schizophrenia. *Comprehensive Psychiatry*, 49(5), 482–488.

Spaulding, W., Sullivan, M., & Poland, J. (2003). *Treatment and Rehabilitation of Severe Mental Illness*. New York, NY: Guilford Press.

Stanghellini, G., & Lysaker, P. H. (2007). The psychotherapy of schizophrenia through the lens of phenomenology: Intersubjectivity and the search for the recovery of first- and second-person awareness. *American Journal of Psychotherapy*, 61(2), 163–179.

Todd, J., Michie, P. T., Schall, U., Ward, P. B., & Catts, S. V. (2012). Mismatch negativity (MMN) reduction in schizophrenia-impaired prediction – Error generation, estimation or salience? *International Journal of Psychophysiology*, 83(2), 222–231.

Yung, A. R., & McGorry, P. D. (1996). The initial prodrome in psychosis: Descriptive and qualitative aspects. *Australian and New Zealand Journal of Psychiatry*, 30(5), 587–599.

Zahavi, D. (2005). *Subjectivity and Selfhood: Investigating the First-person Perspective*. Cambridge, MA: MIT Press.

Chapter

17

Painful incoherence: the self in borderline personality disorder

Giovanni Liotti and Benedetto Farina

According to a well-designed study (Wilkinson-Ryan & Westen, 2000), the key component of the disturbance of the self typical of borderline personality disorder (BPD) is a painful sense of personal incoherence, comprising feelings of unreality, emptiness, and lack of continuity in the experience of self. The hypothesis that this disturbance of the self is the core of BPD is supported by a recent research study evidencing that painful incoherence, rather than other features of the disorder such as mood instability, underpins most of BPD's manifold symptoms (Meares, Gerull, Stevenson, & Korner, 2011). Meares (2012a) argued convincingly that the components of painful incoherence (feelings of unreality, emptiness, and lack of continuity in the experience of self) are the expression of dissociative processes. They should be regarded as primary, in the sense that other typical features of BPD – such as fear of losing the very sense of personal existence if a close relationship is lost, emotional/behavioral dysregulation, tendency to self-injury, and suicidality – are secondary to them.

In this chapter we shall argue that the roots of the painful incoherence characterizing the self-disturbance in BPD can often be traced back to infant attachment disorganization, and that a proper appreciation of these roots helps clinicians in understanding the experience of self of patients with BPD while dealing with it in the psychotherapy process.

Attachment disorganization and borderline personality disorder

An impressive range of theoretical inquiries, clinical studies, and controlled research studies suggest that attachment disorganization plays an important role in borderline psychopathology, although it is not a specific risk factor for BPD (for a review of these studies, see Liotti, 2014). These studies support the idea that the fundamental features of BPD can be explained by a developmental model based on attachment disorganization. Although we lack conclusive research evidence for the hypothesis that the developmental pathways leading to the disorder begin with early attachment disorganization in the majority of BPD cases (Levy, 2005), three controlled studies suggest that this may be the case (Carlson, Egeland, & Sroufe, 2009; Lyons-Ruth, Bureau, Holmes, Easterbrooks, & Brooks, 2012; Lyons-Ruth, Melnick, Patrick, & Hobson, 2007).

Reviewing and summarizing the studies that support the hypothesis of the key role of attachment disorganization in the genesis of BPD is beyond the scope of this chapter. Rather, we shall first provide readers with an overview of the nature and basic features of infant attachment disorganization and of its developmental sequelae, having in mind the final goal of using them in understanding the early developmental roots of painful incoherence in the experience of self in patients with BPD.

Disorganization of infant attachment

About 80% of infants' attachments to the caregivers in low-risk samples can be reliably classified using the Strange Situation procedure (Ainsworth, Blehar, Waters, & Wall, 1978) into three main organized patterns (secure, insecure-avoidant, and insecure-resistant). Most of the remaining attachment styles, being characterized by lack of behavioral and attentional organization, are now classified in the disorganized category (Lyons-Ruth & Jacobvitz, 2008). In samples of families at high risk for psychopathology,

The Self in Understanding and Treating Psychological Disorders, ed. Michael Kyrios, Richard Moulding, Guy Doron, Sunil S. Bhar, Maja Nedeljkovic, and Mario Mikulincer. Published by Cambridge University Press. © Cambridge University Press, 2016.

the percentage of disorganized attachments may be as high as 80% (Lyons-Ruth & Jacobvitz, 2008).

Infants with disorganized attachment manifest bizarre and/or contradictory behavior when reuniting with their caregiver after a brief separation: bizarre behavior such as freezing, hiding, head-banging, abrupt lowering of the muscular tone ending sometimes with the baby collapsing to the ground, and contradictory behavior such as trying to approach the attachment figure with their head averted (Main & Solomon, 1990). Unresolved experiences of losses and traumas, as retrieved through the caregiver's Adult Attachment Interview (AAI; Hesse, 2008), are a frequent precursor of disorganized attachment in the infants, and are significantly less frequent in the caregivers of infants with organized attachment patterns (for a meta-analysis of research on this topic, see Van IJzendoorn, Schuengel, & Bakermans-Kranenbourg, 1999). An important mediating factor between the caregiver's unresolved state of mind and the infant's attachment disorganization is that the infant's fear is increased rather than soothed in the attachment-caregiving interactions. Studies of infant attachment disorganization describe parental behavior, linked by unresolved trauma and loss, that is either frightened and thereby indirectly frightening, or aggressive and directly frightening to the infant (Main & Hesse, 1990; Hesse & Main, 2006). Other adverse influences in the caregivers' past attachment experiences, besides unresolved traumas or losses, have also been evidenced as antecedents of infant attachment disorganization. These antecedents are expressed in hostile and helpless states of mind concerning the attachment-caregiving interaction (Lyons-Ruth, Yellin, Melnick, & Atwood, 2003), and in the "abdication" of the responsibility of caregiving in the face of the infant's expression of attachment needs (Solomon & George, 2011).[1]

Although the type of interaction between the infant and the caregiver plays the key role in infant attachment disorganization, genetic influences exert a moderating influence (Gervai, 2009). Reflections on gene–environment interaction in infant attachment disorganization may contribute to reconciling genetic and attachment-based theories of BPD (Gunderson & Lyons-Ruth, 2008).

Attachment disorganization and dissociative processes

The term "dissociation" in psychopathology is used to signify both a diagnostic category and the pathogenic processes caused by traumatic experiences that, by hindering mental functions involved in the integration of experience and self-perception, generate the dissociative symptoms. These symptoms characterize the dissociative disorders and, according to Meares (2012a) and others (e.g., Farina & Liotti, 2013; Howell, 2008), also BPD. The higher-order integrative functions hindered by dissociative processes are consciousness, self-identity, memory, perception, and those involved in the control of bodily movements (Nijenhuis & Van der Hart, 2011). Many researchers and clinicians have extended the effects of dissociative processes to other integrative mental functions, typically altered in BPD patients, such as affect regulation, metacognitive monitoring, mentalization,[2] and the capacity for coherent autobiographic narratives (Carlson, Yates, & Sroufe, 2009; Farina & Liotti, 2013; Fonagy & Bateman, 2008; Meares, 2012a; Van der Hart, Nijenhuis, & Steele, 2006). This extended view of the potentially wide-ranging effects of trauma on higher mental functions can be seen as the heritage of Pierre Janet's theory of posttraumatic *désagrégation* (Van der Hart & Dorahy, 2006) – Janet's favorite synonym of the word "dissociation," which can be rendered in English as "disintegration."

Liotti's (1992) hypothesis that dissociative processes underpin infant attachment disorganization is supported by two longitudinal controlled research studies (Dutra, Bureau, Holmes, Lyubchik, & Lyons-Ruth, 2009; Ogawa, Sroufe, Weinfield, Carlson, & Egeland, 1997). These studies provide robust evidence that children and adolescents who had been disorganized in their infant attachments are more prone to dissociative mental processes than are their peers who have histories of organized (secure, insecure-avoidant, and insecure-ambivalent) early attachments. The vehicle bringing the dissociative tendencies of infant disorganized attachment into adulthood is, according to attachment theory, the internal working model (IWM: Bowlby, 1969). Let us now have a look at how the kernel of the disorganized IWM can be conceived.

An attachment figure who is neglecting, helpless, frightened, or hostile and straightforwardly frightening to the infant creates a situation in which the source of potential comfort is also, at the same time, the source of fear, even when this caregiver's behavior is not obviously maltreating. This situation has been called fright without solution (Main & Hesse, 1990), because infants cannot find relief from fear in flying from the caregiver nor in approaching her or him. The experience of fright without solution in infant disorganized attachment has been regarded as an early relational trauma (Schore, 2009) because, like other traumatic experiences, it involves powerlessness in the face of an unbearable and inescapable life-threatening situation. Trauma, by definition, involves overwhelming the capacity to cope successfully with a threat through fight or flight defensive responses (supported by the adrenergic arousal of the sympathetic system) so that the only response that remains available is the archaic vagal one – the vasovagal syncope evolved to provide an extreme attempt at self protection under inescapable life-threatening circumstances (Porges, 1997, 2001).[3] The activation of this vagal response causes cataplectic immobility and a shutdown of higher brain connections affording, besides protection from pain, in the case of a predator's attack, the last desperate defense from a predator's attack in the form of feigned death (i.e., the only fugue when no other fugue is possible). The activation of the archaic vagal defense causes disconnection between the different functional levels of the mind, prevents the integration of traumatic memories, and causes discontinuity and fragmentation in the experience of self (Schore, 2009). Such a fragmentation is expressed by the bizarre and contradictory behaviors of disorganized infants in the Strange Situation procedure and, in the AAI, by the incoherence of thought and discourse characterizing the adult mental state related to attachment disorganization.

The clinical relevance of understanding the developmental trajectory that leads from infant disorganized attachment to adult BPD justifies theoretically informed speculations on the features of the contradictory and non-integrated representations stemming from the disorganized IWM. Liotti (2004) suggested that they are akin to the three basic roles of Karpman's (1968) drama triangle: the powerful rescuer, the equally powerful but malevolent persecutor, and the powerless victim. Being at least potentially available and willing to help and comfort the infant, parents and other caregivers are perceived by children as rescuers. At the same time, when they are neglecting, subtly hostile, or prone to episodes of aggression, they are perceived as persecutors. Simultaneously, because they express their helplessness, fear, and suffering (caused by their own unresolved traumatic memories) while taking care of their infants, the parents of disorganized children are perceived as victims. These reciprocally incompatible representational prototypes are the base for construing the behavior of self and others during later attachment interactions. Being constructed

during the first two years of life, these representations pertain to the non-verbal domain of inner representations – that is, they operate at the implicit level of self-knowledge (Amini et al., 1996). In other words, they are aspects of the ongoing implicit relational knowing that characterizes the early phases of personality development and persists throughout the life span (Lyons-Ruth, 1998). Therefore, throughout the developmental years, the multiple and non-integrated representations of the self and of the single caregiver manifest themselves in communication as intersubjective enactments rather than as explicit verbalized structures of memory (Ginot, 2007). No synthesis of these representations in semantic memory and in fully conscious narratives is therefore possible, at least not during childhood. The different, incompatible, simultaneous representations of self-with-other of the disorganized IWM tend to remain compartmentalized throughout the early phases of personality development. Compartmentalization, it should be remembered, is one of the two basic aspects of dissociation (Holmes et al., 2005), the other being detachment (expressed mainly in the manifold symptoms of depersonalization).

The compartmentalized representations of disorganized attachment, together with the dramatic re-experiencing of fear without solution during later attachment interaction, tend to hamper the higher (conscious and regulatory) mental functions during personality development, so that mentalization deficits, emotional dysregulation, and impulsivity may also follow infant attachment disorganization (Bateman & Fonagy, 2004). It should be emphasized that both dissociation among representations of self-with-other and mentalization deficits tend to occur, in people with disorganized attachment, during the experience of attachment needs and wishes rather than in moments where interpersonal behavior is motivated by systems different from attachment (e.g., the competitive, the sexual, the care-giving, or the cooperative systems: Liotti, Cortina, & Farina, 2008; Liotti & Gilbert, 2011).

There is some evidence that a disorganized IWM in infancy may be the first step in the developmental psychopathology of BPD. A longitudinal research study evidenced correlations between early disorganized attachment and adult BPD symptoms (Carlson et al., 2009). A controlled study comparing the AAI coding hostile/helpless (linked to infant attachment disorganization) in samples of dysthymic and borderline female patients shows the expected statistically significant difference (Lyons-Ruth *et al.*, 2007). In the prospective study by Lyons-Ruth and her collaborators (2012), a relational antecedent of attachment disorganization (maternal withdrawal in infancy) significantly predicted borderline symptoms and suicidality/self-injury in late adolescence. Also in keeping with the hypothesis that early attachment disorganization plays a role in BPD are the findings of a neuroscience study evidencing a disintegrative effect of attachment memories on cortical EEG connectivity in adult patients with histories of chronic childhood trauma and a disorganized mental state related to attachment (Farina *et al.*, 2014).

Developmental sequelae of infant attachment disorganization

Remarkably, disorganized attachment in infancy develops into rigid, controlling behavior in middle childhood (Lyons-Ruth & Jacobvitz, 2008). The controlling strategies seem to compensate for disorganization in the child–parent interactions: they allow for organized interpersonal exchanges with the caregivers, thus reducing the likelihood of dissociative processes during these exchanges (Liotti, 2011). There is evidence (Lyons-Ruth & Jacobvitz, 2008) that infants disorganized in their attachments can either become bossy children who strive to obtain dominance by exerting aggressive competitiveness toward the caregiver (controlling–punitive strategy), or become children who invert the attachment relationship and display precocious caregiving toward their parents (controlling–caregiving strategy). A major cause of the controlling caregiving strategy is the relationship with a vulnerable, helpless parent who encourages the child to invert the normal direction of the attachment–caregiving strategy. A parent who perceives the child as powerful and evil may be one particularly malignant condition for the development of a controlling–punitive strategy (for examples, see Hesse, Main, Abrams, & Rifkin, 2003).

The controlling strategies collapse in the face of events (e.g., traumas, pain, threats of separation), that stimulate intensely and durably the child's attachment system (Hesse *et al.*, 2003). During the phases of collapse of the controlling strategies, the child's thoughts and behavior suggest that dissociative processes are at work, presumably because of the reactivation of the disorganized IWM (Hesse *et al.*, 2003; Liotti, 2004, 2011). It is noteworthy, for our understanding of the developmental psychopathology of BPD, that children with a controlling–punitive strategy are more prone than other children to develop externalizing disorders characterized by impulse dyscontrol, while children with a controlling–caregiving strategy tend to develop internalizing disorders, characterized by anxiety and depression (Moss *et al.*, 2006). It can be hypothesized that a controlling–punitive strategy mediates between infant attachment disorganization and adult cluster B personality disorders (including BPD), while a controlling–caregiving strategy is a risk factor for anxiety disorders, mood disorders, or cluster A personality disorders.

While there is no evidence for the hypothesized different pathways of developmental psychopathology toward personality disorders being laid open by the two disorganized/controlling strategies, in the above-quoted longitudinal study of Lyons-Ruth and her collaborators (2012) a disorganized/controlling strategy at age 8 contributed to the prediction of borderline symptoms independently of later traumatic experiences. Borderline personality functioning in adolescence, presumably including painful incoherence in the experience of self, are thus predicted both by disturbed interactions as early as 18 months of age and by later controlling strategies.

In summary, it is reasonable to conclude from the existing data that infant disorganized attachment may lead to adaptational vulnerabilities (e.g., a controlling–punitive strategy developed in middle childhood) which, especially as a consequence of further traumatic experiences, can cause BPD. However, because disorganized attachment can also be an antecedent of other disorders (Levy, 2005; Liotti, 2014), specific developmental pathways must lead to other types of adaptational vulnerabilities linked to adult disorders different from BPD.

Notes on the developmental psychopathology of borderline personality disorder

Borderline psychopathology is the likely consequence of multiple, intertwined relational and mental processes, and is probably influenced by specific temperamental factors. The disintegrative influence of infant attachment disorganization, especially if it is followed by later traumatic experiences, may explain the genesis of the core feature of DBP (painful incoherence in the experience of self), and also the roots of other features: emotional dysregulation, a mentalization deficit, coexisting fears of attachment loss and of affectional closeness (Van der Hart *et al.*, 2006), and the shifting between idealized (attachment figure seen as a powerful rescuer) and aggressively destructive (the same figure perceived as a persecutor) representations of significant others.

Being linked to the disorganized IWM, all these dysfunctions are typically triggered by the relational context in which the patient's attachment system is activated (Liotti *et al.*, 2008; Liotti & Gilbert, 2011). Given this, we should study the peculiarities of these relational contexts for a better understanding of the specific developmental pathways that lead to BPD rather than to other mental disorders whose genesis is potentially linked to infant attachment disorganization. The different responses of the interpersonal environment to the frequent moments of dysfunctional behavior of children who have been disorganized in their infant attachments may influence whether the final result of early disorganized attachment is mental health, BPD or another mental disorder (Liotti, 1992, 2004). For instance, the child's (and later the adolescent's) shifting from the fear of attachment loss to fear of emotional closeness may be met by significant others with a sufficient degree of understanding (facilitating a healthy growth of the personality), by rage or violent aggression leading to severe trauma (a likely antecedent of dissociative identity disorder), or with a rather chaotic admixture of criticism, withdrawal, anger and sometimes oversolicitous attitudes that, in our clinical opinion, is more likely to be found in the personal history of patients with BPD. Such contradictory responses of significant others circularly confirm both the idealization of significant others and the fear of being intruded upon, abandoned, or maltreated – typical features of BPD.

The discovery of untoward ways to shut down the recurring mental suffering linked to the experience of painful incoherence – such as self-injurious behaviors (self-cutting, self-burning, and food or substance abuse) – can also pave the way to a full-blown BPD picture.

Implications for treatment

This understanding of borderline psychopathology has important therapeutic implications. All these implications are consequences of the idea that the activation of the BPD patient's disorganized attachment system in the therapeutic relationship sets into motion the dissociative (disintegrative) processes underpinning painful incoherence in the experience of self. Thus, the prolonged activation of the patient's attachment system is regarded as the main proximate cause of the typical difficulties in the therapeutic relationship with patients with BPD, including premature interruption of the treatment (Liotti *et al.*, 2008; Liotti & Gilbert, 2011). The surfacing of memories of early relational trauma in the care relationships (linked to the disorganized IWM), the related sense of mistrust and powerlessness, the abrupt shifting from fear of loss to fear of attachment, and the increasing experience of painful incoherence of the self in the therapeutic dialogue, are all related to phases of the therapeutic relationship where the patients' attachment (care-seeking) system and the therapists' caregiving system are too strongly and durably activated. The only way for the patient to cope with painful incoherence in the clinical exchange is to resort to a controlling strategy that, in the presence of mentalization deficits, cannot be dealt with easily through transference interpretations.

In order to avoid the formidable obstacles to the treatment posed by the activation of a severely disorganized attachment system, and also to avoid reinforcing the patient's disorganized/controlling strategy based on dominance–submission in the interpersonal exchange (controlling–punitive strategy), it is instrumental to try to base the clinical dialogue on the cooperative motivational system. A cooperative exchange between patient and therapist is the aim of building the therapeutic alliance. Thus, as the consequence of this clinical reasoning, the construction of the therapeutic alliance becomes the first and foremost phase of the treatment. Only after the therapeutic alliance is solidly built, and after its ruptures are repaired, can therapists hope for the success of other interventions (e.g., aimed at fostering emotion regulation and at dealing with dissociative or somatic symptoms). All these other interventions, therefore, must be part of successive phases of the treatment. Thus, this clinical theory is in agreement with the guidelines for the treatment of adult disorders linked to childhood cumulative trauma (including BPD) that prescribe a phase-oriented approach to the psychotherapy (Cloitre *et al.*, 2012; Courtois & Ford, 2013).

The reason for attributing centrality to the therapeutic alliance in the treatment of BPD does not lie only in its being a prerequisite for the successful use of other interventions: it also constitutes the source of corrective relational experiences, paving the way for the difficult task of revising the patient's disorganized IWM in the direction of greater attachment security (Liotti, 2014; Liotti et al., 2008). The process of revising the disorganized IWM is conceived as the core aim when treating BPD, because it is, in turn, a prerequisite for dealing successfully with the painful incoherence in the experience of self (Liotti, 2014; Meares, 2012a).

The construction of the therapeutic alliance, however, is not an easy task with patients with BPD. The strong need for help and soothing can yield a long-lasting activation of the patient's disorganized attachment system, obstructing the activation of the cooperative system. The therapist, therefore, should carefully monitor the activation of the patient's attachment system looking for the cues of a disorganized IWM (e.g., fears of neglect or abandonment and attachment phobia). The patient's negative reactions to the clinical dialogue that is predicted by these cues can adversely affect the therapist. It has been remarked that the main challenge in the treatment of BPD concerns how to deal with the strong counter-transference responses to the patient's tendency to externalize unbearable self-states (Bateman & Fonagy, 2004). Fear, anger, a sense of impotence, and a wish to interrupt the therapy are examples of these counter-transference responses. For instance, the therapist, alarmed due to the patient's self-injurious behaviors, may unwittingly behave as a frightened caregiver, thus re-traumatizing the patient by repeating the interpersonal situation that originally produced the attachment disorganization.

The creation of a good therapeutic alliance and the repair of its ruptures, albeit the primary goal of the first phase of the treatment, must go together with an active engagement of the therapist in alleviating or stabilizing the patient's most disabling symptoms: emptiness, dissociative detachment, rage, panic, helplessness, at-risk behaviors, and the repetition of abusive relations. Even if the success of stabilization procedures is only partial, it allows for the patient to experience the therapeutic relationship as a reasonably safe place – a prerequisite for the therapeutic alliance. The therapist's best efforts, however, may not be enough to build a therapeutic alliance, when they are treating severe borderline pathology. In these cases, it is important to consider a multisetting treatment as a resource.

Multi-setting integrated therapies of BPD

According to the model of BPD based on the idea that painful incoherence is rooted in attachment disorganization and is the core of the disorder, the integration of different but integrated therapy settings involving two or more clinicians helps to prevent or solve many difficulties in the therapeutic alliance that are linked to the activation of the patient's disorganized attachment (Liotti et al., 2008). The adverse influence of a disorganized IWM on the therapeutic alliance can often be counteracted if a second therapist works with the patient in a separate setting (e.g., pharmacotherapy or group therapy). The patient, feeling that there is another source of help available, is less prone to the emotional strain caused by the activation of the attachment system within the first therapeutic relationship (e.g., due to the prospect of the primary therapist's holidays). While the strong activation of the attachment system hinders the patient's mentalization capacity during the clinical dialogue with the primary therapist, the usually lesser involvement of attachment dynamics in the relationship with the secondary therapist may allow for better perspective-taking, so that in the second setting patients may be able to reflect constructively, for instance, on the primary therapist's beliefs and intentions that they have negatively appraised. Reappraising the same interpersonal episode from simultaneous different perspectives improves the capacity for self-reflection and therefore fosters the integration of dissociated internal representations of self-with-others. In turn, this could have a positive feedback effect on the individual's capacity to modulate dysregulated emotions.

The constant cooperating exchange between the different therapists, taking place in scheduled clinical meetings where joint formulation of the clinical case is the goal, could promote another therapeutic effect of multisetting integrated treatments – namely, the patient's experience of two people sharing the same basic reaction to her or his proneness to idealize one of the therapists while aggressively addressing the other. As Bateman and Fonagy (2004) remarked, two or more therapists working as one team when treating a patient with BPD may create the basis for a patient to have a relational experience that is potentially corrective of the tendency to split the representation of others and of the self into exaggeratedly positive and negative pictures.

Finally, another important positive effect is the increased sense of security of the therapist. As noted above, BPD patients, especially those with aggressive impulsive behaviors, quite often evoke negative and sometimes unbearable feelings in their therapists. The involvement of a second, cooperating clinician in the therapy of these severely disturbed patients can reduce the emotional strain on the first therapist, insofar as it allows for the sharing of difficulties, worries, and responsibilities. Thus, the presence of the second therapist is instrumental in avoiding the possibility that the first therapist's counter-transference reactions re-traumatize the patient.

Concluding remarks

One basic assumption underpins the key themes of this chapter: self-constructs and the very experience of self are not a property of the individual mind, but an emergent, intersubjective property of human relatedness. Intellectual giants of philosophical anthropology (e.g., Martin Buber), of sociology (e.g., George Herbert Mead), of developmental psychology (e.g. Daniel Stern), of interpersonal psychiatry (e.g., Harry Stack Sullivan) and of relational psychoanalysis (e.g., Stephen Mitchell) have argued that the experience of self is born of a relational matrix, and can thrive or become disordered according to the quality of interpersonal exchanges. A recent contribution to the relational and social view of the self based on cognitive and developmental neuroscience has been provided by Bruce Hood (2012).

This chapter's inquiry into the disordered experience of self in BPD and its psychotherapy is based as much as possible on the available evidence from controlled research studies or on psychotherapy guidelines suggested by expert consensus. This is the reason for the chapter's focus on the research concerning disorganized attachment and its sequelae rather than on other possible approaches to the relational roots of the painful incoherence in the experience of self that is the core of BPD (e.g., approaches based on self-psychology). This is also the reason for the focus on relational variables of the psychotherapy, such as the therapeutic alliance and the use of parallel integrated interventions, as a way both of coping with the consequences of disorganized attachment followed by relational trauma and dealing with self disturbances – rather than expanding on the particular techniques suggested by the available models of BPD psychotherapy. In our opinion, particular techniques suggested by dialectical-behavior therapy (Linehan, 1993), mentalization-based treatment (Bateman & Fonagy, 2004), transference-focused psychotherapy (Kernberg, Yeomans, Clarkin, & Levy, 2008) and schema therapy (Young, Klosko, & Weishaar, 2003) can all be seen as instrumental in building the therapeutic alliance, repairing its ruptures and providing corrective relational experiences able to gradually correct the patient's attachment disorganization.

The conversational model for the psychotherapy of BPD (Meares, 2012b) is based on this idea, that the self disturbance at the core of BPD can be dealt with successfully with a treatment focused on relational variables. This radically relational approach to the treatment of the core self disturbance of BPD could solve the problem hinted at by an influential Lancet article (Leichsenring, Leibing, Kruse, New, & Leweke, 2011): although the four above-mentioned evidenced-based models of treatment for BPD are based on different conceptualizations of the disorder, there is no evidence that one specific form of treatment is more effective than another. Maybe their different interventions converge in providing the patients with the corrective relational experience necessarily involved in mitigating the painful incoherence in the experience of self-with-others.

Notes

1   The hostile states of mind of a caregiver are assessed in the AAI, according to a coding system proposed by Lyons-Ruth and her collaborators (2005), whenever the persons interviewed report episodes of their childhood where the caregiver has expressed dislike, severe unjustified criticism, or even hate toward the respondent. The coding "helpless state of mind" is attributed to AAI responses where the caregiver is described as powerless or utterly vulnerable. The coding hostile/helpless (HH) of the AAI is statistically related to attachment disorganization. Abdicating attitudes of the caregivers are assessed in a different type of semi-structured interview addressed to the caregivers (Caregiving Interview, CI: George & Solomon, 2008), whenever they describe themselves as incapable or unwilling to take care efficiently of their children. The "abdicating" coding of the CI is also statistically related to disorganization of infant attachment.

2   Mentalization is akin to metacognitive monitoring, but is more focused on monitoring one's own affective mental processes and not mainly concerned with cognition.

3   According to Porges' polyvagal theory, the nucleus of the vagus nerve comprises a myelinated, evolutionarily recent ventral part that is active in conditions of safety, and an evolutionarily older, unmyelinated dorsal part that is active in conditions for extreme, inescapable threat. The dorsal vagus is responsible for a type of immobility characterized by very low muscular tone, bradycardia, superficial slow breath, and numbing of consciousness.

References

Ainsworth, M. D. S., Blehar, M. C., Waters, E., & Wall, S. (1978). *Patterns of Attachment: A Psychological Study of the Strange Situation*. Hillsdale, NJ: Erlbaum.

Amini, F., Lewis, T., Lannon, R., *et al.* (1996). Affect, attachment, memory: Contributions toward psychobiologic integration. *Psychiatry*, 59, 213–239.

Bateman, A. W. & Fonagy, P. (2004).*Psychotherapy for Borderline Personality Disorder: Mentalization Based Treatment*. Oxford: Oxford University Press.

Bowlby, J. (1969). *Attachment and Loss*. Vol. 1. London: The Hogarth Press.

Carlson, E. A., Egeland, B., & Sroufe, L. A. (2009). A prospective investigation of the development of borderline personality symptoms. *Development and Psychopathology*, 21, 1311–1334.

Carlson, E. A., Yates, T. M., & Sroufe, A. (2009). Dissociation and the development of the self. In P. F. Dell & J. A. O'Neill (Eds.), *Dissociation and the Dissociative Disorders* (pp. 39–52). New York, NY: Routledge.

Cloitre, M., Courtois, C. A., Ford, J. D., *et al.* (2012). *The ISTSS Expert Consensus Treatment Guidelines for Complex PTSD in Adults*. Retrieved from http://www.istss.org/

Courtois, C. A. & Ford, J. D. (2013). *Treating Complex Trauma: A Sequenced, Relationship-based Approach*. New York, NY: Guilford

Dutra, L., Bureau, J., Holmes, B., Lyubchik, A., & Lyons-Ruth, K. (2009). Quality of early care and childhood trauma: A prospective study of developmental pathways to dissociation. *Journal of Nervous and Mental Disease*, 197, 383–339.

Farina, B., Speranza, A. M., Dittoni, S., *et al.* (2014). Memories of attachment hampers EEG cortical connectivity in dissociative patients. *European Archives of Psychiatry and Clinical Neurosciences*, 264, 449–458.

Farina, B. & Liotti, G. (2013). Does a dissociative psychopathological dimension exist? A review on dissociative processes and symptoms in developmental trauma spectrum disorders. *Clinical Neuropsychiatry*, 10, 11–18.

Fonagy, P. & Bateman, A. (2008). Attachment, mentalization and borderline personality disorder. *European Psychiatry*, 8, 35–47.

George, C. & Solomon. J. (2008). The caregiving system: A behavioral systems approach to parenting. In J. Cassidy & P. R. Shaver (Eds.), *Handbook of Attachment: Theory, Research and Clinical Applications* (2nd ed., pp. 833–856). New York, NY: Guilford.

Gervai, J. (2009). Environmental and genetic influences on early attachment. *Child and Adolescent Psychiatry and Mental Health*, 3, 25. doi: 10.1186/1753-2000-3-25

Ginot, E. (2007). Intersubjectivity and neuroscience: Understanding enactments and their therapeutic significance within emerging paradigms. *Psychoanalytic Psychology*, 24, 317–332.

Gunderson, J. G. & Lyons-Ruth, K. (2008). BPD's interpersonal hypersensitivity phenotype: A gene–environment–developmental model. *Journal of Personality Disorders*, 22, 22–41.

Hesse, E. (2008). The Adult Attachment Interview: Protocol, method of analysis, and empirical studies. In J. Cassidy & P. R. Shaver (Eds.), *Handbook of Attachment: Theory, Research and Clinical Applications* (2nd ed., pp. 552–598). New York, NY: Guilford.

Hesse, E., Main, M., Abrams, K. Y., & Rifkin, A. (2003). Unresolved states regarding loss or abuse can have "second-generation" effects: Disorganized, role-inversion and frightening ideation in the offspring of traumatized non-maltreating parents. In D. J. Siegel & M. F. Solomon (Eds.), *Healing Trauma: Attachment, Mind, Body and Brain* (pp. 57–106). New York, NY: Norton.

Hesse, E. & Main, M. (2006). Frightened, threatening, and dissociative parental behavior in low-risk samples: Description, discussion, and interpretations. *Development and Psychopathology*, 18, 309–343.

Holmes, E., Brown, R. J., Mansell, W., *et al.* (2005). Are there two qualitatively distinct forms of dissociation? A review and some clinical implications. *Clinical Psychology Review*, 25, 1–23.

Hood, B. (2012). *The Self Illusion: Why There Is No You Inside Your Head*. London: Constable.

Howell, E. (2008). From hysteria to chronic relational trauma disorder: The history of borderline personality disorder and its links with dissociation and psychosis. In A. Moskowitz, I. Schafer, & M. J. Dorahy (Eds.), *Psychosis, Trauma and Dissociation* (pp. 105–116). Oxford: Wiley-Blackwell.

Karpman, S. (1968). Fairy tales and script drama analysis. *Transactional Analysis Bulletin*, 7, 39–43.

Kernberg, O. F., Yeomans, F. E., Clarkin, J. F., & Levy, K. N. (2008). Transference focused psychotherapy: Overview and update. *International Journal of Psychoanalysis*, 89, 601–620.

Leichsenring, F., Leibing, E., Kruse, J., New, A., & Leweke, P. (2011). Borderline personality disorder. *Lancet*, 377, 74–84.

Levy, K. N. (2005). The implications of attachment theory and research for understanding borderline personality disorder. *Development and Psychopathology*, 17, 959–986.

Linehan, M. M. (1993). *Cognitive Behavioral Treatment of Borderline Personality Disorder*. New York, NY: Guilford.

Liotti, G. (1992). Disorganized/disoriented attachment in the etiology of the dissociative disorders. *Dissociation*, 5, 196–204.

Liotti, G. (2004). Trauma, dissociation and disorganized attachment: Three strands of a single braid. *Psychotherapy: Theory, Research, Practice, Training*, 41, 472–486.

Liotti, G. (2011). Attachment disorganization and the controlling strategies: An illustration of the contributions of attachment theory to developmental psychopathology and to psychotherapy integration. *Journal of Psychotherapy Integration*, 21, 232–252.

Liotti, G. (2014). Disorganized attachment in the pathogenesis and the psychotherapy of borderline personality disorder. In A. N. Danquah & K. Berry (Eds.), *Attachment Theory in Adult Mental Health* (pp. 113–128). London: Routledge.

Liotti, G., Cortina, M., & Farina, B. (2008). Attachment theory and the multiple integrated treatment of borderline personality disorder. *Journal of the American Academy of Psychoanalysis and Dynamic Psychiatry*, 36, 293–312.

Liotti, G. & Gilbert, P. (2011). Mentalizing, motivation and social mentalities: Theoretical considerations and implications for psychotherapy. *Psychology and Psychotherapy: Theory, Research and Practice*, 84, 9–25.

Lyons-Ruth, K. (1998). Implicit relational knowing: Its role in development and psychoanalytic treatment. *Infant Mental Health Journal*, 19, 282–289.

Lyons-Ruth, K., Bureau, J., Holmes, B., Easterbrooks, A.,& Brooks, N. H. (2102). Borderline symptoms and suicidality/self-injury in late adolescence: Prospectively observed relationship correlates in infancy and childhood. *Psychiatry Research*, 24, 65–78.

Lyons-Ruth, K., & Jacobvitz, D. (2008). Attachment disorganization: Genetic factors, parenting contexts and developmental transformations from infancy to adulthood. In J. Cassidy & P. R. Shaver (Eds.), *Handbook of Attachment* (2nd ed., pp. 666–697). New York, NY: Guilford.

Lyons-Ruth, K., Melnick, S., Patrick, M., & Hobson, R. P. (2007). A controlled study of hostile–helpless states of mind among borderline and dysthymic women. *Attachment and Human Development*, 9, 1–16.

Lyons-Ruth, K., Yellin, C., Melnick, S., & Atwood, G. (2003). Childhood experiences of trauma and loss have different relations to maternal unresolved and hostile–helpless states of mind on the AAI. *Attachment and Human Development*, 5, 330–352.

Main, M., & Hesse, E. (1990). Parents' unresolved traumatic experiences are related to infant disorganized attachment status: Is frightened and/or frightening parental behavior the linking mechanism? In M. T. Greenberg, D. Cicchetti, & E. M. Cummings (Eds.), *Attachment in the Preschool Years* (pp. 161–182). Chicago, IL: Chicago University Press.

Main, M., & Solomon, J. (1990). Procedures for identifying infants as disorganized/disoriented during the Strange Situation. In M. T. Greenberg, D. Cicchetti, & E. M. Cummings (Eds.), *Attachment in the Preschool Years* (pp. 121–160). Chicago, IL: Chicago University Press.

Meares, R. (2012a). *A Dissociation Model of Borderline Personality Disorder*. New York, NY: Norton.

Meares, R. (2012b) *Borderline Personality Disorder and the Conversational Model: A Clinician's Manual*. New York, NY: Norton.

Meares, R., Gerull, F., Stevenson, J., & Korner, A. (2011). Is self disturbance the core of borderline personality disorder? An outcome study of borderline personality factors. *Australian and New Zealand Journal of Psychiatry*, 45(3), 214–222.

Moss, E., Smolla, N., Cyr, C., et al. (2006). Attachment and behavior problems in middle childhood as reported by adult and child informants. *Development and Psychopathology*, 18, 425–444.

Nijenhuis, E. R & Van der Hart, O. (2011). Dissociation in trauma: A new definition and comparison with previous formulations. *Journal of Trauma and Dissociation*, 12, 416–445.

Ogawa, J. R., Sroufe, L. A., Weinfield, N. S., Carlson, E. A. & Egeland, B. (1997). Development and the fragmented self: Longitudinal study of dissociative symptomatology in a nonclinical sample. *Development and Psychopathology*, 9, 855–879.

Porges, S. W. (1997). Emotion: An evolutionary by-product of the neural regulation of the autonomic nervous system. *Annals of the New York Academy of Sciences*, 807, 62–77.

Porges, S. W. (2001). The polyvagal theory: Phylogenetic substrates of a social nervous system. *International Journal of Psychophysiology*, 42, 123–146.

Schore, A. N. (2009). Attachment, trauma and the developing right brain: Origins of pathological dissociation. In P. F. Dell & J. A. O'Neil (Eds.), *Dissociation and the Dissociative Disorders: DSM-V and Beyond* (pp. 107–141). New York, NY: Routledge.

Solomon, J. & George, C. (2011). Disorganization of maternal caregiving across two generations: The origins of caregiving helplessness. In J. Solomon & C. George (Eds.), *Disorganized Attachment and Caregiving* (pp. 25–51). New York, NY: Guilford.

Van der Hart, O. & Dorahy, M. (2006). Pierre Janet and the concept of dissociation. *American Journal of Psychiatry*, 163, 1646.

Van der Hart, O., Nijenhuis, E. R. S., & Steele, K. (2006). *The Haunted Self: Structural Dissociation and the Treatment of Chronic Traumatization*. New York, NY: Norton.

Van IJzendoorn, M. H., Schuengel, C., & Bakermans-Kranenburg, M. J. (1999). Disorganized attachment in early childhood: Meta-analysis of precursors, concomitants and sequelae. *Development and Psychopathology*, 11, 225–250.

Wilkinson-Ryan, T. & Westen, D. (2000). Identity disturbance in borderline personality disorder: An empirical investigation. *American Journal of Psychiatry*, 157, 528–541.

Young, J. E., Klosko, J. S., & Weishaar, M. (2003). *Schema Therapy: A Practitioner Guide*. New York, NY: Guilford.

Chapter

18

The self in obsessive–compulsive personality disorder

Maja Nedeljkovic, Richard Moulding, Michael Kyrios, and Stephanie Mathews

Introduction

According to the fifth edition of the *Diagnostic and Statistical Manual of Mental Disorders*, personality disorders involve long-standing, persistent, inflexible, and maladaptive ways of experiencing, relating to, and thinking about oneself and the environment, which are associated with impairment in intrapersonal, social, occupational, and academic functioning (American Psychiatric Association [APA], 2013). As such, disturbances in self-concept are key characteristics of personality disorders. Indeed, the alternative DSM-5 model of personality disorders that was proposed to supersede the DSM-4 models – but was moved into Section III of the manual prior to publishing (emerging measures and models) – highlighted this to an even greater degree, with characteristic symptoms described for each personality type within the self (identity and self-direction) and interpersonal (empathy and intimacy) directions (APA, 2013). The personality disorder diagnostic classification embraces a wide variety of personality disorder presentations, with specific types comprising the paranoid, schizoid, schizotypal (cluster A, the "odd, eccentric" disorders); antisocial, borderline, histrionic, narcissistic (cluster B, the "dramatic, emotional, erratic" cluster); and avoidant, dependent, and obsessive–compulsive personality disorders (cluster C, the "anxious, fearful" cluster). This chapter describes the involvement of self within the anxious and fearful cluster, and focuses on the most common and most researched disorder within this cluster – obsessive–compulsive personality disorder (OCPD) – as an exemplar for the impact of self-concept in etiology, maintenance, and treatment

within the cluster C personality disorders. This chapter summarizes and builds on previous theorizing by notable workers in the field, particularly Guidano and Liotti (1983), Beck, Freeman, and Davis (2004), and Millon (2011; Millon & Davis, 1996), along with our own previous theorizing in the area, which integrates and builds on work from these authors (see Kyrios, 1998; Kyrios, Nedeljkovic, Moulding, & Doron, 2007).

Phenomenology of OCPD

OCPD is characterized by eight behavioral or personality traits: rigidity and stubbornness, perfectionism that interferes with task completion, hypermorality and scrupulosity, overattention to detail, miserliness, an inability to discard worn or useless items, excessive devotion to work, and an inability to delegate tasks (APA, 2013). When recast in the alternative model of the DSM-5 as self and other-oriented, these were noted to reflect: difficulties in identity (sense of self derived predominantly from work or productivity; constricted experience and expression of strong emotions), self-direction (difficulty completing tasks and realizing goals, associated with rigid and unreasonably high and inflexible internal standards of behavior; overly conscientious and moralistic attitudes); along with difficulties in empathy (understanding others) and intimacy (work and rigidity interfering with relationships); accompanied by personality traits of rigid perfectionism (must be present), perseveration, intimacy avoidance, and restricted affectivity. The restricted affectivity trait interestingly reflects earlier versions of the DSM criteria for OCPD, but is only considered an associated feature for the working criteria used in the DSM-5.

The Self in Understanding and Treating Psychological Disorders, ed. Michael Kyrios, Richard Moulding, Guy Doron, Sunil S. Bhar, Maja Nedeljkovic, and Mario Mikulincer. Published by Cambridge University Press. © Cambridge University Press, 2016.

Anankastic Personality Disorder in the International Classification of Diseases – 10 (World Health Organization, 1992) is largely consistent with the criteria for OCPD, albeit omitting the miserliness and hoarding criteria in favor of feelings of doubt and caution, and behaviors of excessive pedantry and adherence to social conventions. Indeed, the miserliness and hoarding criteria in DSM-5 can be seen as holdovers from early psychoanalytic descriptions of the anal personality type; Freud considered hoarding behaviors to be a manifestation of the anal stage of development, alongside other characterological aspects now considered to represent OCPD, such as orderliness, obstinancy, and parsimony. However, the hoarding criterion is the least specific and has the lowest positive predictive value of the nine criteria for OCPD in the DSM-IV (Grilo et al., 2001; cf. Pertusa et al., 2008) and now is usually considered to be better accounted for by hoarding disorder, which often shares with OCPD the personality trait of perfectionism (see Moulding, Mancuso, Rehm, & Nedeljkovic, Chapter 13 of this volume, for a discussion of self-concept and structure in hoarding disorder).

OCPD is one of the more common personality disorders, with lifetime prevalence rates of 3–8% (APA, 2013; Diedrich & Voderholzer, 2015; Grant, Mooney, & Kushner, 2012). Individuals with OCPD often present with other mental disorders, including anxiety and affective and substance-related disorders (Grant et al., 2012), as well as eating disorders, hypochondriasis or illness anxiety, and neurological movement disorders (Kyrios, 1998). OCPD accounts for up to 10% of cases in clinical practice (APA, 2013) and represents a major hurdle to successful treatment (Kyrios, 1998). OCPD is not to be confused with obsessive–compulsive disorder (OCD). While earlier psychoanalytic theories placed these two disorders on a continuum, with OCPD on the less severe end and OCD at the more extreme end, there is now research and clinical consensus that there is a distinction between the two disorders (Eisen et al., 2006). However, while a specific relationship between OCPD and OCD is not supported by the data (Black, Noyes, Pfohl, Goldstein, & Blum, 1993; Wu, Clark, & Watson, 2006), they share (non-specific) similarities in their associated characteristics, particularly in the domains of perfectionism and the need for control. Eisen et al. (2006) found that preoccupation with details, hoarding, and perfectionism (i.e., three of the eight criteria for OCPD) were significantly more common in individuals with OCD than in individuals without OCD.

Furthermore, the relationship between these criteria and OCD demonstrated a unique association relative to depressive and other anxiety disorders. Calvo et al. (2009) reported that OCPD was more common in parents of children with OCD, with the same three criteria being more frequent. Therefore, while the OCPD diagnostic classification is not uniquely associated with OCD, certain characteristics of OCPD are associated with OCD. Nevertheless, there has been some confusion, particularly in the earlier literature, with a lack of distinction between these two disorders. Consistent with this, the concept of self-ambivalence discussed in the chapter on OCD (Ahern & Kyrios, Chapter 12 in this volume) takes a prominent role in some of the theoretical approaches to OCPD described below. However, unlike in OCD, where studies have empirically defined and provided support for the role of self-ambivalence (Bhar & Kyrios, 2007), there has been no such empirical research to provide support for the theorized role of self in OCPD. Further, even if there are specific common features that may share common underlying factors, research is also needed to examine the differential etiological pathways that lead to OCPD versus OCD.

In terms of phenomenology, Millon (2011) described eight characteristic patterns of individuals with OCPD: (a) a tendency for them to be highly regulated in their expressiveness and appearance (e.g., tense, restrained, and serious demeanor), which hides an inner ambivalence and insecurity, fear of disapproval, and intense feelings of anger; (b) an overly respectful interpersonal manner characterized by social correctness, formality, a highly developed sense of morality, and a high degree of respect for persons of authority; (c) a highly regulated cognitive style typified by a high adherence to conventional rules, schedule, and hierarchies; (d) a conscientious self-image characterized by a highly disciplined and responsible self, with a dedication to perfection and productivity and that exhibits reservations regarding participating in recreational activities; (e) a high degree of defensiveness against the conscious experience of socially unacceptable thoughts, images, and impulses; (f) activation of a wide range of defenses in response to discomfort associated with emotional responses such as anger, defiance, resentment, and rebelliousness; (g) a compartmentalized morphological organization – that is, a rigid compartmentalization of their inner world, which allows little interaction between drive, memory, and cognition; in order to prevent ambivalent images, feelings, and attitudes spilling into consciousness; and (h) a solemn, overly sensitive, or anhedonic temperament or mood, which could be constitutionally based. Such patterns are said to fall on a continuum ranging from normal and adaptive through to pathological and mal-adaptive, although contextual factors define what con-stitutes dysfunction (Pollak, 1987). The characteristics listed all implicate either implicitly or explicitly the role of self, be it in terms of self-image, self-ambivalence, self in relation to others, and self-regulation.

Numerous OCPD subtypes have been identified which may present different challenges and may there-fore require differential management strategies. Millon and Davis (1996) discuss five adult subtypes: (a) *the conscientious subtype*, characterized by conformity to rules and authority because of a fear of rejection or fail-ure; (b) *the puritanical subtype*, who is characteristically strict and punitive, highly controlled, self-righteous, and extremely judgmental; (c) *the bureaucratic subtype*, who is traditional and who values formality, and who has a powerful identification with bureaucracy, which provides a set of rules, regulations, and firm boundaries to contain feared inner impulses; (d) *the parsimonious subtype*, who protects against the prospect that others might recognize the inner emptiness that they experi-ence, and who is identifiable by a meanness and defen-siveness against loss; and (e) *the bedevilled subtype*, who experiences discord, as their need to conform with the wishes of others clashes with a yearning to assert their own interests, leading to chronic feelings of resentment and conflict. While the identification of these subtypes may be useful, research has yet to establish their valid-ity, the need for idiosyncratic interventions, or even their distinctive etiologies. However, self-concepts are again implicated throughout these types, including an inner emptiness, a fear of inner impulses and a repres-sion of inner wishes, as well as a fear of rejection.

Etiology of OCPD

From an etiological perspective, the role of self is impli-cit across various theoretical models of OCPD, ranging from early psychodynamic approaches to the more modern constructivist approaches of Guidano and Liotti (1983) and of Millon and Davis (1996), which emphasize the concept of self-ambivalence in the eti-ology and maintenance of OCPD, to recent cognitive models by Kyrios (1998; Kyrios et al., 2007) and Beck and colleagues (2004), who incorporate aspects of self-view within the core systems associated with the development and maintenance of the symptoms.

Attachment, post-rationalist and evolutionary perspectives on self in OCPD

Attachment theory (Bowlby, 1969, 1973, 1988) may represent a plausible basis on which to integrate the various approaches to the etiology of personality disor-ders, given the increasingly recognized significance of attachment relationships to psychopathology (Kyrios, 1998; Mikulincer & Doron, Chapter 3, this volume). Based upon the security of an individual's attachment to significant others, basic trust in the world is created which enables the individual to explore their environ-ment and hence to gain a sense of self-control and the ability to deal effectively with difficulty, uncertainty and complexity in the world (Bowlby, 1988). According to Guidano and Liotti (1983), obsessive–compulsive per-sonality reflects an ambivalent attachment style, which developed from parents conveying rejecting attitudes behind an outward facade of attentiveness. Parents of individuals with OCPD are said to be typically emo-tionally undemonstrative and forbid not only the expression of emotion but the feeling of emotion. They tend to set high ethical standards and make unrealistic demands. Positive regard is conditional and rewards are difficult to achieve within this family environment.

Given these early life experiences, post-rationalist approaches such as Guidano and Liotti's (1983) theo-rized that the internalized sense of self is character-ized by a split pattern of self-recognition. That is, individuals simultaneously believe they are loved, accepted, and worthy of love; and unloved, rejected, and unworthy of love. This significantly reduces the possibility of the individual developing a single inte-grated sense of self (Guidano, 1987). The self-concept is ambivalent and incorporates polarized extremes, and self-regard consequently fluctuates between "acceptable" and "unacceptable." Given that any uncer-tainty is perceived as intolerable, to maintain a positive self-image, ambivalence needs to be controlled for and certainty re-established. The commitment to certainty is therefore a commitment to a unified and definite self-identity. Thus the "perception of a unitary iden-tity is equated with the perceived certainty of having control of oneself" (Guidano, 1987, p. 180). It should be noted that, like earlier psychodynamic approaches which viewed OCPD as being on a continuum with OCD, the concept of self-ambivalence has also been applied when describing the cognitive affective structure of those with OCD, albeit with some alterations to the nuance such as how such ambivalence is resolved (see Bhar & Kyrios, 2007; Ahern & Kyrios, Chapter 12, this volume).

Millon's (2011) evolutionary perspective provides an alternative conception of the operation of ambivalence within OCPD. In this model, self-ambivalence is created in OCPD through the struggle between obedience and deviance, and this ambivalence is resolved through inflexible obedience. Oppositional thoughts are repressed in favor of rigid adherence to rules and social expectancies. To illustrate, this can be seen in the relationship of individuals with OCPD to others. The awareness that others do not share their perfectionistic standards can result in individuals with OCPD experiencing internal conflict between fearing social disapproval and expressing feelings of hostility (Millon, 2011). The belief that others' performances are unsatisfactory can result in the perception of increased responsibility and a need for control over feelings of frustration. As such, individuals with OCPD have a strong need to control their social and physical environment, and they find it hard to trust others as they perceive them to be irresponsible and incompetent (Beck *et al.*, 2004; Millon & Davies, 1996). Hostility towards others develops from an assumed coercion that the individual has to accept the standards imposed by others, an assumption that is derived from their early experiences of constraint and discipline in response to times when they had contravened parental rules (Millon & Davis, 1996). Fear of social disapproval evolves from such other-directedness and an assumption that they may be rejected for any possible infringement of such strict and restrictive moral codes. Hence, individuals with OCPD are likely to become preoccupied with perfectionism, control of self and environment, along with order, rules, and regulations, in order to resolve their ambivalence towards others. However, individuals with OCPD also fear revealing their internalized hostility. They experience a fear that these feelings may spiral out of control and reveal their imperfections, resulting in their rejection by others (Millon, 1981). This internal struggle results in further attempts for control, rigidity of behavior, and in affective restriction (McWilliams, 1994).

Individuals with OCPD compartmentalize many aspects of their lives (Millon & Davies, 1996) and rigidly allocate times for every task. In their attempts to maintain control they can disregard their emotional reactions to events and suppress memories. Such efforts for emotional and cognitive control lead to a lack of knowledge regarding the self and difficulties with regulating their emotions. While the compartmentalization may be successful to some extent (e.g., avoiding thinking about relationship issues during weekdays), at other times it may fail (e.g., they may consistently ruminate about these topics during weekends or on vacation times). In addition, a total absorption in the task at hand may result in lashing out at any disturbance. In some cases, such compartmentalization may lead to extreme feelings of detachment from the self, difficulties recalling recent important life events and a continuous sense of never "feeling emotion" or "being in the world." This in turn is likely to further feed into self-ambivalence.

Cognitive perspectives

Cognitive perspectives on OCPD tend to focus closely on characteristic thinking styles and perfectionism. Individuals with OCPD have a rigid cognitive style: with characteristics such as dichotomous (black-or-white) thinking, the use of inflexible rules and on overattentiveness to detail where they "can't see the wood for the trees" (Kyrios, 1998). The sense of autonomy in individuals with OCPD is affected by their central cognitive themes of "should" and the need for control (Beck *et al.*, 2004). This can be seen in their views of self and others, their main beliefs, and the main cognitive strategies they utilize. Cognitive theories note that OCPD is characterized by a conscientious self-image (Beck *et al.*, 2004; Millon, 2011). This includes seeing the self as industrious, reliable, efficient, loyal, disciplined; a fearfulness towards making errors; and dedication to perfection. These aspects of the self are overvalued. Individuals with OCPD hold themselves accountable to their perfectionistic evaluative standards. A lack of self-confidence and indecisiveness can be compensated for through strong conviction to their high standards and disciplined self-restraint (Beck *et al.*, 2004; Millon, 2011). They tend to be as harsh in their self-judgments as they are in their judgments of others. These negative self-evaluations are generally indicative of a self-schema that emphasizes control and order.

Individuals with OCPD are threatened by disorganization and imperfections. To protect against this threat, they utilize cognitive strategies characterized by perfectionistic standards, control, and the application of rules. Beck *et al.* (2004) suggest that individuals with personality disorders demonstrate patterns of behavior that are both under- and overdeveloped. In particular, OCPD is characterized by an overdeveloped sense of control, responsibility, and systemization, while spontaneity and playfulness are underdeveloped. These strategies act as compensatory factors for a vulnerable self-concept. However, while on one hand these strategies are used to protect a vulnerable self-concept, they lead to restriction and a lack of self-complexity. Individuals with OCPD also apply their excessively high standards to others in an attempt to minimize their own weaknesses (Beck *et al.*, 2004). Others are often perceived as incompetent, irresponsible, and self-indulgent. In turn, this can lead to inner hostility and difficulties with relationships.

Individuals with OCPD show an excessive, dysfunctional devotion to achievement, activities of mastery, and work. Their basic insecurity, fear of exploration, and intolerance for uncertainty hinders the development of a range of social roles. Rather than having several social roles, individuals with OCPD overinvest in socially sanctioned, structured social roles such as job competence. This is likely to lead to lower self-complexity, which has been defined as "the number of aspects one uses to cognitively organize knowledge about the self, and the degree of relatedness of these aspects" (Linville, 1985, p. 97). Possessing a greater number of well-developed but disparate areas of self-concept is associated with improved psychological adjustment and a resilience to stressors or disruption within the valued life domains (see Clark, Chapter 5 of this volume for discussion). Conversely, there is extensive evidence from the social-cognitive literature that lower self-complexity is associated with greater affective extremity, greater vulnerability to stressors and failures, more negative self evaluations, a greater level of depression, and poorer adjustment following traumatic experiences (Dixon & Baumeister, 1991; Linville, 1985, 1987; Rafaeli-Mor & Steinberg, 2002).

Perfectionism is a predominant theme characterizing OCPD, and the role of self-concept has been extensively implicated in perfectionism (see e.g., Gregory, Peters & Rapee, Chapter 10, this volume). For example, Flett, Hewitt, and Martin (1995) have suggested that procrastination is a response to a form of social evaluation that involves the perceived imposition of unrealistic expectations on the self. Flett, Hewitt, Davis, and Sherry (2004) suggested that such procrastination is related to a strong fear of failure due to perfectionistic standards. This fear of failure is either associated with, or a byproduct of, feelings of personal inferiority,

inefficacy, and low self-acceptance. While self-oriented perfectionism is sometimes associated with procrastination, socially prescribed perfectionism shows a more robust relationship, reflecting introjected beliefs regarding standards that others require one to meet. Flett and colleagues suggest that this relationship is mediated by automatic cognitions regarding perfectionism, stemming from schemas that the self should be ideal; this conception is similar to conceptions of OCPD as inflexibly adhering to ethical or moral codes with repeated attempts to prove their worth through achieving "perfection" and avoiding "failure" (Guidano & Liotti, 1983). Such avoidant tendencies would serve to place the individual in a high stress position familiar to any student completing assignments, whereby the impending deadline for tasks serves to further pressure the individual, leading to a dysfunctional pattern of avoidance that only serves to increase the stress. Clinical descriptions of individuals with perfectionism or OCPD note that such individuals may never complete their assigned tasks. Such failure to perform tasks would feed into the affected individual's trust of others.

Accompanying such perfectionistic standards, there is a strong belief in achieving correct solutions and that mistakes should be avoided, with any failure being viewed as intolerable (Beck *et al.*, 2004; Kyrios, 1998). "Shoulds" and "musts" are characteristic of individuals with OCPD, with individuals setting up unrealistic expectations of themselves and others. If these expectations are not met, extreme personal criticism results. Consequently, the individual's self-worth suffers; this is particularly the case as the characteristic dichotomous thinking associated with perfectionism, which is rife in OCPD, leads individuals to think that any deviation from what is "right" is automatically "wrong." In essence, their goal is to eliminate mistakes in an attempt to have total control over themselves and their environment.

Integrative perspective

From an integrative perspective incorporating cognitive theory along with the above post-rationalist, evolutionary, and attachment orientations, Kyrios (1998; Kyrios *et al.*, 2007) identified a range of etiological factors relevant to OCPD, including: evolutionary instincts, biological dispositions, and temperament; experiences during developmental stages; and dysfunctional schemas regarding the self, others, and the world. According to Kyrios, ambivalent early attachment experiences were theorized as contributing to the development of five interrelated core cognitive domains that are associated with strong affect and polarities of beliefs. In addition to (a) an ambivalent sense of self worth and defectiveness, as noted by Guidano and Liotti (1983), Kyrios also theorized about resultant impacts upon (b) trust in oneself and others; (c) sense of control over oneself and the external environment; (d) the acquisition of various roles and identities; and (e) the specific role adopted, which emphasizes the ethical, religious, and moral aspects of the self.

Kyrios (1998) suggested that an ambivalent structure of self has flow-on effects on the ability to trust others in individuals with OCPD. That is, trust requires, as a prerequisite, the ability to feel one is truly worthy of love and that other individuals are capable of providing such love. Such trust also has flow-on effects to an individual's sense of control and self-efficacy with respect to the external world, as a consequence of trust in one's ability to elicit care from others in the world (i.e., as one needs a secure base in order to explore the environment and build experiences of mastery). For instance, research suggests that securely attached children are more likely to explore their environment, facilitating the development of cognitive and social skills (Cassidy, Kirsh, Scolton, & Parke, 1996; Jacobsen & Hofmann, 1997; Verschueren & Marcoen, 1999). The lack of trust may then lead to strategies to compensate for such lack of trust – either through the individual becoming extremely dependent or independent; through their setting perfectionistic and unattainable goals; through testing self or others; and through adhering to inflexible rules and regulations. The net result is often procrastination and a lack of creative freedom and problem-solving options, the development of which relies on building a body of experiences upon which to draw.

Kyrios (1998) further suggested that, as a consequence of the limited development of self-efficacy, which is due to a lack of exploration and of trust, the individual with OCPD comes to fear disorganization and uncertainty, and overcompensates through establishing unrealistic, unattainable, and/or unsustainable control strategies over themselves and the world. The lack of exploration also leads to a limitation upon the roles that the individual with OCPD may undertake within the world – a notion similar to that in acceptance and commitment therapy, which posits that avoidance behavior leads individuals to a lack of roles due to its limiting of actions that would be consistent

with valued domains of self (see Zettle, Chapter 6 in this volume). Kyrios suggests that the lack of acquisition of various social roles means the individual does not achieve a normal balance between autonomy and dependence, which in normal development can allow for a sense of social security and confidence in one's ability to deal with challenging situations. Ultimately, the individual with OCPD may adopt Eriksonian (1950, 1959) extremes of either role cohesion (due to an obsession with control) or role diffusion (through procrastination). However, existing at either extreme is not adaptive.

Finally, with respect to morality, Kyrios (1998) suggested that the vulnerable sense of self in OCPD may be bolstered for those who obtain social roles via the adherence to rules and regulations that is apparent in OCPD – particularly the prototypical hypermorality and sense of responsibility. The use of rigid rules and morality enables the individual with OCPD to avoid the complexity and confusion of the world, and to paint for themselves a black-and-white world that in reality exists in shades of gray. The individual feels such a need as their uncertain and unstable self-image, based on their ambivalence, leads to self-doubt. This is developmentally derived from the noted likelihood of parents of individuals with OCPD to adhere to extreme standards and moral codes (Guidano & Liotti, 1983). Kyrios suggests that by taking to the moral high ground, the individual with OCPD can compensate for their ambivalent and unsure self-image through identifying with an external moral authority, abating the need for the individual's normal defenses.

In summary, the above review, and particularly the integrative model of Kyrios (1998), suggests that early attachment experiences and life experiences (particularly significant or recurrent events) play an important role in the development of dysfunctional internal working models and schemas about self, others, and the world, and defenses against such unstable or unsure self-images. While cognitive behavioral therapy techniques addressing beliefs and thinking biases might then be effective in treating OCPD (albeit that OCPD is notoriously difficult to treat), such work also suggests that consideration of underlying schemas and self-representations will also be of importance. A failure to address such constructs may lead to the missing of important drivers of OCPD behavior, or – in a nod to the terminology of psychoanalytically based therapy – to removing defenses without removing the underlying self dysfunction.

Treatment

There has been a dearth of research into the effectiveness of treatments for OCPD, largely because OCPD is less likely to be the presenting issue for treatment (Mancebo, Eisen, Grant, & Rasmussen, 2005). The ego-syntonic nature of the symptoms, the self-imposed high standards, and the potential loss of control and exposure of a vulnerable self-concept may present as barriers to the individual seeking treatment. However, in many cases, the increasingly unachievable standards or failure and interpersonal problems are likely to lead to significant distress and to be associated with a range of other problems including anxiety, depression, OCD, or health problems. Cognitive-behavioral strategies may be useful in addressing some of the presenting symptoms (e.g., anxiety, mood problems, stress, relationship difficulties) and may be used to address the inconsistencies between the client's perceptions and expectations and reality. However, as noted by Kyrios (1998) and supported by Clark (Chapter 5, this volume), traditional cognitive-behavioral frameworks need to be extended to account for the impact of attachment and self-related issues not only on the individual's symptomatology but also on the client's response and engagement in treatment. Indeed, studies have shown that treatments that incorporate work on self-esteem and therapeutic alliance are associated with improved outcomes (Cummings, Hayes, Cardaciotto, & Newman, 2012; Strauss *et al.*, 2006) and that changes in self-construals are associated with better treatment outcomes and lower relapse rates (Kyrios, Hordern, & Fassnacht, 2015).

Treatment protocols for the most common personality trait within OCPD – perfectionism – exist (Egan, Wade, Shafran, & Antony, 2014; Shafran, Egan, & Wade, 2010) and there is some evidence that they are effective (Egan & Hine, 2008; Riley, Lee, Cooper, Fairburn, & Shafran, 2007), particularly those within the CBT modality (for review, see Egan, Wade, & Shafran, 2011). CBT protocols typically emphasize cognitive distortions such as black-and-white thinking; high standards and should statements; overgeneralizing, and catastrophic thinking. Notably, some of these treatment approaches also implicate self-concept. For example, "should" statements are evaluative standards that can be considered to represent one's failure to have actual self meet the standards of ideal self, when considered from the viewpoint of Higgins' (1987) self-discrepancy theory. As a client once told us, "If you use 'shoulds', you are 'shoulding' all over yourself." Equally, in exploring overgeneralization, Egan and colleagues recommend a number of questions related to self-definition; for example, "How does it follow that someone's worth as a person can be judged from one mistake or one instance of not meeting a goal?", "What is the universal definition that people in society would hold of a 'failure?' How do you compare to that definition? In what ways are you similar or different?", and "How does your belief that 'even one small mistake makes me a complete failure' impact on your self-esteem and mood?"

In addition, mindfulness techniques (Segal, Williams, & Teasdale, 2002), whereby the client is required to refocus attention on the present moment, could be quite useful in decreasing intense mood states, but also may allow the client to be able to expose themselves to feeling states as an observer and thereby increasing tolerance of mild negative affective states, and avoiding rumination over past mistakes and errors. A recent study in a college sample found that mindfulness may impact on the relationship between socially prescribed perfectionism and negative affect, by removing the mediating effects of rumination (Short & Mazmanian, 2013). Mindfulness intervention can be undertaken in conjunction with cognitive techniques that involve challenging of faulty beliefs surrounding the expression of emotions (e.g., "emotions can and should be controlled"). Gestalt techniques (e.g., the empty chair technique) can also be useful in bringing the client's emotions to "here-and-now" and to integrate polarized self views.

Activity scheduling is a behavioral strategy that can be particularly useful in improving mood in OCPD through engagement in a range of rewarding activities in the short term, but also from a preventative perspective in addressing the OCPD-related aversion for recreational activities, overemphasis on work, and job overinvolvement. From an alternative viewpoint, values-based exercises from acceptance and commitment therapy may achieve a similar outcome, in terms of expanding commitment to a variety of domains of life (see Zettle, Chapter 6, this volume). Clearly, one of the most important aspects of mental well-being is the ability "to gain satisfaction from a variety of sources" (Speller, 1989). More importantly, however, these strategies also have the potential of increasing self-complexity. As noted previously, individuals with OCPD are likely to engage or derive satisfaction from a restricted range of activities, often in those they perceive as productive. Increasing the range of activities, particularly in areas or domains unrelated to existing interests, is important to both increase the number and decrease overlap of domains, the two aspects contributing to self-complexity (Linville, 1985). These activities may be scheduled initially in a structured manner with assistance of the therapist, particularly as many of them (e.g., relaxation, mindfulness) may be viewed by the individual with OCPD as unproductive and unnecessary.

Such strategies counter the narrow and closed attention of the individual with OCPD to particular work-based domains of self-concept through providing experiences outside their usual routines, while increasing their ability to manage and tolerate affective states. Indeed, the ability for emotional regulation and distress tolerance is becoming increasingly recognized as important across a range of areas of dysfunction, including interpersonal relationships, study, and the workplace (Aldao & Nolen-Hoeksema, 2010; Aldao, Nolen-Hoeksema, & Schweizer, 2010; Kyrios et al., 2007). This will be particularly important as individuals with OCPD start to increasingly encounter situations that are novel and subjectively threatening and that may have been previously avoided. Individuals with OCPD may require support in dealing with their internal emotional states and the appropriate identification and expression of emotion, particularly with respect to hostility and anger. For instance, assertiveness training and anger management are useful strategies for dealing with the internalized hostility that often threatens to break out in affected individuals, along with interventions aimed at increasing distress tolerance (Barlow, Allen, & Choate, 2004; Bornovalova, Gratz, Daughters, Hunt, & Lejuez, 2012; Boswell et al., 2013; Linehan, 1993). Furthermore, training in appropriate interpersonal skills (e.g., social skills, sensitivity, and empathy training) can also be useful in circumventing the build-up of hostility.

Further, given the high need for control, it is important for difficulties and fears to be confronted in a structured and graded manner and in the presence of unconditional and consistent support. Identification of "high-risk" situations, expected outcomes and responses, gradual exposure to the identified situation in an order of increasing risk, and testing out the individual's predictions and coping levels would all likely be of assistance. Emphasis should be placed on the collaborative nature of the relationship, through provision of consistent support and encouragement for a client-led treatment agenda. Ultimately, individuals would develop skills in dealing with anxiety and discomfort in specific situations and, in addition, build up a sense of confidence in their ability to deal with threat and ambivalence. Indeed, the lack of trust suggested to be developmentally important within OCPD would indicate that it is vital to provide a therapeutic relationship following basic Rogerian principles of strong positive regard and a consistent and responsive therapist.

Conclusion

The above review suggests that individuals with OCPD hold restricted self-views as defined by work-related competence, alongside extreme perfectionistic traits and an attempt to assert complete control over their lives or environment. These attempts are doomed to failure; as a result, some individuals are likely to report becoming overwhelmed. The focus of individuals with OCPD on particular areas of their lives leads to a general neglect of other domains, with the self defined with respect to excellence and achievement within such areas. Even within the individual with OCPD's focus on work, they may focus on areas of their workload in which they feel a degree of control or that they find more black-and-white (e.g., tasks requiring attention to detail, solo tasks) to the detriment of tasks requiring creativity, flexibility, and group interaction. We have suggested potential developmental pathways to such dysfunction, following earlier theoretical work by Kyrios (1998), which particularly implicates as relevant the areas of ambivalence in self, lack of trust, low self-efficacy, role limitation, and ethical/moral inflexibility. In addition to treatment protocols focusing on cognitive distortions within perfectionism, the attuned therapist should be aware of opportunities to challenge such self-domains and expand some limited conceptualizations of self, which we believe to be important for the functioning of individuals with OCPD in the world.

In general, this is an area needing much future empirical work to support the theoretical discourse. Specifically, as concepts such as self-ambivalence have now been empirically validated (Bhar & Kyrios, 2007), the relationship to OCPD and potential points of differentiation with OCD can now be examined empirically. Further, future research needs to examine the potential neurocognitive bases of such self-conceptions and potential links to OCPD cognitions and behaviors. There is an emerging body of research indicating that specific neural mechanisms are associated with hypomorality and hypermorality, the latter of which is characteristic of individuals with OCPD (Blair, Marsh, Finger, Blair, & Luo, 2006; Braun, Lévellé, & Guimond, 2008). The relationship between self perceptions, cognitions, and behaviors with the function in these areas needs to be an area of future research.

References

Aldao, A., & Nolen-Hoeksema, S. (2010). Specificity of cognitive emotion regulation strategies: A transdiagnostic examination. *Behaviour Research and Therapy*, 48(10), 974–983.

Aldao, A., Nolen-Hoeksema, S., & Schweizer, S. (2010). Emotion-regulation strategies across psychopathology: A meta-analytic review. *Clinical Psychology Review*, 30(2), 217–237.

American Psychiatric Association. (2013). *Diagnostic and Statistical Manual of Mental Disorders (DSM-5®)*. Washington, DC: American Psychiatric Publishing.

Barlow, D. H., Allen, L. B., & Choate, M. L. (2004). Toward a unified treatment for emotional disorders. *Behavior Therapy*, 35(2), 205–230.

Beck, A. T., Freeman, A., & Davis, D. D. (2004). *Cognitive Therapy of Personality Disorders* (2nd ed.). New York, NY: Guilford.

Bhar, S. S., & Kyrios, M. (2007). An investigation of self-ambivalence in obsessive–compulsive disorder. *Behaviour Research and Therapy*, 45(8), 1845–1857.

Black, D. W., Noyes, R., Pfohl, B., Goldstein, R. B., & Blum, N. (1993). Personality disorder in obsessive–compulsive volunteers, well comparison subjects, and their first-degree relatives. *The American Journal of Psychiatry*, 150(8), 1226–1232.

Blair, J., Marsh, A. A., Finger, E., Blair, K. S., & Luo, J. (2006). Neuro-cognitive systems involved in morality. *Philosophical Explorations: An International Journal for the Philosophy of Mind and Action*, 9, 13–27.

Bornovalova, M. A., Gratz, K. L., Daughters, S. B., Hunt, E. D., & Lejuez, C. (2012). Initial RCT of a distress tolerance treatment for individuals with substance use disorders. *Drug and Alcohol Dependence*, 122(1), 70–76.

Boswell, J. F., Farchione, T. J., Sauer-Zavala, S., *et al.* (2013). Anxiety sensitivity and interoceptive exposure: A transdiagnostic construct and change strategy. *Behavior Therapy*, 44(3), 417–431.

Bowlby, J. (1969). *Attachment and Loss, Volume I: Attachment*. New York, NY: Basic Books.

Bowlby, J. (1973). *Attachment and Loss: Separation: Anxiety and Anger* (Vol. 2). New York, NY: Basic Books.

Bowlby, J. (1988). *A Secure Base: Parent–Child Attachment and Healthy Human Development*. New York, NY: Basic Books.

Braun, C. M. J., Levelle, C., & Guimond, A.(2008). An orbitofrontostriatopallidal pathway for morality: Evidence from postlesion antisocial and obsessive compulsive disorder. *Cognitive Neuropsychiatry*, 13, 296–337.

Calvo, R., Lázaro, L., Castro-Fornieles, J., *et al.* (2009). Obsessive–compulsive personality disorder traits and personality dimensions in parents of children with obsessive–compulsive disorder. *European Psychiatry*, 24(3), 201–206.

Cassidy, J., Kirsh, S. J., Scolton, K. L., & Parke, R. D. (1996). Attachment and representations of peer relationships. *Developmental Psychology*, 32(5), 892.

Cummings, J. A., Hayes, A. M., Cardaciotto, L., & Newman, C. F. (2012). The dynamics of self-esteem in cognitive therapy for avoidant and obsessive–compulsive personality disorders: An adaptive role of self-esteem variability? *Cognitive Therapy and Research*, 36(4), 272–281.

Diedrich, A., & Voderholzer, U. (2015). Obsessive–compulsive personality disorder: A current review. *Current Psychiatry Reports*, 17(2), 1–10.

Dixon, T. M., & Baumeister, R. F. (1991). Escaping the self: The moderating effect of self-complexity. *Personality and Social Psychology Bulletin*, 17(4), 363–368.

Egan, S. J., & Hine, P. (2008). Cognitive behavioural treatment of perfectionism: A single case experimental design series. *Behaviour Change*, 25(4), 245–258.

Egan, S. J., Wade, T. D., & Shafran, R. (2011). Perfectionism as a transdiagnostic process: A clinical review. *Clinical Psychology Review*, 31(2), 203–212.

Egan, S. J., Wade, T. D., Shafran, R., & Antony, M. M. (2014). *Cognitive-Behavioral Treatment of Perfectionism*. New York, NY: Guilford Publications.

Eisen, J. L., Coles, M. E., Shea, M. T., *et al.* (2006). Clarifying the convergence between obsessive compulsive personality disorder criteria and obsessive compulsive disorder. *Journal of Personality Disorders*, 20(3), 294–305.

Erikson, E. H. (1950). *Childhood and Society*. New York, NY: WW Norton & Co.

Erikson, E. H. (1959). Growth and crises of the "healthy personality." In G. S. Klein (Ed.), *Psychological Issues*. New York, NY: International University Press.

Flett, G. L., Hewitt, P. L., Davis, R. A., & Sherry, S. B. (2004). Description and counseling of the perfectionistic procrastinator. In H. C. Schouwenburg, C. H. Lay, T. A. Pychyl, & J. R. Ferrari (Eds.), *Counseling the Procrastinator in Academic Settings* (pp. 181–194). Washington, DC: American Psychological Association.

Flett, G. L., Hewitt, P. L., & Martin, T. R. (1995). Dimensions of perfectionism and procrastination. In *Procrastination and Task Avoidance* (pp. 113–136). New York, NY: Springer.

Grant, J. E., Mooney, M. E., & Kushner, M. G. (2012). Prevalence, correlates, and comorbidity of DSM-IV obsessive–compulsive personality disorder: Results from the National Epidemiologic Survey on Alcohol and Related Conditions. *Journal of Psychiatric Research*, 46(4), 469–475.

Grilo, C. M., McGlashan, T. H., Morey, L. C., *et al.* (2001). Internal consistency, intercriterion overlap and diagnostic efficiency of criteria sets for DSM-IV schizotypal, borderline, avoidant and obsessive–compulsive personality disorders. *Acta Psychiatrica Scandinavica*, 104(4), 264–272.

Guidano, V. F. (1987). *Complexity of the Self*. New York, NY: Guilford.

Guidano, V. F., & Liotti, G. (1983). *Cognitive Processes and Emotional Disorders: A Structural Approach to Psychotherapy*. New York, NY: Guilford Press.

Higgins, E. T. (1987). Self-discrepancy: A theory relating self and affect. *Psychological Review*, 94(3), 319.

Jacobsen, T., & Hofmann, V. (1997). Children's attachment representations: Longitudinal relations to school behavior and academic competency in middle childhood and adolescence. *Developmental Psychology*, 33(4), 703–710.

Kyrios, M. (1998). A cognitive-behavioral approach to the understanding and management of obsessive–compulsive personality disorder. In C. Perris & P. McGorry (Eds.), *Cognitive Psychotherapy of Psychotic and Personality Disorders: Handbook of Theory and Practice* (pp. 351–378). New York, NY: Wiley.

Kyrios, M., Hordern, C., & Fassnacht, D. B. (2015). Predictors of response to cognitive behaviour therapy for obsessive–compulsive disorder. *International Journal of Clinical and Health Psychology*, 15(3), 181–190.

Kyrios, M., Nedeljkovic, M., Moulding, R., & Doron, G. (2007). Problems of employees with personality disorders: The exemplar of obsessive–compulsive personality disorder (OCPD). In J. Langan-Fox, C. L. Cooper, & R. J. Klimoski (Eds.), *Research Companion to the Dysfunctional Workplace: Management Challenges and Symptoms* (pp. 40–57). Cheltenham: Elgar.

Linehan, M. (1993). *Cognitive-Behavioral Treatment of Borderline Personality Disorder*. New York, NY: Guilford Press.

Linville, P. W. (1985). Self-complexity and affective extremity: Don't put all of your eggs in one cognitive basket. *Social Cognition*, 3(1), 94–120.

Linville, P. W. (1987). Self-complexity as a cognitive buffer against stress-related illness and depression. *Journal of Personality and Social Psychology*, 52(4), 663.

Mancebo, M. C., Eisen, J. L., Grant, J. E., & Rasmussen, S. A. (2005). Obsessive compulsive personality disorder and obsessive compulsive disorder: Clinical characteristics, diagnostic difficulties, and treatment. *Annals of Clinical Psychiatry*, 17(4), 197–204.

McWilliams, N. (1994). *Psychoanalytic Diagnosis*. New York, NY: Guilford Press.

Millon, T. (1981). *Disorders of Personality: DSM-III, Axis II*. New York, NY: John Wiley & Sons.

Millon, T. (2011). *Disorders of Personality: Introducing a DSM/ICD Spectrum from Normal to Abnormal*. New York, NY: John Wiley & Sons.

Millon, T., & Davis, R. O. (1996). *Disorders of Personality: DSM-IV and Beyond*. New York, NY: John Wiley & Sons.

Pertusa, A., Fullana, M., Singh, S., *et al.* (2008). Compulsive hoarding: OCD symptom, distinct clinical syndrome, or both? *The American Journal of Psychiatry*, 165(10), 1289.

Pollak, J. (1987). Obsessive–compulsive personality: Theoretical and clinical perspectives and recent research findings. *Journal of Personality Disorders*, 1(3), 248–262.

Rafaeli-Mor, E., & Steinberg, J. (2002). Self-complexity and well-being: A review and research synthesis. *Personality and Social Psychology Review*, 6(1), 31–58.

Riley, C., Lee, M., Cooper, Z., Fairburn, C. G., & Shafran, R. (2007). A randomised controlled trial of cognitive-behaviour therapy for clinical perfectionism: A preliminary study. *Behaviour Research and Therapy*, 45(9), 2221–2231.

Segal, Z. V., Williams, J. M. G., & Teasdale, J. D. (2002). *Mindfulness-based Cognitive Therapy for Depression: A New Approach to Relapse Prevention*. New York, NY: Guilford Press.

Shafran, R., Egan, S., & Wade, T. (2010). *Overcoming Perfectionism: A Self-help Guide using Cognitive Behavioral Techniques*. London: Robinson.

Short, M. M., & Mazmanian, D. (2013). Perfectionism and negative repetitive thoughts: Examining a multiple mediator model in relation to mindfulness. *Personality and Individual Differences*, 55(6), 716–721.

Speller, J.L. (1989). *Executives in Crisis: Recognizing and Managing the Alcoholic, Drug-addicted, or Mentally Ill Executive*. San Francisco, CA: Jossey-Bass.

Strauss, J. L., Hayes, A. M., Johnson, S. L., *et al.* (2006). Early alliance, alliance ruptures, and symptom change in a nonrandomized trial of cognitive therapy for avoidant and obsessive–compulsive personality disorders. *Journal of Consultations in Clinical Psychology*, 74(2), 337.

Verschueren, K., & Marcoen, A. (1999). Representation of self and socioemotional competence in kindergartners: Differential and combined effects of attachment to mother and to father. *Child Development*, 70(1), 183–201.

World Health Organization. (1992). *The ICD-10 Classification of Mental and Behavioural Disorders: Clinical Descriptions and Diagnostic Guidelines*. Geneva: World Health Organization.

Wu, K., Clark, L. E., & Watson, D. (2006). Relations between obsessive–compulsive disorder and personality: Beyond axis i–axis ii comorbidity. *Journal of Anxiety Disorders,* 20, 695–717.

Chapter

19

The self in chronic fatigue syndrome

Stefan Kempke, Eline Coppens, Patrick Luyten, and
Boudewijn Van Houdenhove

Introduction

Chronic fatigue syndrome (CFS) is a chronic and disabling condition that closely resembles Beard's description of neurasthenia (or nervous exhaustion) in the nineteenth century (Wessely, Hotopf, & Sharpe, 1998). Today, CFS is considered part of a larger group of functional somatic syndromes that are characterized by persistent somatic symptoms (e.g., musculoskeletal pain, fatigue, gastrointestinal problems), which cannot be fully explained by a medical or psychiatric condition (Wessely et al., 1998; Wessely, Nimnuan, & Sharpe, 1999). The syndrome is most commonly diagnosed in women between the ages of 40 and 49 (Boneva et al., 2011), and is usually associated with high personal costs (e.g., job loss, social isolation; Assefi, Coy, Uslan, Smith, & Buchwald, 2003). Prevalence rates of the illness remain unclear, but according to Reeves et al. (2007) are estimated at 2.5% of the adult population. The diagnosis of CFS is by exclusion: it is based on consensus criteria developed by experts and involves an extensive medical and psychiatric examination to exclude other disorders that could explain the symptoms. According to current diagnostic criteria, the core symptoms of CFS are unexplained and prolonged fatigue, and effort intolerance (i.e., post-exertional malaise or extreme exhaustion following physical or mental efforts; Carruthers et al., 2011; Fukuda et al., 1994). Additional symptoms include muscle pain, headaches, sore throat, tender lymph nodes, substantial impairment of short-term memory or concentration, and unrefreshing sleep (Fukuda et al., 1994). In most cases, the symptoms are triggered by acute physical and/or emotional stressors (e.g., after a viral infection or after a psychological loss experience; Van

Houdenhove & Egle, 2004; Van Houdenhove, Luyten, & Kempke, 2013; see also below) and the illness onset gradually develops over months or years (Boneva et al., 2011; Van Houdenhove, Van Hoof, et al., 2009).

Several studies in CFS have shown that comorbidity is the rule rather than the exception (Van Houdenhove, Kempke, & Luyten, 2010). For instance, there is a high rate of comorbidity between CFS and other functional somatic syndromes, most notably fibromyalgia (FM) syndrome (i.e., chronic widespread pain in muscles and joints), leading researchers to propose that CFS and FM are part of one spectrum of pain and fatigue disorders that are interrelated through common etiopathogenic mechanisms (Ablin et al., 2012; Van Houdenhove et al., 2010, 2013). Moreover, CFS has been associated with elevated rates of both lifetime and current psychiatric disorders – particularly depression (Van Houdenhove et al., 2010; Van Houdenhove & Luyten, 2006). According to a population-based study by Nater et al. (2009), for instance, almost 60% of patients with CFS had at least one current psychiatric diagnosis.

Although the etiology of CFS is considered to be multifactorial (Van Houdenhove & Luyten, 2008), there is accumulating evidence that life stress – probably in combination with genetic factors – may play a role in the illness via disturbances in the stress response system (Nater, Maloney, Heim, & Reeves, 2011; Van Houdenhove et al., 2013). Specifically, recent evidence strongly suggests that at least in a subgroup of patients, CFS may reflect a fundamental dysregulation – or, more specifically, a loss of resilience – of the hypothalamic–pituitary–adrenal (HPA) axis, the main human stress response system (Van Houdenhove & Luyten, 2010; Van Houdenhove et al., 2013; Van

The Self in Understanding and Treating Psychological Disorders, ed. Michael Kyrios, Richard Moulding, Guy Doron, Sunil S. Bhar, Maja Nedeljkovic, and Mario Mikulincer. Published by Cambridge University Press. © Cambridge University Press, 2016.

Houdenhove, Van Den Eede, & Luyten, 2009). The HPA axis is responsible for the production of the stress hormone cortisol, which enables an individual to adequately adapt to various stressors (Claes & Nemeroff, 2005). In terms of McEwen's allostatic load concept (i.e., the cumulative wear and tear on the body resulting from chronic stress; McEwen, 1998), CFS seems to be associated with an "allostatic crash" after a prolonged period of hyperactivity of the HPA axis due to chronic stress or overexertion, as evidenced by, for instance, lower cortisol activity, enhanced negative feedback, and blunted cortisol reactivity to stress, compared to non-fatigued controls (Cleare, 2003; Papadopoulos & Cleare, 2011; Tak *et al.*, 2011; Tomas, Newton, & Watson, 2013; Van Houdenhove, Van Den Eede, *et al.*, 2009). This may explain why patients with CFS do not adequately respond to and recover from mental and/or physical stressors ("effort intolerance"), which is one of the most important diagnostic characteristics of the illness (Van Houdenhove & Luyten, 2010; Van Houdenhove *et al.*, 2013). Importantly, dysregulation of the HPA axis has been shown to affect various other biological systems, such as neurotransmitter systems, the immune system as well as pain regulatory systems (Van Houdenhove & Egle, 2004). For instance, CFS has been associated with increased immune activity, generating typical post-exertional flu-like malaise and "sickness-behavior" (Silverman, Heim, Nater, Marques, & Sternberg, 2010).

From a psychological point of view, there is increasing evidence that in at least a subgroup of patients with CFS, a strong achievement orientation, a self-critical attitude, and a perfectionistic lifestyle are key factors contributing to chronic stress/overload and the ensuing neurobiological alterations that underlie the illness (Kempke *et al.*, 2013a; Kempke, Luyten, Mayes, Van Houdenhove, & Claes, in press; Luyten *et al.*, 2011; Van Houdenhove *et al.*, 2013). Moreover, we and others have argued that excessive achievement strivings and self-critical perfectionism may reflect disruptions in normal personality development, i.e., be compensatory strategies to defend against negative self-feelings and to prove one's self-worth (Kempke *et al.*, 2013a; Van Houdenhove, Neerinckx, Onghena, Lysens, & Vertommen, 2001). Indeed, behind the image of self-sufficiency and resilience (whereby patients present themselves in relation to others as self-reliant and strong) often lies extreme vulnerability, particularly due to unresolved trauma. In this chapter, we discuss findings showing that a lack of integration of (opposing) self-experiences or mental representations may contribute to a dysregulation of the central stress mechanisms in CFS. We take a dialectic perspective on the emergence and experience of the self in health and disease, rooted in Sidney Blatt's two-configurations theory of normal and pathological development (e.g., Blatt, 2004). First, we give an overview of theory and research concerning the role of self-critical perfectionism (SCP) and its correlates in CFS. Next, we discuss the role of attachment insecurities in CFS within the context of empirical research on early adverse experiences. Finally, we consider the implications of the above-mentioned theory and research for treatment programs for CFS.

Case example

Catherine, a 41-year-old secretary, has suffered for three years from severe mental and physical fatigue combined with widespread muscle pain. Lately, she feels weak and tired after minimal effort (e.g., reading a book or going for a walk), and it seems she will not be able to continue her full-time job. She has been through a very stressful period – a difficult and painful divorce from her husband. After a comprehensive examination at the local hospital, she was diagnosed with CFS because of unexplained fatigue lasting for more than six months. She has always been very critical and demanding of herself, pushing herself beyond her limits and ignoring bodily signals (e.g., recurrent throat infections, unrefreshing sleep). She wanted to do everything perfectly, both in her job as a secretary but also at home. Last year she was awarded as the best secretary of the company; now she cannot even do simple household activities. She felt she had failed both as a wife and as a secretary. She says she does not want any help, especially not from her mother. The relationship with her mother has always been problematic; Catherine described her mother as very critical, pragmatic, and rather unemotional. Catherine was named after her mother's first daughter who passed away after birth. She always had the feeling of being unwanted.

Self-critical perfectionism and overload in CFS

As illustrated by the story of Catherine, many patients with CFS are characterized by high achievement orientation and perfectionistic personality traits (Kempke *et al.*, 2013a). Following Blatt's theory, maladaptive personality development in CFS may reflect a disruption of the normal dialectical interaction between two fundamental developmental lines, i.e., an anaclitic, relatedness or attachment line that normally leads to increasingly mature, complex, and mutually satisfying interpersonal relations, on the one hand, and an introjective or self-definitional line that normally leads to the development of a stable, realistic, and essentially positive self and identity on the other hand (Luyten & Blatt, 2013; Luyten *et al.*, 2011). Disruption in this dialectic, however, leads to an overemphasis on or exaggeration of one developmental line to the neglect of the other. Self-critical perfectionism (SCP), which shows similarities with Beck's description of "autonomy" and the concept of attachment avoidance (Blatt & Levy, 2003; Luyten, Blatt, & Corveleyn, 2005; Shahar, 2001; Sibley, 2007), thus includes an overemphasis on the self-definition line and a defense against dependency needs – also termed "counterdependency" (Gregory, Manring, & Wade, 2005). This personality configuration is characterized by a harsh ego ideal leading to overly critical self-evaluations and feelings of guilt when not meeting standards (Blatt, 2004; Luyten *et al.*, 2005). Hence, self-representations in patients with CFS are often fragmented and extremely dependent on the approval of others. In order to protect the self from "negative introjects" – often experienced as a threat to the self – and to prove one's self-worth, self-critical patients with CFS primarily use higher order (counteractive) defense mechanisms, in particular reaction formation and overcompensation in terms of mental and/or physical overexertion, leading to a "false" self that is self-reliant and strong (Cuykx, Van Houdenhove, & Neerinckx, 1998; Van Houdenhove, Neerinckx, Onghena, *et al.*, 2001). In the same vein, CFS has been associated with excessive self-sacrificing tendencies (e.g., compulsive caregiving), reflecting the underlying search for acceptance and recognition (Van Houdenhove, Neerinckx, Lysens, *et al.*, 2001). This is reminiscent of Blumer and Heilbronn's (1982, p. 387) classical description of the core issues of the pain-prone disorder in terms of "strong needs to be accepted and to depend on others, as well as marked needs to receive affection and to be cared for."

Empirical research has supported the important role of overcompensation in the development and maintenance of CFS. In an interesting qualitative study, Wentz and colleagues (Wentz, 2005; Wentz, Lindberg, & Hallberg, 2004) identified an unprotected self in fibromyalgia (FM) patients, reflecting high levels of stress during childhood (due to lack of protection in relation to stimuli and affects) and emotion regulation difficulties in adulthood, promoting the use of so-called compensating strategies, such as "hypomanic repair" (i.e., meeting the needs of others to an extreme extent), conflict handling through action, and demonstrating strength/being in control. According to Wentz (2005), extreme helpfulness to other people and intense activity has become a way for these individuals to compensate for psychological vulnerability. In the same vein, Pemberton and Cox (2014), using semi-structured interviews, reported a pre-morbid state of constant motion among patients with CFS and a tendency towards negative feelings and beliefs about "doing nothing." Similar findings have been reported in a population-based study consisting of 4779 participants who were followed for the first 53 years of their life (Harvey, Wadsworth, Wessely, & Hotopf, 2008). Results of this study showed that increased pre-morbid levels of exercise were associated with an increased risk of developing CFS.

Moreover, both cross-section and longitudinal studies suggest that SCP is implicated in CFS (Dittner, Rimes, & Thorpe, 2011; Kempke *et al.*, 2013a; Kempke, Van Houdenhove, *et al.*, 2011; Magnusson, Nias, & White, 1996; Moss-Morris, Spence, & Hou, 2011). For instance, Kempke, Van Houdenhove, *et al.* (2011), in an attempt to replicate previous findings on the nature of perfectionism (Dunkley, Blankstein, Masheb, & Grilo, 2006), demonstrated a distinction between adaptive and maladaptive (i.e., concern over mistakes, doubts about actions) perfectionism in CFS in that only the maladaptive (or self-critical) component was significantly related to fatigue. More recently, we showed that SCP predicted increased levels of fatigue and pain over the 14-day period and this was independent of the severity of depression, and was probably mediated by its impact on stress and activity levels, as discussed in greater detail below (Kempke *et al.*, 2013a). Using a prospective design, Moss-Morris *et al.* (2011) showed that maladaptive perfectionism predicted the onset of CFS in patients suffering from glandular fever. Recently, we investigated whether SCP in CFS may reflect disruptions in normal personality development, i.e., be a compensatory strategy to defend against negative self-feelings, or be associated with broader personality disturbances. In a controlled study, we demonstrated elevated levels of maladaptive personality features (notably obsessive–compulsive personality disorder features) that are related to negative perfectionism, but found no evidence for increased prevalence rates of personality disorders (16.3%) in patients with CFS (Kempke, Van Den Eede, *et al.*, 2013). Finally, a number of studies have demonstrated higher levels of maladaptive or unhealthy perfectionism in CFS as compared to normal controls and non-fatigued patients (Deary & Chalder, 2010; Sirois & Molnar, 2014; White & Schweitzer, 2000). Of particular interest is a study by Luyten, Van Houdenhove, Cosyns, and Van den Broeck (2006) showing that patients with CFS retrospectively reported both higher pre- and post-morbid levels of perfectionism compared to normal controls. Most recently, Sirois and Molnar (2014) found higher levels of maladaptive perfectionism among patients with CFS compared to healthy controls and patients with irritable bowel syndrome or fibromyalgia/arthritis. It is important to note here that although SCP is more closely related to exhaustion and chronic fatigue, studies have also demonstrated a link between high self-criticism and chronic pain (Lerman, Rudich, & Shahar, 2010; Lerman, Shahar, & Rudich, 2011; Rudich, Lerman, Gurevich, Weksler, & Shahar, 2008).

Several mechanisms may explain the observed relationship between SCP and chronic fatigue. SCP may increase stress sensitivity and lead to the "active" generation of stress (i.e., experiences of failure because of having unrealistic high expectations) as well as the "degeneration" of protective factors (e.g., positive affect, social support), resulting in an exacerbation of symptoms (Blatt & Shahar, 2005; Luyten & Blatt, 2013; Luyten, Blatt, Van Houdenhove, & Corveleyn, 2006; Shahar, 2001). Recently, our group replicated these findings in patients with CFS by showing that SCP was associated with increased stress sensitivity and more daily hassles, which in turn predicted increased levels of depression (Luyten et al., 2011). This fits with our previous findings showing that maladaptive perfectionism, because of high self-criticism, may give rise to negative self-perceptions (i.e., low self-esteem), which, in turn, increase the chance of depression and even more self-criticism (Kempke, Luyten, et al., 2011; Kempke, Van Houdenhove, et al., 2011).

As noted above, we and others have hypothesized that SCP may be associated with hypofunctioning of the HPA axis in CFS because of the "wear and tear" on the body due to chronic or repeated high stress levels (Kempke, Luyten, De Coninck et al., 2015; Kempke, Luyten, Mayes et al., in press; Luyten et al., 2011). In line with this reasoning, we recently demonstrated that SCP was related to increased levels of subjective (self-reported) stress, but with decreased (blunted) HPA axis reactivity (i.e., lower cortisol responses)

following acute experimental stress induced by the Trier Social Stress Test (Kempke, Luyten, Mayes et al., in press). These findings provide preliminary evidence that SCP in CFS may be associated with loss of "adaptability" of the neurobiological stress system (Van Houdenhove et al., 2013).

Further, SCP has been related to specific maladaptive cognitions and behaviors – or dominant coping strategies – to compensate for feelings of inferiority and low self-esteem, including high "action-proneness" (i.e., a tendency toward direct action leading to periodic overactivity; Van Houdenhove, Bruyninckx, & Luyten, 2006), high "persistence" (i.e., a tendency to persevere despite frustration and fatigue; Fukuda et al., 2010; Van Campen et al., 2009), and "all-or-nothing" behavior (Moss-Morris et al., 2010), leading to physical and/or mental overexertion and lack of acceptance of functional limitations (Brooks, Rimes, & Chalder, 2011; Van Houdenhove, Neerinckx, Onghena, et al., 2001). Importantly, the tendency towards overactivity often persists after illness onset, as illustrated by periodic "outbursts of activity" when feeling better followed by complete rest/inactivity (a "boom-and-bust" activity pattern), which may perpetuate symptoms and impede recovery (Kempke et al., 2013a; Luyten et al., 2011; Moss-Morris et al., 2010).

Driver (2005), in her analysis of a young woman suffering from chronic fatigue, argued that the swings between overactivity and underactivity in CFS may reflect an underlying "fight–flight" response demonstrating a fundamental inability to regulate internal states. Indeed, patients with CFS, and highly self-critical patients in particular, have been shown to have impaired emotion regulation strategies, such as with respect to the suppression of emotions, emotional avoidance, and the tendency to express negative beliefs about emotions (e.g., emotions are a sign of "weakness," "others will negatively react to displays of emotions"; Hambrook et al., 2011; Oldershaw et al., 2011; Rimes & Chalder, 2010; see also Van Middendorp et al., 2008), thereby increasing stress sensitivity and overload. Interestingly, Nemiah and Sifneos, in the early 1970s, coined the term "alexithymia" to describe a similar personality style in psychosomatic patients characterized by difficulty describing feelings and distinguishing them from bodily sensations (Sifneos, 1973; Taylor, Bagby, & Parker, 1991). A few years earlier, theorists from the Paris School of Psychosomatics introduced the notion of operational or concrete thinking (pensée opératoire), which is closely related to the concept of alexithymia (Aisenstein, 2006). Taerk and Gnam (1994, p. 320), in turn, from an object-relations perspective, stated that CFS vulnerability results from "poorly developed capacity for regulating internal states in response to certain types of stressors, namely disturbances in object relations."

More recently, Luyten and colleagues (Luyten, van Houdenhove, Lemma, Target, & Fonagy, 2012; Luyten, Van Houdenhove, Lemma, Target, & Fonagy, 2013) have argued that CFS is related to impaired mentalization (i.e., the metacognitive ability to reflect on internal processes) and, in particular, dysfunctions in "embodied mentalization" – referring to difficulties in identifying and transforming bodily sensations into mental states (i.e., the "embodied" self). This may explain patients' tendencies to ignore affective signals of being stressed or overburdened. Of particular interest in this regard is a study by Oldershaw et al. (2011), showing that CFS is associated with difficulties in emotion recognition and inferring own emotions. Comparable findings have been reported in somatoform disorders. Subic-Wrana and colleagues (Subic-Wrana, Beutel, Knebel, & Lane, 2010; Subic-Wrana, Bruder, Thomas, Lane, & Kohle, 2005) showed decreased emotional awareness and deficits in emotion recognition in these patients.

Developmentally, impairments in mentalization have been linked to a history of early adversity and insecure attachment (Bateman & Fonagy, 2006), as discussed later in this chapter. Indeed, impaired mentalization has been implicated in trauma-related psychopathology (e.g., borderline disorders) (Bateman & Fonagy, 2006). Yet, impairments in mentalization in CFS might also be exacerbated by the illness itself, because of being chronically invalidated and feeling dismissed or not understood. Moreover, the overwhelming fatigue and pain may be felt like an attack on the self and is often experienced as a "bad" internal object threatening one's identity, leading to a dissociation between the (suffering) body and the self (Osborn & Smith, 2006; Schattner, Shahar, & Abu-Shakra, 2008; Smith & Osborn, 2007; Van Damme & Kindermans, 2015). In this regard, Sachs (2001) has argued that the (medical) diagnosis of CFS may transform the patient's lived (subjective) body into a medicalized (real) body.

Childhood adversity and attachment insecurity in CFS

In this section, we will show that the premorbid overactive lifestyle and "counterdependency" observed in

many patients with CFS may reflect attempts to compensate for low self-esteem and narcissistic injuries associated with early negative experiences and disruptive attachment experiences (Van Houdenhove, 2005; Van Houdenhove, Neerinckx, Lysens, et al., 2001). As Van Houdenhove and colleagues (2001, p. 574) have noticed, "particularly those with childhood victimisation experiences often show a tendency to exceed physical limits (in work or sports) as a way of coping, i.e., to maintain self-esteem, stabilise the affective equilibrium and prevent anxiety and depression."

Indeed, a number of studies have demonstrated elevated rates of adverse childhood experiences in patients with CFS, with a considerable subgroup of patients reporting multiple trauma (for an overview, see Kempke et al., 2013b), congruent with the notion of an "unprotected" self in chronic pain and fatigue conditions (Wentz et al., 2004, 2005). These findings are also in keeping with more basic research showing that a history of abuse and maltreatment, especially during critical periods of development, may lead to increased stress sensitivity and impairments in social cognition, thereby increasing the risk for stress-related disorders in genetically susceptible individuals (Heim, Ehlert, & Hellhammer, 2000; Lupien, McEwen, Gunnar, & Heim, 2009).

More than a decade ago, Van Houdenhove et al. (2001) reported for the first time elevated levels of early adversity in a mixed sample of CFS and FM patients (i.e., 64.1% experienced adversity) as compared to controls. Interestingly, emotional neglect (48.4%) appeared to be one of the most important trauma domains among CFS/FM patients. Moreover, patients in this study were more likely to experience re-victimization in later life (e.g., living in an abusive relationship), which might be related to impaired mentalization capacities within the context of attachment relationships. These findings have been replicated in a number of other studies in CFS. For instance, Heim et al. (2006, 2009), in a population-based study in the USA, demonstrated that early childhood trauma was associated with a three- to eightfold increased risk for CFS. In keeping with these findings, in a sample of 90 well-screened patients with CFS, Kempke et al. (2013b) showed that more than half of the patients (54.4%) had experienced at least one type of early childhood trauma. Importantly, prevalence rates were particularly high for emotional trauma (i.e., emotional abuse and/or emotional neglect: 46.7%). Furthermore, we found that early adversity directly influenced the course of CFS in terms of levels of pain and fatigue over a period of 14 days, probably due to its impact on stress sensitivity, stress generation, and interpersonal distress in particular, as well as on maladaptive cognitive-perceptual factors such as catastrophizing and somatic hypervigilance (Luyten et al., 2011; Van Houdenhove & Luyten, 2008; Van Houdenhove et al., 2013; Van Houdenhove, Neerinckx, Lysens, et al., 2001).

Although early adversity has been implicated in a wide range of functional somatic syndromes, including FM and irritable bowel syndrome (Afari et al., 2014), the findings seem to converge that CFS is more closely linked to "emotional" adverse experiences rather than more "objective" or physical types of trauma. This fits with the trauma studies reviewed above, and suggests that emotional disturbances and dysfunctions in embodied mentalization may be particularly prominent in patients with CFS (Luyten et al., 2012, 2013). In fact, emotional childhood adversities in CFS can include a wide range of negative experiences, such as early parentification, being abandoned, or growing up in an emotionally unresponsive or highly critical environment (Van Houdenhove, Neerinckx, Lysens, et al., 2001; Van Houdenhove, Neerinckx, Onghena, et al., 2001). According to Wentz et al. (2004; Wentz, 2005), many patients prone to CFS/FM were overstrained as a child; that is, unsupported or overexposed to mental load.

Turning to attachment insecurity, childhood adversity may have a profound effect on the development of mental representations or internal working models (IWM) of the self in relation to significant others (Mikulincer & Shaver, 2007). Specifically, CFS has been associated with insecure attachment or the use of so-called "secondary" attachment strategies to seek an inner sense of security, most notably dismissive–avoidant attachment strategies; this is further reinforced by the current scientific controversy and even overt societal disbelief surrounding CFS (Luyten et al., 2012, 2013). As a result, these patients often lack a basic sense of trust in others and tend to deactivate the attachment system (i.e., denial of attachment needs, self-reliance and independence) to regulate affective states by distancing themselves from others, leading to isolation and loneliness, thereby decreasing the stress-buffering effects of social support (Luyten et al., 2013). Moreover, it is recognized that patients who rely on dismissive attachment strategies are prone to alexithymia, less emotional awareness, and, most importantly, "deactivating" emotion regulation strategies (e.g., suppression of negative emotions),

leading to increased levels of stress and "allostatic load" in the long run (Mikulincer & Shaver, 2007). Also, these patients tend to deny the impact of psychosocial factors (e.g., life stress, early attachment relationships) on the course of their illness and typically do not seek help for their problems unless there is a "medical" cure (Luyten et al., 2013). Indeed, as described by Muller (2009, 2010), deactivation reflects "minimization" of painful attachment-related experiences. It should be noted, however, that not all CFS (or FM) patients are characterized by deactivating attachment strategies. Some patients may have a predominant hyperactivating (preoccupied) attachment pattern (e.g., these patients try to elicit support through clinging and claiming behavior, leading to hostility in others and subsequent rejection), while others may show a combination of hyperactivating and deactivating attachment strategies (Luyten et al., 2013). Moreover, not all behavior is "deactivated" in avoidant attached patients (Muller, 2010). In fact, only intimacy is avoided, because the attachment figure was often the source of distress and the patient has learnt that it is safer to be self-reliant (Muller, 2010). Although empirical research on attachment in patients with CFS is largely lacking, findings in somatoform and chronic pain patients have shown a higher (relative) incidence of insecure-dismissive attachment, unresolved states of mind, and narrative incoherence – or the inability to construct a coherent self-narrative (Maunder & Hunter, 2008; Neumann, Nowacki, Roland, & Kruse, 2011; Pedrosa Gil, Scheidt, Hoeger, & Nickel, 2008; Subic-Wrana et al., 2005; Waller & Scheidt, 2006; Waller, Scheidt, & Hartmann, 2004).

Conclusions

As shown throughout this chapter, there is good evidence to suggest that CFS is associated with conflicting self-experiences leading to impairments in stress regulation and long-term neurobiological alterations, i.e., a pseudo-independent and resilient self as a way to compensate for a vulnerable and highly dependent self. Indeed, studies have amply demonstrated that self-critical perfectionism and related traits such as "persistence" and "action proneness" may be implicated in CFS, leading to chronic stress and overload. Yet, beneath this image of perfection, there is much psychological vulnerability, as evidenced by research showing elevated rates of childhood adversity and severe emotion regulation difficulties in these patients.

As reviewed in Luyten and Van Houdenhove (2013), there is an urgent need to identify treatment approaches based on etiological, developmental factors, especially because existing merely symptom-based treatments have shown only limited success (Price, Mitchell, Tidy, & Hunot, 2008). Several attempts have been made to develop a more integrated treatment approach for functional somatic conditions, focused on representations of self and others and how these schemas may become (re)activated in the therapeutic relationship (Beutel, Michal, & Subic-Wrana, 2008; Maunder & Hunter, 2004; Nickel, Ademmer, & Egle, 2010; Sattel et al., 2012; Stuart & Noyes, 2006). For instance, Nickel et al. (2010) developed a psychodynamic–interactional group treatment for chronic pain patients, focusing on the role of attachment patterns and insecure psychological defenses. Beutel et al. (2008), in turn, described the long tradition in Germany of a psychoanalytic-oriented treatment setting for patients with somatoform disorders, using a framework that is focused on symbolization of affect, restoring mentalization and changing underlying defenses. In a randomized controlled trial, Sattel et al. (2012) demonstrated the long-term efficacy of brief psychodynamic interpersonal therapy (PIT) for patients with multisomatoform disorder (defined as a disorder characterized by severe and disabling bodily symptoms including pain-related symptoms). Similarly, Luyten and colleagues (2012, 2013), recognizing the importance of attachment processes in understanding chronic pain and fatigue conditions, developed dynamic interpersonal therapy (DIT), a brief and focused psychodynamic treatment aimed at restoring the capacity to regulate affect and stress in patients with functional somatic syndromes by using techniques borrowed from traditional mentalization-based treatment (MBT). Similarly, so-called third-wave cognitive approaches, i.e., acceptance and commitment therapy (ACT) and mindfulness-based cognitive therapy (MBCT), have been recommended for the treatment of functional somatic syndromes (van Ravesteijn et al., 2013; Wicksell et al., 2013).

Overall, research findings suggest that treatment of CFS should include strategies that enhance the metacognitive ability to reflect on how specific mental representations or cognitive-affective schemas associated with self-criticism/attachment avoidance (e.g., excessive need for control, search for acceptance and recognition) and early negative experiences (e.g., "I am worthless as a person") may affect stress regulation and daily functioning in these patients. Importantly, clinicians should invest enough time to build a secure relationship, especially in highly self-critical patients (see also Blatt, 2004; Luyten et al., 2005), because only a secure therapeutic relationship may promote change of so-called "compensating strategies" into new and more adequate behavior. In the case of Catherine, treatment focused on helping her to accept her "vulnerable" self. She learned to tolerate her "weaknesses" and was able to let go of her self-criticism. Ultimately, such interventions may help patients to integrate different self-experiences into a coherent and "real" self, which may lead to a more balanced lifestyle and increased long-term resilience of the neurobiological stress response system (Van Houdenhove et al., 2013).

References

Ablin, J. N., Buskila, D., Van Houdenhove, B., et al. (2012). Is fibromyalgia a discrete entity? *Autoimmunity Reviews*, 11(8), 585–588.

Afari, N., Ahumada, S. M., Wright, L. J., et al. (2014). Psychological trauma and functional somatic syndromes: A systematic review and meta-analysis. *Psychosomatic Medicine*, 76(1), 2–11.

Aisenstein, M. (2006). The indissociable unity of psyche and soma: A view from the Paris Psychosomatic School. *International Journal of Psychoanalysis*, 87(Pt 3), 667–680.

Assefi, N. P., Coy, T. V., Uslan, D., Smith, W. R., & Buchwald, D. (2003). Financial, occupational, and personal consequences of disability in patients with chronic fatigue syndrome and fibromyalgia compared to other fatiguing conditions. *Journal of Rheumatology*, 30(4), 804–808.

Bateman, A., & Fonagy, P. (2006). *Mentalization-based Treatment for Borderline Personality Disorder. A Practical Guide*. Oxford: Oxford University Press.

Beutel, M. E., Michal, M., & Subic-Wrana, C. (2008). Psychoanalytically-oriented inpatient psychotherapy of somatoform disorders. *Journal of the American Academy of Psychoanalysis and Dynamic Psychiatry*, 36(1), 125–142.

Blatt, S. J. (2004). *Experiences of Depression: Theoretical, Clinical and Research Perspectives*. Washington, DC: APA.

Blatt, S. J., & Levy, K. N. (2003). Attachment theory, psychoanalysis, personality development, and psychopathology. *Psychoanalytic Inquiry*, 23, 104–152.

Blatt, S. J., & Shahar, G. (Eds.). (2005). *A Dialectic Model of Personality Development and Psychopathology: Recent Contributions to Understanding and Treating Depression.*

Leuven/New York, NY: Leuven University Press/ Lawrence Erlbaum.

Blumer, D., & Heilbronn, M. (1982). Chronic pain as a variant of depressive disease: The pain-prone disorder. *Journal of Nervous and Mental Disease*, 170(7), 381–406.

Boneva, R. S., Maloney, E. M., Lin, J. M., *et al.* (2011). Gynecological history in chronic fatigue syndrome: A population-based case-control study. *Journal of Women's Health*, 20(1), 21–28.

Brooks, S. K., Rimes, K. A., & Chalder, T. (2011). The role of acceptance in chronic fatigue syndrome. *Journal of Psychosomatic Research*, 71(6), 411–415.

Carruthers, B. M., van de Sande, M. I., De Meirleir, K. L., *et al.* (2011). Myalgic encephalomyelitis: International Consensus Criteria. *Journal of Internal Medicine*, 270(4), 327–338.

Claes, S., & Nemeroff, C. B. (2005). Corticotropin releasing factor (CRF) and major depression: Towards an integration of psychology and neurobiology in depression research. In J. Corveleyn, P Luyten & S. J. Blatt (Eds.), *The Theory and Treatment of Depression: Towards a Dynamic Interactionism Model* (pp. 227–252). Leuven/Mahwah, NJ: Leuven University Press/Lawrence Erlbaum Associates.

Cleare, A. J. (2003). The neuroendocrinology of chronic fatigue syndrome. *Endocrine Reviews*, 24(2), 236–252.

Cuykx, V., Van Houdenhove, B., & Neerinckx, E. (1998). Childhood abuse, personality disorder and chronic fatigue syndrome. *General Hospital Psychiatry*, 20(6), 382–384.

Deary, V., & Chalder, T. (2010). Personality and perfectionism in chronic fatigue syndrome: A closer look. *Psychology and Health*, 25(4), 465–475.

Dittner, A. J., Rimes, K., & Thorpe, S. (2011). Negative perfectionism increases the risk of fatigue following a period of stress. *Psychology and Health*, 26(3), 253–268.

Driver, C. (2005). An under-active or over-active internal world? An exploration of parallel dynamics within psyche and soma, and the difficulty of internal regulation, in patients with Chronic Fatigue Syndrome and Myalgic Encephalomyelitis. *Journal of Analytical Psychology*, 50(2), 155–173.

Dunkley, D. M., Blankstein, K. R., Masheb, R. M., & Grilo, C. M. (2006). Personal standards and evaluative concerns dimensions of "clinical" perfectionism: a reply to Shafran *et al.* (2002, 2003) and Hewitt *et al.* (2003). *Behavior Research and Therapy*, 44(1), 63–84.

Fukuda, K., Straus, S. E., Hickie, I., *et al.* (1994). The chronic fatigue syndrome: A comprehensive approach to its definition and study. International Chronic Fatigue Syndrome Study Group. *Annals of Internal Medicine*, 121(12), 953–959.

Fukuda, S., Kuratsune, H., Tajima, S., *et al.* (2010). Premorbid personality in chronic fatigue syndrome as determined by the Temperament and Character Inventory. *Comprehensive Psychiatry*, 51(1), 78–85.

Gregory, R. J., Manring, J., & Wade, M. J. (2005). Personality traits related to chronic pain location. *Annals of Clinical Psychiatry*, 17(2), 59–64.

Hambrook, D., Oldershaw, A., Rimes, K., *et al.* (2011). Emotional expression, self-silencing, and distress tolerance in anorexia nervosa and chronic fatigue syndrome. *British Journal of Clinical Psychology*, 50(3), 310–325.

Harvey, S. B., Wadsworth, M., Wessely, S., & Hotopf, M. (2008). Etiology of chronic fatigue syndrome: Testing popular hypotheses using a national birth cohort study. *Psychosomatic Medicine*, 70(4), 488–495.

Heim, C., Ehlert, U., & Hellhammer, D. H. (2000). The potential role of hypocortisolism in the pathophysiology of stress-related bodily disorders. *Psychoneuroendocrinology*, 25(1), 1–35.

Heim, C., Nater, U. M., Maloney, E., *et al.* (2009). Childhood trauma and risk for chronic fatigue syndrome: Association with neuroendocrine dysfunction. *Archives of General Psychiatry*, 66(1), 72–80.

Heim, C., Wagner, D., Maloney, E., *et al.* (2006). Early adverse experience and risk for chronic fatigue syndrome: Results from a population-based study. *Archives of General Psychiatry*, 63(11), 1258–1266.

Kempke, S., Luyten, P., Claes, S., *et al.* (2013a). Self-critical perfectionism and its relationship to fatigue and pain in the daily flow of life in patients with chronic fatigue syndrome. *Psychological Medicine*, 43(5), 995–1002.

Kempke, S., Luyten, P., Claes, S., *et al.* (2013b). The prevalence and impact of early childhood trauma in Chronic Fatigue Syndrome. *Journal of Psychiatric Research*, 47(5), 664–669.

Kempke, S., Luyten, P., De Coninck, S., *et al.* (2015). Effects of early childhood trauma on hypothalamic–pituitary–adrenal (HPA) axis function in patients with chronic fatigue syndrome. *Psychoneuroendocrinology*, 52, 14–21.

Kempke, S., Luyten, P., Mayes, L., Van Houdenhove, B., & Claes, S. (in press). Self-critical perfectionism predicts lower cortisol response to experimental stress in patients with chronic fatigue syndrome. *Health Psychology*.

Kempke, S., Luyten, P., Van Houdenhove, B., *et al.* (2011). Self-esteem mediates the relationship between maladaptive perfectionism and depression in chronic fatigue syndrome. *Clinical Rheumatology*, 30(12), 1543–1548.

Kempke, S., Van Den Eede, F., Schotte, C., *et al.* (2013). Prevalence of DSM-IV personality disorders in patients with chronic fatigue syndrome: A controlled study. *International Journal of Behavioral Medicine*, 20(2), 219–228.

Kempke, S., Van Houdenhove, B., Luyten, P., *et al.* (2011). Unraveling the role of perfectionism in chronic fatigue syndrome: Is there a distinction between adaptive and maladaptive perfectionism? *Psychiatry Research*, 186(2–3), 373–377.

Lerman, S. F., Rudich, Z., & Shahar, G. (2010). Distinguishing affective and somatic dimensions of pain and depression: A confirmatory factor analytic study. *Journal of Clinical Psychology*, 66(4), 456–465.

Lerman, S. F., Shahar, G., & Rudich, Z. (2011). Self-criticism interacts with the affective component of pain to predict depressive symptoms in female patients. *European Journal of Pain*, 16(1), 115–22.

Lupien, S. J., McEwen, B. S., Gunnar, M. R., & Heim, C. (2009). Effects of stress throughout the lifespan on the brain, behaviour and cognition. *Nature Reviews Neuroscience*, 10(6), 434–445.

Luyten, P., & Blatt, S. J. (2013). Interpersonal relatedness and self-definition in normal and disrupted personality development: retrospect and prospect. *American Psychologist*, 68(3), 172–183.

Luyten, P., & Van Houdenhove, B. (2013). Common versus specific factors in the treatment of functional somatic disorders. *Journal of Psychotherapy Integration*, 23, 14–27.

Luyten, P., Blatt, S. J., & Corveleyn, J. (2005). The convergence among psychodynamic and cognitive-behavioral theories of depression: Theoretical overview. In J. Corveleyn, P. Luyten & S. J. Blatt (Eds.), *The Theory and Treatment of Depression: Towards a Dynamic Interactionism Model* (pp. 67–94). Leuven/Mahwah, NJ: Leuven University Press/Lawrence Erlbaum Associates.

Luyten, P., Blatt, S. J., Van Houdenhove, B., & Corveleyn, J. (2006). Depression research and treatment: Are we skating to where the puck is going to be? *Clinical Psychology Review*, 26(8), 985–999.

Luyten, P., Kempke, S., Van Wambeke, P., *et al.* (2011). Self-critical perfectionism, stress generation, and stress sensitivity in patients with chronic fatigue syndrome: Relationship with severity of depression. *Psychiatry*, 74(1), 21–30.

Luyten, P., Van Houdenhove, B., Cosyns, N., & Van den Broeck, A.-L. (2006). Are patients with chronic fatigue syndrome perfectionistic – Or were they? A case-control study. *Personality and Individual Differences*, 40(7), 1473–1483.

Luyten, P., van Houdenhove, B., Lemma, A., Target, M., & Fonagy, P. (2012). A mentalization-based approach to the understanding and treatment of functional somatic disorders. *Psychoanalytic Psychotherapy*, 26(2), 121–140.

Luyten, P., Van Houdenhove, B., Lemma, A., Target, M., & Fonagy, P. (2013). Vulnerability for functional somatic disorders: A contemporary psychodynamic approach. *Journal of Psychotherapy Integration*, 23(3), 250–262.

Magnusson, A. E., Nias, D. K., & White, P. D. (1996). Is perfectionism associated with fatigue? *Journal of Psychosomatic Research*, 41(4), 377–383.

Maunder, R., & Hunter, J. (2004). An integrated approach to the formulation and psychotherapy of medically unexplained symptoms: Meaning- and attachment-based intervention. *American Journal of Psychotherapy*, 58(1), 17–33.

Maunder, R. G., & Hunter, J. J. (2008). Attachment relationships as determinants of physical health. *Journal of the American Academy of Psychoanalysis and Dynamic Psychiatry*, 36(1), 11–32.

McEwen, B. S. (1998). Stress, adaptation, and disease. Allostasis and allostatic load. *Annals of the New York Academy of Sciences*, 840, 33–44.

Mikulincer, M., & Shaver, P. R. (2007). *Attachment in Adulthood: Structure, Dynamics, and Change.* New York, NY: Guilford Press.

Moss-Morris, R., Spence, M. J., & Hou, R. (2011). The pathway from glandular fever to chronic fatigue syndrome: Can the cognitive behavioural model provide the map? *Psychological Medicine*, 41 (5), 1099–1107.

Muller, R. T. (2009). Trauma and dismissing (avoidant) attachment: Intervention strategies in individual psychotherapy. *Psychotherapy: Theory, Research, Practice, Training*, 46(1), 68–81.

Muller, R. T. (2010). *Trauma and the Avoidant Client: Attachment-Based Strategies for Healing.* New York, NY: Norton & Company.

Nater, U. M., Lin, J. M., Maloney, E. M., *et al.* (2009). Psychiatric comorbidity in persons with chronic fatigue syndrome identified from the Georgia population. *Psychosomatic Medicine*, 71(5), 557–565.

Nater, U. M., Maloney, E., Heim, C., & Reeves, W. C. (2011). Cumulative life stress in chronic fatigue syndrome. *Psychiatry Research*, 189(2), 318–320.

Neumann, E., Nowacki, K., Roland, I. C., & Kruse, J. (2011). Attachment and somatoform disorders: Low coherence and unresolved states of mind related to chronic pain. *Psychotherapie, Psychosomatik, Medizinische Psychologie*, 61(6), 254–261.

Nickel, R., Ademmer, K., & Egle, U. T. (2010). Manualized psychodynamic-interactional group therapy for the treatment of somatoform pain disorders. *Bulletin of the Menninger Clinic*, 74(3), 219–237.

Oldershaw, A., Hambrook, D., Rimes, K. A., *et al.* (2011). Emotion recognition and emotional theory of mind in chronic fatigue syndrome. *Psychology and Health*, 26(8), 989–1005.

Osborn, M., & Smith, J. A. (2006). Living with a body separate from the self. The experience of the body in chronic benign low back pain: An interpretative phenomenological analysis. *Scandinavian Journal of Caring Sciences*, 20, 216–222.

Papadopoulos, A. S., & Cleare, A. J. (2011). Hypothalamic–pituitary–adrenal axis dysfunction in chronic fatigue syndrome. *Nature Reviews Endocrinology*, 8(1), 22–32.

Pedrosa Gil, F., Scheidt, C. E., Hoeger, D., & Nickel, M. (2008). Relationship between attachment style, parental bonding and alexithymia in adults with somatoform disorders. *International Journal of Psychiatry in Medicine*, 38(4), 437–451.

Pemberton, S., & Cox, D. L. (2014). Experiences of daily activity in chronic fatigue syndrome/myalgic encephalomyelitis (CFS/ME) and their implications for rehabilitation programmes. *Disability and Rehabilitation*, 36(21), 1790–1797.

Price, J. R., Mitchell, E., Tidy, E., & Hunot, V. (2008). Cognitive behaviour therapy for chronic fatigue syndrome in adults. *Cochrane Database of Systematic Review*, 2008, issue 3, CD001027.

Reeves, W. C., Jones, J. F., Maloney, E., *et al.* (2007). Prevalence of chronic fatigue syndrome in metropolitan, urban, and rural Georgia. *Population Health Metrics*, 5, 5.

Rimes, K. A., & Chalder, T. (2010). The Beliefs about Emotions Scale: Validity, reliability and sensitivity to change. *Journal of Psychosomatic Research*, 68(3), 285–292.

Rudich, Z., Lerman, S. F., Gurevich, B., Weksler, N., & Shahar, G. (2008). Patients' self-criticism is a stronger predictor of physician's evaluation of prognosis than pain diagnosis or severity in chronic pain patients. *Journal of Pain*, 9(3), 210–216.

Sachs, L. (2001). From a lived body to a medicalized body: Diagnostic transformation and chronic fatigue syndrome. *Medical Anthropology*, 19(4), 299–317.

Sattel, H., Lahmann, C., Gundel, H., *et al.* (2012). Brief psychodynamic interpersonal psychotherapy for patients with multisomatoform disorder: Randomised controlled trial. *British Journal of Psychiatry*, 200(1), 60–67.

Schattner, E., Shahar, G., & Abu-Shakra, M. (2008). 'I used to dream of lupus as some sort of creature': Chronic illness as an internal object. *American Journal of Orthopsychiatry*, 78(4), 466–472.

Shahar, G. (2001). Personality, shame, and the breakdown of social bonds: The voice of quantitative depression research. *Psychiatry*, 64(3), 228–239.

Sibley, C. G. (2007). The association between working models of attachment and personality: Toward an integrative framework operationalizing global relational models. *Journal of Research in Personality*, 41(1), 90–109.

Sifneos, P. E. (1973). The prevalence of 'alexithymic' characteristics in psychosomatic patients. *Psychotherapy and Psychosomatics*, 22(2), 255–262.

Silverman, M. N., Heim, C. M., Nater, U. M., Marques, A. H., & Sternberg, E. M. (2010). Neuroendocrine and immune contributors to fatigue. *PM & R*, 2(5), 338–346.

Sirois, F. M., & Molnar, D. (2014). Perfectionism and maladaptive coping styles in chronic fatigue syndrome: A comparative analysis with well controls and individuals with irritable bowel syndrome, and fibromyalgia/arthritis. *Psychotherapy and Psychosomatics*, 83(6), 384–385.

Smith, J., & Osborn, M. (2007). Pain as an assault on the self: An interpretative phenomenological analysis. *Psychology and Health*, 22(5), 517–34.

Stuart, S., & Noyes, R., Jr. (2006). Interpersonal psychotherapy for somatizing patients. *Psychotherapy and Psychosomatics*, 75(4), 209–219.

Subic-Wrana, C., Beutel, M. E., Knebel, A., & Lane, R. D. (2010). Theory of mind and emotional awareness deficits in patients with somatoform disorders. *Psychosomatic Medicine*, 72(4), 404–411.

Subic-Wrana, C., Bruder, S., Thomas, W., Lane, R. D., & Kohle, K. (2005). Emotional awareness deficits in inpatients of a psychosomatic ward: A comparison of two different measures of alexithymia. *Psychosomatic Medicine*, 67(3), 483–489.

Taerk, G., & Gnam, W. (1994). A psychodynamic view of the chronic fatigue syndrome. The role of object relations in etiology and treatment. *General Hospital Psychiatry*, 16(5), 319–325.

Tak, L. M., Cleare, A. J., Ormel, J., *et al.* (2011). Meta-analysis and meta-regression of hypothalamic–pituitary–adrenal axis activity in functional somatic disorders. *Biological Psychology*, 87(2), 183–194.

Taylor, G. J., Bagby, R. M., & Parker, J. D. (1991). The alexithymia construct: A potential paradigm for psychosomatic medicine. *Psychosomatics*, 32(2), 153–164.

Tomas, C., Newton, J., & Watson, S. (2013). A review of hypothalamic–pituitary–adrenal axis function in chronic fatigue syndrome. *ISRN Neuroscience*, 2013, 784520.

Van Campen, E., Van Den Eede, F., Moorkens, G., *et al.* (2009). Use of the Temperament and Character Inventory (TCI) for assessment of personality in chronic fatigue syndrome. *Psychosomatics*, 50(2), 147–154.

Van Damme, S., & Kindermans, H. (2015). A self-regulation perspective on avoidance and persistence behaviour in chronic pain: New theories, new challenges? *Clinical Journal of Pain*, 31(2), 115–122.

Van Houdenhove, B. (2005). Premorbid "overactive" lifestyle and stress-related pain/fatigue syndromes. *Journal of Psychosomatic Research*, 58(4), 389–390.

Van Houdenhove, B., Bruyninckx, K., & Luyten, P. (2006). In search of a new balance. Can high "action-proneness" in patients with chronic fatigue syndrome be changed by a multidisciplinary group treatment? *Journal of Psychosomatic Research*, 60(6), 623–625.

Van Houdenhove, B., & Egle, U. T. (2004). Fibromyalgia: A stress disorder? Piecing the biopsychosocial puzzle together. *Psychotherapy and Psychosomatics*, 73(5), 267–275.

Van Houdenhove, B., Kempke, S., & Luyten, P. (2010). Psychiatric aspects of chronic fatigue syndrome and fibromyalgia. *Current Psychiatry Reports*, 12(3), 208–214.

Van Houdenhove, B., & Luyten, P. (2006). Stress, depression and fibromyalgia. *Acta Neurologica Belgica*, 106(4), 149–156.

Van Houdenhove, B., & Luyten, P. (2008). Customizing treatment of chronic fatigue syndrome and fibromyalgia: The role of perpetuating factors. *Psychosomatics*, 49(6), 470–477.

Van Houdenhove, B., & Luyten, P. (2010). Chronic fatigue syndrome reflects loss of adaptability. *Journal of Internal Medicine*, 268(3), 249–251.

Van Houdenhove, B., Luyten, P., & Kempke, S. (2013). Chronic fatigue syndrome/fibromyalgia: A 'stress-adaptation' model. *Fatigue: Biomedicine, Health & Behavior*, 1(3), 137–147.

Van Houdenhove, B., Neerinckx, E., Lysens, R., et al. (2001). Victimization in chronic fatigue syndrome and fibromyalgia in tertiary care: A controlled study on prevalence and characteristics. *Psychosomatics*, 42(1), 21–28.

Van Houdenhove, B., Neerinckx, E., Onghena, P., Lysens, R., & Vertommen, H. (2001). Premorbid "overactive" lifestyle in chronic fatigue syndrome and fibromyalgia. An etiological factor or proof of good citizenship? *Journal of Psychosomatic Research*, 51(4), 571–576.

Van Houdenhove, B., Van Den Eede, F., & Luyten, P. (2009). Does hypothalamic–pituitary–adrenal axis hypofunction in chronic fatigue syndrome reflect a 'crash' in the stress system? *Medical Hypotheses*, 72(6), 701–705.

Van Houdenhove, B., Van Hoof, E., Becq, K., et al. (2009). A comparison of patients with chronic fatigue syndrome in two "ideologically" contrasting clinics. *Journal of Nervous and Mental Disease*, 197(5), 348–353.

Van Middendorp, H., Lumley, M. A., Jacobs, J. W., et al. (2008). Emotions and emotional approach and avoidance strategies in fibromyalgia. *Journal of Psychosomatic Research*, 64(2), 159–167.

van Ravesteijn, H., Lucassen, P., Bor, H., van Weel, C., & Speckens, A. (2013). Mindfulness-based cognitive therapy for patients with medically unexplained symptoms: A randomized controlled trial. *Psychotherapy and Psychosomatics*, 82(5), 299–310.

Waller, E., & Scheidt, C. E. (2006). Somatoform disorders as disorders of affect regulation: A development perspective. *International Review of Psychiatry*, 18(1), 13–24.

Waller, E., Scheidt, C. E., & Hartmann, A. (2004). Attachment representation and illness behavior in somatoform disorders. *Journal of Nervous and Mental Disease*, 192(3), 200–209.

Wentz, K. A. (2005). *Fibromyalgia and self-regulatory patterns. Development, maintenance or recovery in women.* PhD dissertation, Göteborg University, Göteborg.

Wentz, K. A., Lindberg, C., & Hallberg, L. R. (2004). Psychological functioning in women with fibromyalgia: A grounded theory study. *Health Care for Women International*, 25(8), 702–729.

Wessely, S., Hotopf, M., & Sharpe, M. (1998). *Chronic Fatigue and its Syndromes.* Oxford: Oxford University Press.

Wessely, S., Nimnuan, C., & Sharpe, M. (1999). Functional somatic syndromes: One or many? *Lancet*, 354(9182), 936–939.

White, C., & Schweitzer, R. (2000). The role of personality in the development and perpetuation of chronic fatigue syndrome. *Journal of Psychosomatic Research*, 48(6), 515–524.

Wicksell, R. K., Kemani, M., Jensen, K., et al. (2013). Acceptance and commitment therapy for fibromyalgia: A randomized controlled trial. *European Journal of Pain*, 17(4), 599–611.

Chapter

20

The self in eating disorders

Christopher Basten and Stephen Touyz

Anorexia Nervosa is fundamentally both a cognitive disorder and a disorder of the self.

Vitousek and Ewald (1993; p. 288)

DSM-5 (American Psychiatric Association, 2013) offers criteria to diagnose anorexia nervosa (AN), bulimia nervosa (BN), binge-eating disorder (BED) and other specified eating disorders (EDs). Within DSM-5, one of the defining and diagnostic features of both AN and BN is the "undue influence of body weight and shape on self-evaluation" (APA, 2013, p. 345). This phrase is a small glimpse into the vast influence of issues of self-worth, self-definition, and self-management in the EDs. In this chapter, the term *eating disorders* is taken to include BN and AN, and their minor variations characterized as "other specified." BED is rarely included in research investigations or theoretical discussions on issues of the self. However, BED has many commonalities with BN, with the exception of compensating behaviors such as vomiting (Sanchez-Oritz & Schmidt, 2010), and so any comments made about BN are equally applicable to BED. This chapter builds on the extensive literature that already exists on the way that "the self" intersects with EDs. An ED is never simply about losing weight or looking better – it usually emerges in the context of some form of significant distress and in an effort to deal with that distress in some way. The body is the locus of the self and the corporeal manifestation of the self. In an ED, it simultaneously becomes the object of change and the vehicle of transforming the self. Not everyone who is distressed develops an ED – indeed, relatively few do – indicating that further consideration of how distress leads to ED is important. Two broad and apparently divergent theoretical perspectives are reviewed before an integration is attempted with treatment recommendations in mind. The main theoretical domains under consideration are psychodynamic and cognitive–behavioral. The key unifier is the widely acknowledged concept that each ED is a "functional illness." That is to say that the disorder (and its symptoms, consequences, and maintaining behaviors) serve powerfully reinforcing roles for the affected person.

Psychodynamic theories

Disturbances of the self are central to psychodynamic theories of psychopathology, and for decades now these theories have been specifically tailored in efforts to account for the EDs. It is misleading and unhelpful to discuss "the psychodynamic model," as there exists a range of theories that seem more divergent than they are based on a common theme (see Shahar & Schiller, Chapter 4 in this volume). This seems to reflect the natural evolution of psychoanalytic thinking over several decades.

In the 1970s the work of Klein (1975) and Mahler (Mahler, Pine, & Bergman, 1975) became the dominant accepted models of how a healthy *self* grows through infant–mother interactions, and when this is thwarted, how potentially severe problems emerge in feelings of self-worth, sense of identity, and emotion self-regulation. It was in this intellectual milieu that Bruch (1973, 1978) documented her own extensive and insightful observations of emotional and behavioral functioning in her female patients with EDs. Building on this, Ewell, Smith, Karmel, and Hart (1996) have also offered an account of how sense of self develops naturally and how its disturbances can easily create a vulnerability to EDs. In their analysis

The Self in Understanding and Treating Psychological Disorders, ed. Michael Kyrios, Richard Moulding, Guy Doron, Sunil S. Bhar, Maja Nedeljkovic, and Mario Mikulincer. Published by Cambridge University Press. © Cambridge University Press, 2016.

of what comprises sense of self, these authors emphasize a tripartite structure of the self: subjective self-consciousness, reflective awareness, and a sense of agency. The subjective self-consciousness is the sense of "I" that we have and this can reflect on the "me" through awareness. A sense of agency refers to the sense of knowing that one is effective in the world as an individual. They show how disruptions in the development of sense of self at various ages can render a person vulnerable to developing an ED – such as through needing to regain a sense of agency through oral control or by managing strong feelings of falseness by aligning their self-behavior with the clear ideal of thinness (Ewell *et al.*, 1996). The notion of falseness or "the false-self" is central to many psychodynamic theories of personality and emotional disturbance and is the counterpoint to a coherent, stable, healthy self (Kohut, 1971; Winnicott, 1965).

Following Klein and Mahler and colleagues, the work of Bowlby (1988) on attachment and its relationship to psychopathology has been incorporated into psychodynamic theory and has informed many who see ED pathology emerging from core attachment deficits (Bruch, 1978; Goodsitt, 1985; Zerbe, 2010). This may be why interpersonal psychotherapy, which is rooted firmly in attachment theory, is as effective for some eating disorders as is CBT (Tanofsky-Kraff & Wilfley, 2010).

Another dimension of psychoanalytic theory came with object relations theory (Winnicott, 1965) and then Kohut's *self psychology* (Kohut, 1971; Kohut & Wulf, 1978). Kohut's extensive and influential work focused on the patients presenting with persisting lack of vitality and with other manifestations of weak identity, such as is seen in the narcissistic and borderline personality structures, as well as in the EDs. In the self psychology approach, the self refers to a tripartite structure: (a) a system of largely unconscious goals, drive or motives, emotions, and cognition; (b) a subjective aspect of the self; and (c) the self-regulatory structure, which refers to the capacity to regulate tensions and moods and to maintain feelings of vitality, self-worth, and cohesiveness (Kohut, 1971; Strober, 1991; Westen, 1992). With regards to the subjective sense of self, it has been documented that many clients with EDs state that, especially over time, they do not know who they would be without their ED – their identity and substance depends on this (Bruch, 1978; Schupak-Neuberg & Nemeroff, 1993; Garner, Vitousek, & Pike, 1997).

Bruch (1973, 1978) was among the first to write extensively of the sense of emptiness and poor self-definition that many women with EDs describe. She suggested that much of the overt pathology (such as relentless pursuit of thinness) and associated features (such as perfectionism and obsessionality) seen in EDs stems from a need to compensate for an impoverished self and constitute a maladaptive "search for selfhood and self-respecting identity" (Bruch, 1978, p. 255). This thinking has influenced many recently evolved permutations of therapy for EDs (Goodsitt, 1985; Strober, 1991). Goodsitt argues that other variations of psychoanalytic thinking (specifically drive-conflict and object relations approaches) do not adequately account for the observations of those with EDs, while the "self psychology" model does: "The symptoms of anorexia nervosa represent both a disruption of the self and the defensive adaptive measures against further disruption" (Goodsitt, 1985, p. 55). Strober offers a very similar account of the idea of the fractured or underdeveloped self as a vulnerability to developing an ED in particular. Lerner (1993) has offered a similar but less coherent psychodynamic account of the role of self-disturbance in the generation of EDs.

Many of these theories have sound face validity and seem to account for what the clinician sees in the consulting room. However, some of the psychodynamic theories are open to the problem of being unfalsifiable and most have never been empirically investigated. There have been a few attempts to experimentally measure any link between impaired sense of self and EDs. Stein and Corte (2007) compared controls with patients with EDs in terms of self-descriptions designed to assess "identity impairment." They concluded that those with an ED have an "overall identity impairment" (p. 68) and that this impairment was likely etiologically relevant to the ED. Schupak-Neuberg and Nemeroff (1993) tried to test the hypothesis that women with BN lack a clearly defined "sense of self" or "identity confusion, defined as a sense of confusion and inconsistency in one's idea of who one is" (Schupak-Neuberg & Nemeroff, 1993, p. 339). Using a novel (psychometrically untested) set of questions, they found that women with BN had greater levels of "identity confusion," "enmeshment with others," and "overall instability in self-concept" (p. 335) compared to non-ED controls. In a recent attempt to measure subjective sense of self, a questionnaire was developed and validated to examine the parts of the self, including feelings of cohesion, vitality, completeness, personhood or identity and self-regulation (Basten, 2008). Compared to a non-clinical sample, those being treated for an ED responded on this questionnaire in a way that indicated a weaker sense of self. The measure of sense of self correlated with the severity of ED, as measured by (a) a composite score on the Eating Disorders Inventory, and (b) frequency of eating-disordered behaviors, such as fasting, vomiting, and compulsive exercise (Basten, 2008).

Feminist perspectives have added to the psychodynamic literature on EDs. Feminist theories suggest that EDs emerge from a combination of several factors beyond obvious social pressures. Key issues that are commonly cited as potentially causally relevant include the role of the mother in socializing gender roles in society, sociocultural messages about the importance of appearance for women and the central role of thinness in physical beauty, and social and commercial conspiracies that are designed to reinforce these messages and narrow the measure of worth and attractiveness to available products and procedures (Fallon, Katzman, & Wooley, 1993; Striegel-Moore, 1995). Similarly, the role that the body plays in Western culture has been noted as problematic for women. The well-known and documented cultural pressures about conformity of body-image become internalized and interact with the other private struggles that each young woman is already having, and in doing so the struggle to find and be comfortable with one's authentic self becomes even more impossible (Orbach, 1985; Zerbe, 2010).

In summary, psychodynamic theories are very varied and have evolved over time. More modern permutations have emphasized (a) issues of attachment and failure to individuate, and (b) impaired self-functioning and the notion of "disorder of the self." This raises core treatment implications that are taken up later.

Cognitive model

The cognitive or cognitive–behavioral model of EDs is also a multifaceted and evolving effort to account for all the clinical observations and experimental research on the EDs. Certain authors in this area have their own emphases, but the model is much more homogeneous than is the range of psychodynamic theories proffered over the years. The major components of the cognitive model are mentioned below and formulated together in Figure 20.1.

Centrality of importance placed on weight and shape

This has been noted by several authors (Garner *et al.*, 1997; Vitousek & Ewald, 1993), but is most commonly associated with Fairburn's CBT model of EDs (Fairburn, 2008; Fairburn, Cooper, & Shafran, 2003). Fairburn refers to this as the "over-evaluation" of weight and shape, by which he means that the person's self-evaluation system is almost exclusively based on weight and shape and on the ability to control these aspects of the self. Fairburn suggests that all the disturbances of AN and BN stem from "the core psychopathology" of excessively valuing weight and shape and their control. There is considerable support for the importance that those with EDs have this feature in their self-evaluation system and that this is a powerful maintaining factor. On the other hand, there is only modest support that this self-evaluation system exists before the onset of the ED. Moreover, Fairburn explicitly limits his CBT model to the processes that *maintain* psychopathology, rather than those responsible for its development (Cooper & Fairburn, 2010). As a model to help understand and explain EDs, this is a remarkable shortcoming, although integrative models are emerging and will be discussed below. Suffice it to say that additions are required to the cognitive model concerning the pre-existing psychological vulnerabilities that lead a person to develop this self-esteem structure.

Internalizing the thin-ideal

Thin-ideal internalization refers to the processes and outcomes when a person accepts the messages from those around them about ideals of attractiveness and then engages in behaviors designed to approximate those ideals (Thompson, Heinberg, Altabe, & Tantleff-Dunn, 1999). These messages can come from broader society (such as media), one's immediate subculture (sport or school friends), and also family (Stice, 2001; Thompson *et al.*, 1999). This model helps understanding of why women are much more likely to develop AN than men, whose body discontent around muscle morphology is more likely to lead them away from severe restriction and its biological consequences. Body dissatisfaction blooms in the presence of engaging with the thin-ideal, especially because the ideal is effectively unattainable for most females (Hausenblas *et al.*, 2013; Thompson *et al.*, 1999). Stice (2001) has identified how bulimic symptoms (not just

AN) develop from the thin-ideal, via its promotion of negative affect, shame, and restriction.

The tripartite influence model incorporates the thin-ideal internalization. This theory is designed to account for body-image and eating disturbances via three direct sources (parental, peer, and media) and two moderating variables (thin-ideal internalization and appearance comparisons) (Hardit & Hannum, 2012; Keery, van den Berg, & Thompson, 2004; van den Berg, Thompson, Obremski-Brandon, & Coovert, 2002). While the tripartite influence model may apply to those with EDs, to date, the research has been limited to student and community samples.

The concept of thin-ideal internalization helps us to understand the question why some people might come to over-value weight and shape. Yet other questions still remain, such as what might make one person more vulnerable to internalizing the thin-ideal. A partial answer may exist in the normal tendency for adolescents to bend in order to conform to social norms (Slade, 1982). Other measurable cognitive traits also make some people more prone to arriving at a fixed over-valuing of weight and shape and these are discussed in the next two sections.

Self-discrepancy

According to Higgins (1987), there are three major domains of the self: (a) the *actual* self, which is one's representation that the person (or others) believe they possess; (b) the *ideal* self, which is a representation of the attributes that one believes are ideal in the eyes of others; and (c) the *ought* self, which relates to the attributes that someone – that person or another – believes that the person ought to possess. *Ideal* attributes are typically personal aspirations, while *ought* attributes embody a sense of obligation or duty. Higgins (1987) aimed to account for negative mood states. Since then, various researchers have found that types of self-discrepancies have a role in accounting for body dissatisfaction (Stauman, Vookles, Berenstein, Chaiken, & Higgins, 1991) and ED symptoms (Sawdon, Cooper & Seabrook, 2007; Stauman *et al.*, 1991). Studies have also shown that high self-discrepancies have a mediating influence on the impact that thin-ideal images have on women (Bessenoff, 2006), including the impact on disordered eating (Harrison, 2001). This echoes the research supporting the tripartite influence model, which has shown that the degree to which a person compares their body to other people mediates the

impact of messages that they receive about the body and self-acceptance (Keery *et al.*, 2004; Thompson *et al.*, 1999; van den Berg *et al.*, 2002).

Cognitive functioning and neurocognitive changes

The processes that occur with starvation have long been documented (Keys, Brozek, Henschel, Mickelson, & Taylor, 1950): people become more rigid and obsessional, which can strengthen any informational processing errors and entrench ideas about dieting into "rules." More recent research led by Tchanturia has identified two main clusters of neurocognitive differences seen in those with AN compared to those without EDs: (a) excessively detailed information-processing style, also known as "weak central coherence" (Lopez *et al.*, 2008; Southgate, Tchanturia, & Treasure, 2008); and (b) cognitive inflexibility, also known as "poor set-shifting" (Roberts, Tchanturia, Stahl, Southgate, & Treasure, 2007; Tchanturia, Campbell, Morris, & Treasure, 2005).

With regards to the excessive attention to detail, this means that one's ability to perceive a whole issue or a "bigger picture" is impaired, while the same person's natural cognitive style is to process a task or information piecemeal (Lopez *et al.*, 2008). This can help us understand how a person who decides to lose weight in order to be happier and healthier soon ends up unhealthy and depressed as they pursue this bigger picture by blindly following rules. With regard to cognitive inflexibility, those with AN – even after weight restoration (Tchanturia *et al.*, 2004) – show a much lower ability to shift cognitive focus. This makes it harder for such people to be flexible with the rules and guidelines that we acquire and then live by, and so such people become progressively more reliant on rules to function (including rules that one's appearance is essential, that thinness determines attractiveness, and myriad rules about what to eat and what not to eat and when). Crane, Roberts and Treasure (2007) noted in their review that this trait does seem to be associated with ED pathology and poorer treatment outcome.

Cognitive style and information-processing errors

It is a strong feature of many cognitive models of psychopathology that affected individuals are subject to information-processing errors, most notably in

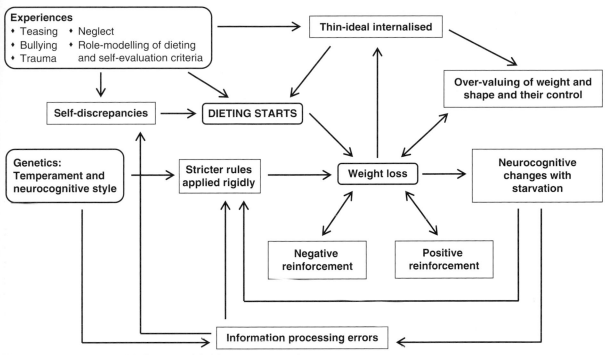

Figure 20.1 Cognitive model of AN: A model of the cognitive contributors to anorexia nervosa.

anxiety (McNally & Reese, 2008). The common automatic cognitive and information-processing errors include filtering and selective memory, selective attention, illusory correlation, and personalizing or egocentric bias (McNally & Reese, 2008; Vitousek & Hollon, 1990). The information-processing errors in EDs have been investigated experimentally in both subclinical samples and patients in treatment (Lee & Shafran, 2004), and the same paradigms are used as in the anxiety disorders (modified Stroop test and dot probe). Findings support that people who are dieting are more likely to have attentional biases to both threat and reward stimuli when using weight and shape stimuli (Lee & Shafran, 2004).

Vitousek and Hollon (1990) have argued that there is a broader, underlying set of biases in cognitive style and information processing that helps to explain the origin and maintenance of EDs. In particular, they note a propensity for oversimplifying material, a preference for certainty, and simplistic, dichotomous thinking in the way that goals are set. These processes are highly automatic and not always a conscious choice or within the awareness of the person. Because the dieting and its consequences can be so reinforcing, they take on a conscious value. Consequently, some of the cognitive and information-processing errors are not automatic;

some are available to conscious awareness and rather than being suppressed may actually be amplified and kept for their functional utility (Garner *et al.*, 1997; Schmidt & Treasure, 2006; Vitousek & Ewald, 1993).

Reinforcement principles

Garner *et al.* (1997) have described the ways that both negative reinforcement and positive reinforcement serve to strengthen and maintain an ED once dieting has commenced. This important part of the cognitive model of EDs has also been a theme in the models presented by Crisp's (1980) individual psychodynamic perspective of AN and Slade's (1982) account of the development of both anorexia and bulimia nervosa. Negative reinforcement refers to the way that the removal or diminution of a negative stimulus following a particular behavior leads to reinforcement of that behavior. Most commonly, the person with an ED discovers over time that their weight loss or their restricting, purging, or bingeing behaviors are reinforcing in this way. This occurs through the effective removal of negative affect about the self or the past, or indeed many ways that a feared stimulus can be avoided, as a consequence of their disordered eating behaviors. However, what if the threat object is inescapable?

Vitousek and Ewald (1993) write: "in anorexia nervosa, the most frightening stimulus is the *self* at unacceptable weight levels" (p. 234). If we keep in mind that the modal patient with anorexia is often biased towards rigid thinking and narrow rule abstraction, it is almost inevitable that their pursuit of thinness then becomes the main cognitive theme they let themselves entertain seriously.

There is a broad range of ways that dieting behaviors and weight loss can be negatively reinforcing and the study of these factors not only gives rise to a greater understanding of a person with an ED, but guides individually tailored treatment. There are several well-documented negative reinforcers: emotional numbing through binge-eating (Stice, 2001), emotional numbing through starvation (Garner & Bemis, 1982; Wildes, Ringham, & Marcus, 2010), flight from sexual maturity (Crisp, 1980), flight from adult responsibilities, and reducing complexities and uncertainties down to elegant (but pathological) simplicity. Bruch (1978) identified in her patients a common thread that they had found "the perfect solution to all their problems" (p. 137). The layers of negative reinforcement multiply over time, as the patient adds extra rules designed to avoid the negative states that afflict them simply because they have broken their own impossible rules.

Positive reinforcement is also typically present, and this can be even more powerful in terms of why a "disorder" becomes egosyntonic and avidly pursued by the affected person (Bruch, 1978; Garner & Bemis, 1985; Garner *et al.*, 1997; Schmidt & Treasure, 2006; Slade, 1982; Vitousek & Ewald, 1993; Vitousek & Hollon, 1990). Briefly, the rewards potentially felt by people as they develop an ED include increased autonomy and personal agency, a sense of competitive superiority (morally, aesthetically, behaviorally), feelings of personal success and attainment, and reward through getting people to notice their emotional needs. For all these reasons, "individuals with anorexia nervosa do not experience their disorder as an affliction but as an accomplishment, in which they feel a complete emotional and moral investment" (Vitousek & Ewald, 1993, p. 233).

This is not to say that a severe ED is a choice exercised because the person finds it rewarding. They often experience a compelling need to continue even if they can see the damage that is being wrought on their bodies and social functioning. The typical patient who has had the disorder for several years is severely depressed

(Touyz *et al.*, 2013). Furthermore, not all these reinforcing factors (negative or positive) are consciously available to the affected person, even if they can be brought to awareness through therapy.

Summary of the elements of a cognitive model

The "cognitive model" of EDs is necessarily multifaceted and encompasses self-discrepancies, internalizing of the thin-ideal, the central over-importance placed on weight and shape, the reinforcements that ensue upon dieting, the errors in information processing, and the neurocognitive changes that also occur. The model is sensitive to the cognitive, personality and emotional vulnerabilities that certain individuals have. Figure 20.1 attempts to capture these major components in a sequence that makes sense for an "average" patient with anorexia. Binge-eating is not included here, but usually follows from efforts to lose weight (Fairburn, 2008). Some important and well-documented features of EDs are not included in Figure 20.1, as they are not "cognitive" in nature (e.g., having an inability to individuate; a fear of maturity; being unsure of one's identity; having feelings of emptiness or utter worthlessness). This raises a desire to see how these known aspects of an ED can be combined with the cognitive issues and processes in a unified model.

An integrated theoretical model

A useful model would be one that accounts for the various clinical and experimental observations that have been documented (such as a preponderance of females being afflicted; the adolescent onset; the comorbid anxiety, perfectionism and obsessionality; and certain neurocognitive traits). A helpful integrated model would also guide treatments that work. This is immediately problematic because the treatment outcome studies for adults have produced a range of treatments that all have some moderate support. In bulimia nervosa, cognitive-behavior therapy (CBT), or its enhanced version (Fairburn, 2008) remains the treatment of choice, while interpersonal psychotherapy (IPT) has been shown to have slightly better outcomes after more than one year follow-up after a slower initial response compared with CBT (Agras, Walsh, Fairburn, Wilson & Kraemer, 2000; Tannofsky-Kraff & Wilfley, 2010). Various treatments have been found to have some degree of effectiveness for AN: specialist supportive clinical management has emerged as an effective treatment (McIntosh *et al.*, 2005; McIntosh, Jordan & Bulik, 2010; Touyz *et al.*, 2013), as has focal, brief psychodynamic therapy (Zipfel *et al.*, 2014), but CBT has had mixed results (Pike, Carter, & Olmstead, 2010). The fact that a variety of therapies have equivalent outcomes suggests that no one approach is "right," but there are some common factors that get addressed through therapeutic engagement with a professional who knows about EDs and offers caring treatment.

In each effort to provide a comprehensive model of the EDs, the common thread is that EDs are egosyntonic conditions that confer powerful adaptive functions for the affected individual. Here is where the commonality lies – in providing a sensitive formulation of the initial vulnerability factors and triggers and then the maintaining factors that are relevant for each individual. Such a formulation must necessarily welcome *psychodynamic* input (vulnerabilities such as an enmeshed maternal relationship, or fears of sexual maturation), *neurocognitive* aspects (as a predisposing factor and then as a maintaining factor with weight loss), *beliefs and attitudes* about one's self worth and the reliance on thinness to feel adequate, as well as *reinforcement* issues once the dieting starts.

Some notable efforts have already been made to incorporate cognitive-behavioral and psychodynamic perspectives into the one treatment-oriented formulation. Garner and Bemis (1982), Garner *et al.* (1997), Schmidt and Treasure (2006), and Vitousek, Watson, and Wilson (1998) have each outlined how CBT is effective when each patient is understood in terms of their underlying personal and interpersonal needs and how the ED serves an adaptive function to meet that need. Guidano and Liotti (1983, 1985) have made an important contribution to the cognitive model of psychopathology by highlighting the role of early development and especially attachment in infancy. One's schemas, or tacit rules, about the world are formed as one relates to others and one's basic fabric of self-knowledge is constructed from early patterns of caregiving. Thereafter, "any information about the outside world always and inevitably corresponds to information about the self" (Guidano & Liotti, 1985, p. 108). Thus attachment influences fundamental tacit self-knowledge which, in turn, drives how we filter all future experiences. They argue that specific attachment experiences and schemas make a person vulnerable to specific conditions later in life, and these include eating disorders (Guidano & Liotti, 1983). Ward, Ramsay, and Treasure (2000) have summarized some of the research into attachment issues as they impact on eating disorders. Hardit and Hannum (2012) also had a focus on attachment when examining the tripartite influence model, finding that anxious attachment was a significant moderator of the effects of sociocultural attitudes on one's body dissatisfaction.

We emphasize the need for a thorough and longitudinal assessment of every patient, with a careful developmental, family, genetic, personal, and social history. The sort of generic model presented in Figure 20.1 cannot readily be used in therapy, as each sketched formulation will necessarily be different for each client. For instance, what makes weight loss so incredibly reinforcing for one person will be different for another, and their personal self-discrepancies will also differ and may (or may not) be very relevant in the start or maintenance of their ED. What makes the weight loss so reinforcing may be a *sociocultural* factor (being involved in a certain subculture, such as dance), or may relate to early trauma and a *damaged self* (e.g. from a punitive and critical but enmeshed parent). Beyond undertaking a thorough assessment of each person, several other treatment implications arise from the literature reviewed above.

Treatment implications

Work with the egosyntonicity

As has been highlighted throughout this chapter, the EDs (especially AN but also binge-eating disorders such as BN) are egosyntonic. That is, the affected person finds that the symptoms and consequences of the disorder serve powerfully helpful functions in their life that feel valued and "right" to them. This has long been understood by clinicians when confronted by the difficulties that their patients encounter as they engage in recovery. Bruch (1973, 1978) highlighted the need for and the exalted valuing of their symptoms, as has Vitousek (Garner & Bemis, 1982; Garner *et al.*, 1997; Vitousek *et al.*, 1998). This can only be done if a thorough and curious assessment of each patient is undertaken by a clinician who is aware of the common adaptive functions that EDs often embody.

The principles and practices of motivational interviewing have been advocated as a means to work with the egosyntonicity of EDs (Garner *et al.*, 1997; Schmidt & Treasure, 2006; Treasure & Schmidt, 2008; Vitousek *et al.*, 1998). The common recommendations that these various authors make include: voicing an understanding of how the ED has indeed been adaptive for that person; timing interventions with regard for the person's readiness for change; using respectful questions about costs, benefits, and whether the ED is truly adaptive; and engaging in a close collaborative relationship in which alternative, healthier ways to meet emotional needs can be taught and experimented with.

Be willing to work deeply

The therapist needs to take time to peel back layers of self-awareness. Some clients are aware of the underlying seed from which the ED grew (such as a fear of developing sexuality or an impossibly enmeshed relationship with an emotionally powerful parent) but will not share that in therapy (e.g., until they trust the therapist to deal with it sensitively or until their assumed hopelessness for a healthy resolution has been assuaged). Other patients do not have conscious access to older psychological issues that help explain the onset and then maintenance of their condition. In such cases, it takes time to explore that together. This exploration is helped if the therapist is aware of the common adaptive functions that EDs can serve. It is often advised that therapy can take well over a year and the chronicity of illness correlates strongly with required duration of treatment (Touyz *et al.*, 2013). However, working "deeply" does not mean very long-term therapy with no requirement to change. A lot of work on self-deficiencies and underlying motivation can be done relatively briefly when the therapy is focused. Fairburn (2008) advocates for 20 sessions for bulimia and 40 for AN when using CBT-E. Zipfel *et al.* (2014) compared CBT-E to focused psychodynamic therapy over 10 months, finding roughly equivalent results. Waller (2012) points out that engagement and motivation increase when early behavioral changes are emphasized and achieved in therapy.

Use "non-negotiables"

The form of therapy advocated above can take some time and the therapist must tolerate anxiety-provoking behaviors in their patient (vomiting and weight loss are objectively dangerous and EDs have a high mortality rate). This necessitates clear non-negotiables for the therapy. Geller has outlined a clinically useful guide in this regard (Geller & Srikameswaran, 2006). The therapist must be clear about when treatment

would pause – perhaps for an inpatient admission, or to address some comorbidity. The involvement of medical practitioners who will monitor and treat any biological disturbances and communicate with the therapist is also advised. Having non-negotiables not only establishes a safe way to proceed, but also helps access core schemas of undeservedness or worthlessness in the client and can repair past experiences of neglect (Geller & Srikameswaran, 2006). Their therapist's actions affirm to the client that they are indeed worth looking after well, and they may then learn how to care for themselves.

Use the parallel-track approach to target the core over-valuing of weight and shape

Addressing the overemphasis on weight and shape in self-evaluation is an almost universal recommendation by clinicians (Garner & Bemis, 1982; Fairburn, 2008; Fairburn *et al.*, 2003; Waller *et al.*, 2007). If the approach was purely psychological (addressing emotional needs and cognitive processes) then one could devote all the therapy time to issues such as self-evaluation, reinforcing a broader base of identity (or ego-strength), meeting the client's interpersonal needs, or managing their emotional deficits. However, when this is done to the exclusion of attending to weight restoration and the normalizing of eating behaviors, then less progress is made (Garner *et al.*, 1997; Waller *et al.*, 2007). The person with an ED often pleadingly requests just to work on their affective distress or self-esteem or identity issues first – which will then enable them to eat more easily. This rarely works and fails to address the medical morbidity. The alternative is to do both roughly at the same time, as the vehicle of therapy moves down two "parallel tracks" (Garner *et al.*, 1997). One cannot repair unhealthy or diminished self-evaluation while hanging on to a single dominant method of feeling adequate or safe (dieting). Furthermore, while the various reinforcing effects of dietary restriction and weight loss are present and while the neurocognitive effects of the same are having sway, then the capacity for and likelihood of therapeutic change is very low.

Identify and modify neurocognitive style

The findings of cognitive rigidity and difficulty in shifting set or seeing a bigger picture appear to be reliable. The importance lies in helping the individual to see how automatic cognitive processes have led them to form and become attached to certain "rules." Cognitive remediation therapy (CRT) has been manualized by the developers of this approach (Tchanturia & Hambrook, 2010). It may not be possible to significantly change how a person's brain processes tasks and information; however, respectfully raising insight into a person's strengths and weaknesses in their cognitive style of information processing and into their capacity for cognitive flexibility may enable them to engage better in recovery.

Cognitive-behavioral therapy

Once this is all done, CBT can work remarkably effectively. There is certainly a role for classic behavioral and cognitive interventions even when the illness was triggered and then maintained by early dynamic processes. Once a patient is able to see objectively the early causal and maintaining factors, then they are better able to consider meeting their needs in healthier ways than through ED symptoms. Even then, they may still lack the insight or skills required to change all the habitual, forceful thoughts, rules, and urges that are the residue of years of ED. This is when the core interventions outlined by many, notably including Fairburn (2008), Garner et al. (1997) and Waller et al. (2007), can be most helpful. These strategies include self-monitoring of eating and its relationship with thoughts and feelings, using a collaborative case-formulation approach, and using goal-setting, hypothesis-testing, thought-challenging, and cognitive defusion. For many patients it is necessary to identify and work with the core beliefs around worth, defectiveness, and likelihood of rejection (Garner et al. 1997; Guidano & Liotti, 1983).

Conclusion

When it is said that EDs are disorders of the self, it means that the disorder reflects the nature of distress that the individual experiences and is manifest in their efforts to change or perfect those aspects of the self. Furthermore, aspects of the self change as the ED becomes more severe and chronic, and these changes reinforce the disorder, making it harder for the affected person to see the need for or benefit of recovery. If one abandons allegiances to any one model, then the psychodynamic and cognitive models can be integrated in clinical application. This integration is centered on the crucial observation that EDs come to serve functions in the person's life that are sometimes desperately needed and at other times valued and prized. These functions can be unconscious needs emerging from early attachment failures, or deficits in coping or emotional damage. They could equally be conscious avoidance of an aversive state (such as sexual maturation) or pursuit of a positive state (such as competitive sense of achievement or moral superiority). Clinical observations require us to accept that there are broad psychodynamic and cognitive-behavioral factors in the development of an ED; and that these factors are present in various combinations and in varying intensities in each patient. As a result, the therapy must be individually tailored in its planning and execution and must offer sensitivity to the psychological needs of the individual, while providing a safe, knowledgeable, and structured pathway to recovery. The emerging success of Specialist Supportive Clinical Management (McIntosh et al., 2010) even for those with longstanding AN (Touyz et al., 2013) is an example of this in action. We all eagerly await the pending results of new large studies that will shed more light on what works for whom.

References

Agras, W. S., Walsh, B. T., Fairburn, C. G., Wilson, G. T., & Kraemer, H. C. (2000). A multicenter comparison of cognitive-behavioral therapy and interpersonal psychotherapy for bulimia nervosa. *Archives of General Psychiatry*, 5, 459–466.

American Psychiatric Association. (2013). *Diagnostic and Statistical Manual of Mental Disorders: DSM-5.* Washington, DC: American Psychiatric Association.

Basten, C. J. (2008). *The Development and Validation of a Questionnaire Measuring Sense of Self.* Unpublished thesis manuscript. University of Sydney.

Bessenoff, G. R. (2006). Can the media affect us? Social comparison, self-discrepancy, and the thin ideal. *Psychology of Women Quarterly*, 30, 239–251.

Bowlby, J. (1988). *A Secure Base: Clinical Applications of Attachment Theory.* London: Routledge.

Bruch, H. (1973). *Eating Disorders: Obesity, Anorexia Nervosa and the Person Within.* New York, NY: Basic Books.

Bruch, H. (1978). *The Golden Cage: The Enigma of Anorexia Nervosa.* Cambridge, MA: Harvard University Press.

Cooper, Z., & Fairburn, C. G. (2010). Cognitive behavior therapy for bulimia nervosa. In C. M. Grilo & J. E. Mitchell (Eds.), *The Treatment of Eating Disorders: A Clinical Handbook.* New York, NY: Guilford Press.

Crane, A. M., Roberts, M. E., & Treasure, J. (2007). Are obsessive–compulsive personality traits associated with a poor outcome in anorexia nervosa? A systematic review of randomised control trials and naturalistic outcome studies. *International Journal of Eating Disorders*, 40, 581–588.

Crisp, A. H. (1980). *Anorexia Nervosa: Let Me Be*. London: Academic Press.

Ewell, S., Smith, F., Karmel, M., & Hart, D. (1996). The sense of self and its development: a framework for understanding eating disorders. In L. Smolak, M. P. Levine, & R. Striegel-Moore (Eds.), *The Developmental Psychopathology of Eating Disorders: Implications for Research, Prevention and Treatment*. Mahwah, NJ: Erlbaum.

Fallon, P., Katzman, M. A., & Wooley, S. C. (1993). *Feminist Perspectives on Eating Disorders*. New York, NY: Guilford Press.

Fairburn, C. G. (2008). *Cognitive Behavior Therapy and Eating Disorders*. New York, NY: Guilford Press.

Fairburn, C. G., Cooper, Z., & Shafran, R. (2003). Cognitive-behaviour therapy for eating disorders: A "transdiagnostic" theory and treatment. *Behavior Research and Therapy*, 4, 509–528.

Garner, D. M. & Bemis, K. M. (1982). A cognitive-behavioral approach to anorexia nervosa. *Cognitive Therapy and Research*, 6, 123–150.

Garner, D. M. & Bemis, K. M. (1985). Cognitive therapy for anorexia nervosa. In D. M. Garner & P. E. Garfinkel (Eds.), *Handbook of Psychotherapy for Anorexia Nervosa and Bulimia*. New York, NY: Guilford Press.

Garner, D. M., Vitousek, K. M., & Pike, K. M. (1997). Cognitive-behavioral therapy for anorexia nervosa. In D. M. Garner & P. E. Garfinkel (Eds.), *Handbook of Treatment for Eating Disorders* (2nd edn). New York, NY: Guilford Press.

Geller, J. & Srikameswaran, S. (2006). Treatment non-negotiables: Why we need them and how to make them work. *European Eating Disorders Review*, 14, 212–217.

Goodsitt, A. (1985). Self psychology and the treatment of anorexia nervosa. In D. M. Garner & P. E. Garfinkel (Eds.), *Handbook of Psychotherapy for Anorexia Nervosa and Bulimia*. New York, NY: Guilford Press.

Guidano, V. F., & Liotti, G. (1983). *Cognitive Processes and Emotional Disorders*. New York, NY: Guilford.

Guidano, V. F., & Liotti, G. (1985). A constructivist foundation for cognitive therapy. In M. Mahoney & A. Freeman (Eds.), *Cognition and Psychotherapy*. New York, NY: Plenum.

Hardit, S. K. & Hannum, J. W. (2012). Attachment, the tripartite influence model and the development of body dissatisfaction. *Body Image*, 9, 469–475.

Harrison, K. (2001). Ourselves, our bodies: Thin-ideal media, self-discrepancies, and eating disorder symptomatology in adolescents. *Journal of Social and Clinical Psychology*, 20, 289–323.

Hausenblas, H. A., Campbell, A., Menzel, J. E., *et al.* (2013). Media effects of experimental presentation of the ideal physique on eating disorder symptoms: A meta-analysis of laboratory studies. *Clinical Psychology Review, 33*, 168–181.

Higgins, E. T. (1987). Self-discrepancy: A theory relating self and affect. *Psychological Review*, 94, 319–340.

Keery, H., van den Berg, P., & Thompson, J. K. (2004). An evaluation of the Tripartite Influence Model of body dissatisfaction and eating disturbance with adolescent girls. *Body Image*, 1, 237–251.

Keys, A., Brozek, J., Henschel, H., Mickelson, O., & Taylor, H. I. (1950). *The Biology of Human Starvation*. Minneapolis: University of Minnesota Press.

Klein, M. (1975). *Love, Guilt and Reparation and Other Works 1921–1945*. London: Hogarth Press.

Kohut, H. (1971). *The Analysis of the Self*. New York, NY: International University Press.

Kohut, H. & Wulf, E. S. (1978). The disorders of the self and their treatment: An outline. *International Journal of Psychoanalysis*, 59, 423–425.

Lee, M. & Shafran, R. (2004). Information Processing Biases in eating disorders. *Clinical Psychology Review*, 24, 215–238.

Lerner, H. D. (1993). Self-representation in eating disorders: A psychodynamic perspective. In Z. V. Segal & S. J. Blatt (Eds.), *The Self in Emotional Distress: Cognitive and Psychodynamic Perspectives*. New York, NY: Guilford Press.

Lopez, C., Tchanturia, K., Stahl, D., *et al.* (2008). An examination of the concept of central coherence in women with anorexia nervosa. *International Journal of Eating Disorders*, 41, 143–152.

Mahler, M., Pine, F., & Bergman, A. (1975). *The Psychological Birth of the Human Infant*. New York, NY: Basic Books.

McIntosh, V. V., Jordan, J., Carter, F. A., *et al.* (2005). Three psychotherapies for anorexia nervosa: A randomized control trial. *American Journal of Psychiatry*, 162, 741–747.

McIntosh, V. V., Jordan, J., & Bulik, C. M. (2010). Specialist supportive clinical management for anorexia nervosa. In C. M. Grilo & J. E. Mitchell (Eds.), *The Treatment of Eating Disorders: A Clinical Handbook*. New York, NY: Guilford Press.

McNally, R. J. & Reese, H. E. (2008). Information-processing approaches to understanding anxiety disorders. In M. M. Antony & M. B. Stein (Eds.), *Oxford Handbook of Anxiety and Related Disorders*. Oxford: Oxford University Press.

Orbach, S. (1985). Accepting the symptom: A feminist psychoanalytic treatment of anorexia nervosa. In D. M. Garner & P. E. Garfinkel (Eds.), *Handbook of Psychotherapy for Anorexia Nervosa and Bulimia*. New York, NY: Guilford Press.

Pike, K. M., Carter, J. C., & Olmsted, M. P. (2010). Cognitive-behavioral therapy for anorexia nervosa. In C. M. Grilo & J. E. Mitchell (Eds.), *The Treatment of Eating Disorders: A Clinical Handbook*. New York, NY: Guilford Press.

Roberts, M., Tchanturia, K., Stahl, D., Southgate, H., & Treasure, J. (2007). A systematic review and meta-analysis of set-shifting ability in eating disorders. *Psychological Medicine*, 37, 1075–1084.

Sanchez-Oritz, V. C. & Schmidt, U. (2010). Self-help approaches for bulimia nervosa and binge-eating disorder. In C. M. Grilo & J. E. Mitchell (Eds.), *The Treatment of Eating Disorders: A Clinical Handbook*. New York, NY: Guilford Press.

Sawdon, A. M., Cooper, M., & Seabrook, R. (2007). The relationship between self-discrepancies, eating disorder and depressive symptoms in women. *European Eating Disorders Review*, 15, 207–212.

Schmidt, U. & Treasure, J. (2006). Anorexia nervosa: Valued and visible. A cognitive-interpersonal maintenance model and its implications for research and practice. *British Journal of Clinical Psychology*, 45, 343–366.

Schupak-Neuberg, E. & Nemeroff, C.J. (1993). Disturbances in identity and self-regulation in bulimia nervosa: Implications for a metaphorical perspective of "body as self". *International Journal of Eating Disorders*, 13, 335–347.

Slade, P. (1982). Towards a functional analysis of anorexia nervosa and bulimia nervosa. *British Journal of Clinical Psychology*, 21, 167–179.

Southgate, L., Tchanturia, K., & Treasure, J. (2008). Information processing bias in anorexia nervosa. *Psychiatry Research*, 160, 221–227.

Stauman, T. J., Vookles, J., Berenstein, V., Chaiken, S. & Higgins, E. T. (1991). Self-discrepancies and vulnerability to body dissatisfaction and disordered eating. *Journal of Personality and Social Psychology*, 61, 946–956.

Stein, K. F. & Corte, C. (2007). Identity impairment and the eating disorders: Content and organization of the self-concept in women with anorexia nervosa and bulimia nervosa. *European Eating Disorders Review*, 15, 58–69.

Stice, E. (2001). A prospective test of the dual pathway model of bulimic pathology: Mediating effects of dieting and negative affect. *Journal of Abnormal Psychology*, 110, 124–135.

Striegel-Moore, R. H. (1995). A feminist perspective on the etiology of eating disorders. In K. D. Brownell & C. G. Fairburn (Eds.), *Eating Disorders and Obesity: A Comprehensive Handbook*. New York, NY: Guilford Press.

Strober, M. (1991). Disorders of the self in anorexia nervosa: An organismic-developmental paradigm. In C. Johnson (Ed.), *Psychodynamic Treatment of Anorexia Nervosa and Bulimia*. New York, NY: Guilford Press.

Tanofsky-Kraff, M. & Wilfley, D. E. (2010). Interpersonal psychotherapy for bulimia nervosa and binge-eating disorder. In C. M. Grilo & J. E. Mitchell (Eds.), *The Treatment of Eating Disorders: A Clinical Handbook*. New York, NY: Guilford Press.

Tchanturia, K., Brecelj, M., Sanchez, P., *et al.* (2004). Cognitive flexibility in anorexia nervosa and bulimia nervosa. *Journal of the International Neuropsychological Society*, 10, 513–520.

Tchanturia, K., Campbell, I. C., Morris, R., & Treasure, J. (2005). Neuropsychological studies in anorexia nervosa. *International Journal of Eating Disorders*, 37, S72–S76.

Tchanturia, K. & Hambrook, D. (2010). Cognitive remediation therapy for anorexia nervosa. In C. M. Grilo & J. E. Mitchell (Eds.), *The Treatment of Eating Disorders: A Clinical Handbook*. New York, NY: Guilford Press.

Thompson, J. K., Heinberg, L. J., Altabe, M. N., & Tantleff-Dunn, S. (1999). *Exacting Beauty: Theory, Assessment and Treatment of Body Image Disturbance*. Washington, DC: American Psychological Association.

Touyz, S., Le Grange, D., Lacey, H., *et al.* (2013). Treating severe and enduring anorexia nervosa: A randomized control trial. *Psychological Medicine*, 43, 2501–2511.

Treasure, J. & Schmidt, U. (2008). Motivational Interviewing in the management of eating disorders. In H. Arkowitz, H. A. Westra, W. R. Miller, & S. Rollnick (Eds.), *Motivational Interviewing in the Treatment of Psychological Disorders*. New York, NY: Guilford Press.

van den Berg, P., Thompson, J. K., Obremski-Brandon, K., & Coovert, M. (2002). The tripartite influence model of body dissatisfaction and eating disturbance: A covariance structure modeling investigation testing the mediational role of appearance comparison. *Journal of Psychosomatic Research*, 53, 1007–1020.

Vitousek, K. & Ewald, L. S. (1993). Self-representation in eating disorders: A cognitive perspective. In Z. V. Segal & S. J. Blatt (Eds.), *The Self in Emotional Distress: Cognitive and Psychodynamic Perspectives*. New York, NY: Guilford Press.

Vitousek, K. & Hollon, S. D. (1990). The investigation of schematic content and processing in eating disorders. *Cognitive Therapy and Research*, 14, 191–214.

Vitousek, K., Watson, S., & Wilson, G. T. (1998). Enhancing motivation for change in treatment-resistant eating disorders, *Clinical Psychology Review*, 18, 391–420.

Waller, G., Dordery, H., Corstorphine, E., *et al.* (2007). *Cognitive Behavioral Therapy for Eating Disorders: A Comprehensive Treatment Guide.* Cambridge: Cambridge University Press.

Waller, G. (2012). The myths of motivation: Time for a fresh look at some received wisdom in the eating disorders? *International Journal of Eating Disorders*, 45, 1–16.

Ward, A., Ramsay, R., & Treasure, J. (2000). Attachment research in eating disorders. *British Journal of Medical Psychology*, 73, 35–51.

Westen, D. (1992). The cognitive self and the psychoanalytic self: Can we put our selves together? *Psychological Inquiry: An International Journal for the Advancement of Psychological Theory*, 3, 1–13.

Wildes, J. E., Ringham, R. M., & Marcus, M. D. (2010). Emotion avoidance in patients with anorexia nervosa: Initial test of a functional model. *International Journal of Eating Disorders*, 43(5), 398–404.

Winnicott, D. W. (1965). *The Maturational Processes and the Facilitating Environment.* New York, NY: International Universities Press.

Zerbe, K. J. (2010). Psychodynamic therapy for eating disorders. In C. M. Grilo & J. E. Mitchell (Eds.), *The Treatment of Eating Disorders: A Clinical Handbook.* New York, NY: Guilford Press.

Zipfel, S., Wild, B., Groß, G., *et al.* (2014). Focal psychodynamic therapy, cognitive behaviour therapy, and optimised treatment as usual in outpatients with anorexia nervosa (ANTOP study): Randomised controlled trial. *The Lancet*, 383, 127–137.

Chapter

21

The self in dementia

Lisa S. Caddell

Introduction

Dementia is a neurodegenerative condition that mostly affects older adults. Prevalence increases with age, although a small proportion of cases affect people before the age of 65 and are classified as "early-onset" (Tindall & Manthorpe, 1997). It is estimated that currently at least 35 million people worldwide have a form of dementia, and this is expected to rise to over 115 million people by the year 2050 (Welsh Assembly Government, 2011). There are several types of dementia; Alzheimer's Disease accounts for approximately 62% of all cases of dementia, vascular dementia for 17%, mixed dementia for 10%, and the remaining 11% includes fronto-temporal dementia and dementia with Lewy Bodies (Dementia UK, 2007). Diagnostic criteria vary across different types of dementia, but memory difficulties are commonly observed through objective memory testing, while other cognitive impairments such as aphasia (problems with speech, such as word-finding) or executive impairment (such as issues with planning or problem-solving) may also be present. Such cognitive difficulties are severe enough to result in impairments in daily living and represent a significant decline from a higher level of functioning. The course of the disease varies according to the type of dementia; some types have a gradual onset and a continuing cognitive decline, such as Alzheimer's Disease, whereas other types tend to have a more sudden onset and a step-wise deterioration, such as vascular dementia (Groves et al., 2000).

Why is 'the self' important in dementia?

Much research has been undertaken to support policy guidelines concerning the care of people with dementia, and these have evolved from concentrating on physical needs to also considering relevant psychological and social needs. The National Institute for Health and Clinical Excellence guidelines (NICE, 2011) suggested that non-pharmacological therapies should be considered for people with dementia who exhibit challenging behavior such as aggression or agitation, or for those who show signs of depression. Policy writers have recently started to recognize the importance of "person-centered" care for people with dementia, which has been heavily influenced by the work of Kitwood (1997) and Fazio (2008), who strongly believed that maintaining the self was key to maximizing the well-being of individuals with dementia. The NICE guidelines (2011) state that the principles of person-centered care underpin good practice in supporting people with dementia, and that these principles reflect the value and individuality of each individual, including his/her unique personality and life history. The guidelines also highlight the importance of relationships and interactions with others, a person's individual biography, including religious or spiritual beliefs and cultural identity, and other psychosocial factors for good quality person-centered care. A substantial amount of research has focused on "the self" (or "identity") in people with dementia, and a range of

The Self in Understanding and Treating Psychological Disorders, ed. Michael Kyrios, Richard Moulding, Guy Doron, Sunil S. Bhar, Maja Nedeljkovic, and Mario Mikulincer. Published by Cambridge University Press. © Cambridge University Press, 2016.

definitions of these terms has been used, as will be discussed in this chapter. Research has also examined the implications of maintaining identity for high-quality care and optimal well-being of the person with dementia (e.g. Clarke, Hanson, & Ross, 2003; George, 1998; Harrison, 1993; Ronch, 1996).

How is 'the self' conceptualized with respect to people with dementia?

Researchers have described "the self" in various ways. Some of these definitions overlap while others appear to be based on completely different theoretical frameworks. One of the earliest distinctions to be made was between consciousness and self-awareness, which was addressed by both Mead (1934) and James (1950), who described "the self" according to whether attention is directed outwards through an ongoing stream of consciousness or directed inwards towards traits, characteristics, and preferences ("self-awareness"). Other researchers went on to elaborate on this distinction (e.g. Brown, 1976; Farthing, 1992) by defining various "levels" of consciousness.

More recently, models have been put forward where the complexity of information about the self is more detailed and can be accessed at differing levels of consciousness (Morin, 2006). There has often been a distinction between perceptual information about the self, such as information available directly through the senses, and conceptual information about the self, which is not immediately available through the senses and is therefore represented mentally at an abstract level (e.g. Neisser, 1988; Newen & Vogeley, 2003). Further research has used a level or "component" of the self identified by such models as the basis for measurements of the self for the purpose of quantification. For example, Caddell and Clare (2012, 2013) recently used Neisser's model of self as a framework for their research with people with dementia. This is constructed from five different components: the "ecological self," which represents the self with respect to the physical environment; the "interpersonal self," which represents the self as engaged in social interaction; the "extended self" is the self as it is experienced across time and can involve personal memories; the "private self," which is based on conscious experiences not available to anyone else (e.g. thoughts, feelings, dreams); and the "conceptual self," which is made up of abstract representations about oneself such as traits, characteristics and autobiography,

and is effectively a drawing together of the other four types of self.

Neisser's model of self has also been used in research concerning other disorders, and the components of the model may be impacted upon differently according to the features of the disorder. For example, the hallucinations and delusions that can be a feature of schizophrenia may interfere with the "ecological self," in that the person may believe that they are elsewhere, and the "private self," because thoughts and feelings may be disturbed. In autism, the "interpersonal self" is likely to be affected, because there are differences in how the person responds to other people. Because the main feature of many types of dementia is memory loss, the "extended self" is likely to be compromised, which in turn would impact upon the "conceptual self" (Neisser, 1997).

Other researchers have based their work on a range of models, many of which overlap with one or more of the components of Neisser's model. Examples include the social constructionist model, which posits that language is of fundamental importance in the creation of the self (Fazio & Mitchell, 2009; Li & Orleans, 2002; Sabat & Harre, 1992), and embodied selfhood (Kontos, 2004), which suggests that the body itself is an important source of selfhood, thus challenging the notion that the self is based solely on cognitive abilities. Various interactionist models have been used to study the self in people with dementia, based on the theory that the self is constructed within the context of social interactions and relationships (e.g. Fontana & Smith, 1989; Hubbard, Cook, Tester & Downs, 2002; Saunders, 1998). Other studies have focused on autobiographical memory as the basis for the self (Addis & Tippet, 2004) or the ability to put together a narrative drawing together a combination of significant life experiences (Mills, 1997; Usita, Hyman, & Herman, 1998). A number of qualitative studies have been conducted with people with dementia, with the aim of understanding people's thoughts and feelings about their own selves using interview techniques (e.g. Beard, 2004; Caddell & Clare, 2011a; Clare, 2003; Gillies & Johnston, 2004; Li & Orleans, 2002). Numerous other studies have asked participants to rate what the researchers believe to be features of the self, such as role identities (e.g. Caddell & Clare, 2012, 2013; Cohen-Mansfield, Golander & Arnheim, 2000), or personality traits (Klein, Cosmides, & Costabile, 2003; Rankin, Baldwin, Pace-Savitsky, Kramer, & Miller, 2005; Ruby *et al.*, 2007), which have often then been compared with parallel ratings from a carer to derive a measure of how accurately a person can describe him/herself. Finally, a number of studies have used self-recognition (for example, in mirrors, photographs, or videos) as a representation of how intact a person's sense of self is (e.g. Biringer & Anderson, 1992; Bologna & Camp, 1995; Fazio & Mitchell, 2009, Grewal, 1994; Hehman, German, & Klein, 2005).

The persistence of self in dementia

It is challenging to draw firm conclusions regarding the self in individuals with dementia due to the range of theoretical frameworks described above, and also because of the resulting disparity in methods and participant samples used to measure aspects of the self. Thus, to date, there is limited agreement regarding the maintenance of the self in people with dementia.

Much of the older research concluded that participants experienced a "loss of self" (Cohen & Eisdorfer, 1986), an "unbecoming of self" (Fontana & Smith, 1989), or the "loss of all those qualities by which we have come to define our humanness" (Robertson, 1991). The basis for this argument tends to rest on the decline in cognitive abilities, particularly memory functioning, observed in people with dementia. However, a review by Caddell and Clare (2010) included 33 studies of people with a diagnosis of dementia, using the search terms "self," "identity," "personhood," and "selfhood," and came to several preliminary conclusions. The review suggested that almost all of the qualitative studies provided evidence to suggest that the self was preserved in people with dementia – it concluded that, during speech, participants could use personal pronouns and talk about their physical and mental attributes, as well as demonstrate their multiple personae and construct their identities in social interactions (e.g. Fazio & Mitchell, 2009; Hubbard, Cook, Tester & Downs, 2002; Li & Orleans, 2002; Sabat & Harre, 1992; Saunders, 1998; Small, Geldart, Gutman, & Scott, 1998; Tappen, Williams, Fishman, & Touhy, 1999). The only qualitative study to contradict this finding is that of Fontana and Smith (1989), who controversially contended that the self erodes until only "emptiness" is left. The review also examined the quantitative studies, and concluded that many of these studies presented evidence for the persistence of self, but simultaneously suggested that some results pointed to a deterioration in the self, or proposed aspects of the self, such as role-identities (e.g. Cohen-Mansfield et al., 2000), self-recognition (e.g. Biringer & Anderson, 1992; Grewal, 1994) and

self-knowledge (e.g. Klein et al., 2003; Rankin et al., 2005; Ruby et al., 2009). Overall, the review concluded that the majority of existing studies found evidence for the persistence of self, at least to some degree, but that there may be a deterioration in various components of the self, possibly linked to the stage or severity of the illness. However, these conclusions are based on evidence that is limited in several respects and is therefore rather disparate and difficult to interpret.

Despite evidence for the persistence of self in people with dementia, many existing studies also highlight a deterioration in some aspects of self, as mentioned above (e.g. Caddell & Clare, 2010; Fontana & Smith, 1989; Mills, 1997; Small et al., 1998). A recent study (Caddell & Clare, 2012) measured levels of anxiety, depression, and quality of life as well as aspects of identity (self-concept, role-identities, self-knowledge, and autobiographical memory functioning) in their sample of 50 people with dementia. In general, higher scores on measures of identity, indicating a stronger sense of self, were associated with lower levels of anxiety and depression, and a better quality of life.

The role of self for well-being in individuals with dementia remains to be examined. Further, there are very few research studies on the whether interventions that target the self in people with dementia improve well-being in such populations (also see a review by Caddell & Clare, 2011b).

Interventions developed to support the self in people with dementia

This section will review the interventions conducted as part of research studies where the researchers were specific about the aim of the study (or one of them) being to support self or identity in participants who had a diagnosis of dementia, or the intervention is at least discussed with reference to its impact upon self or identity. These interventions have been broken down into several groups according to their features. It is important to note that in much of this literature, the terms "self," "identity," and "personhood" have been used interchangeably.

Firstly, there have been three group interventions that aimed to support self or identity in participants but failed to use outcome measures (Harlan, 1993; Jensen & Wheaton, 1997; Johnson, Lahey, & Shore, 1992). These three studies were all based around the use of art materials. One of the studies also included a variety of music and movements at the beginning of each class before the participants began using the art materials, and often allowed time for discussion at the end of each class (Jensen & Wheaton, 1997). Of these studies, only Johnson *et al.* referred to a specific framework or concept of self, by referring to memory as playing an important role in the maintenance of identity. There was little information available about the participants in these interventions, such as the number of people involved or the severity of the dementia of those who participated, which again made it challenging to draw very specific conclusions from these studies. This difficulty is exacerbated by a lack of detail about the intervention, such as the time spent participating by each person. However, the researchers were able to draw some conclusions from these studies. Jensen and Wheaton (1997) reported improvements in activity level and self-esteem during weekly 90-minute sessions in a nursing home, which included music, movement, and visual art. They suggested that the classes acted as a reminder of participants' healthier, more productive selves such that remote memory was stimulated. Harlan (1993) noted that the intervention provided an opportunity for communication and enhanced motivation, confidence, and feelings of identity, and suggested that this might partly be due to the group nature of the sessions. Johnson *et al.* provided regular creative art therapy sessions and focused on remaining strengths and abilities to increase self-esteem, as well as offering opportunities for expression and spontaneity. Although there were no comparison groups or outcome data for these three studies, therapists reported a variety of positive results, and no drawbacks were noted.

A further three intervention studies have been conducted where supporting self or identity was not specified as a direct aim of the study, but the researchers explained why the intervention might be expected to be supportive of self or identity (Irish *et al.*, 2006; Sherratt, Thornton & Hatton, 2004; Yasuda, Kuwabara, Kuwahara, Abe, & Tetsutani, 2009). Yasuda *et al.* and Irish *et al.* believed that using reminders of a person's life to stimulate autobiographical memory (i.e., photos or music) could lead to an improved sense of identity, while Sherratt *et al.* also believed that listening to music has the potential to maintain personhood. Thus, these studies all involved participants listening to music, but each study involved more than one condition. One intervention involved participants watching a personalized reminiscence photo video, with music and narration added, before or after which they

would also watch two other types of TV show, so that the researchers could compare responses across conditions (Yasuda *et al.*, 2009). Yasuda *et al.* noted that the participants' concentration scores were highest while their personalized reminiscence photo video was being shown. Irish *et al.* (2006) used music as a background stimulus while 10 participants completed measures of anxiety and autobiographical memory, which were also completed by each participant in a silent condition at another time. They found that in the music condition people with dementia (but not control participants) reported lower levels of anxiety and a significantly better score on the measure of autobiographical memory. Sherratt *et al.* (2004) compared the effects of live music and taped music on well-being in 24 people in the moderate to severe stages of dementia, and found improved lengths of responding and higher levels of well-being during the live music condition compared to the other conditions. Thus, the researchers from all interventions noted some benefits of one specific condition over others, highlighting the benefits of certain types of activity over others. However, no outcomes specifically related to the self or identity were reported.

There were four further studies that were very specific about the aim of the intervention being to support self or identity, and which used outcome measures for at least some variables, which enabled more precise conclusions to be drawn from each study. As the studies were rather diverse, they will be discussed separately. An intervention based on the concept of "self-maintenance therapy" was developed by Romero and Wenz (2001), who conceptualized the self as a cognitive schema which can store and update information about the person and his/her environment. The intervention consisted of a four-week residential programme that was attended by both the person with dementia and their primary caregiver. The intervention attempted, among other objectives, to maintain personal identity and continuity in people with dementia. The aim was to achieve this through four different components of the programme: psychotherapy, training in self-knowledge, the facilitation of everyday activities, and communication in caregiving. A range of measures were completed by the 43 participants with moderate-stage dementia before and after the intervention; these showed a reduction in depression, psychopathological symptoms, and disturbances in social behavior. No significant changes were found in memory functioning, activities of daily living or self-care. As no measures specifically targeting aspects of self or identity were included in the study, it is difficult to assess whether improvements in these variables occurred.

Cohen-Mansfield, Parpura-Gill, and Golander (2006) tested an individualized treatment based on role identities, whereby each participant was assessed to determine their most prominent identity role using the Self-Identity in Dementia Questionnaire (SID; Cohen-Mansfield *et al.*, 2006). An activity related to this specific identity role was then developed and was delivered to participants for 30 minutes each day for 5 days. The researchers defined identity as the roles that people take on throughout their lives, which are demonstrated through both speech and behavior, and four main roles were defined: occupational roles, family roles, leisure activities, and attributes. A control group was also used in this study, where participants received the usual activities and care. Measures were completed before and after the intervention by research assistants and care staff. A greater awareness of identity was recorded in the treatment group post-intervention by the research assistants but not by participants themselves, and greater pleasure and interest in activities were observed in the treatment group relative to the control group. No changes in anxiety or depression were seen post-intervention.

Haight, Gibson, and Michel (2006) created a life review/life storybook intervention in which 15 people in care homes participated, as well as 15 people in the control group who did not receive the intervention. The researchers believed that it would be possible to "preserve personhood" by reinforcing personal identity both through conversation and also through retaining tangible reminders of experiences from a person's lifetime. Those in the intervention group participated in weekly life review sessions for eight weeks and also created a life storybook with help from care staff, using photographs and captions. A variety of measures were used, pre- and post-intervention, and significant improvements were recorded on cognition, depression, positive mood, and communication in the intervention group. No differences were seen in independence, memory, or behavioral problems between the two groups, and again, no specific measures of aspects of self or identity were used, making it difficult to ascertain whether actual changes in self or identity occurred.

The final study was conducted with a single participant in the moderate stages of Alzheimer's disease and involved developing and installing an in-home display of the participant's life history on a screen called a "biography theatre" (Massimi *et al.*,

2008). The participant spent eight sessions with the researcher, selecting photographs and arranging them into themes, which were then displayed on a touch-screen computer in the participant's own home which was permanently left on and was accessible at all times. Measures were completed at baseline, after collection of the biographical material, and four weeks after installation of the biography theater. Researchers noted an improvement in identity on the interim and final assessments, which was recorded on the Self Image Profile–Adult (Butler & Gasson, 2004).

Thus, these latter studies have been clearer about their aim of supporting self or identity, but as with some of the studies described earlier, measures of self/identity have not always been used. Often studies have focused on various aspects of well-being, and it appears that a sense of identity is automatically being equated with well-being in some studies. While it is of interest to see whether the intervention is responsible for changes in the well-being in participants, without a specific measure of identity it is not possible to determine whether there have been changes in self or identity, or whether such changes did in fact mediate any changes in well-being. This makes it challenging to evaluate the intervention in terms of its stated aims.

Summary/characteristics of the above research studies

The 10 interventions described above are clearly diverse with respect to the content of the intervention itself, as well as the manner in which efficacy has been investigated. This section will summarize the various aspects of the interventions discussed.

All studies explain the rationale behind the intervention, at least to some extent, and there are similarities and differences with respect to the reasoning. The primary aim of the interventions described tended to be to maintain the self, with the secondary aim of improving well-being in some way. Two main themes emerged concerning the rationale for the intervention. Several interventions were based on the premise that stimulating memory would support a person's sense of self, and therefore presented participants with reminders of their past (e.g. Haight *et al.*, 2006; Massimi *et al.*, 2008; Yasuda *et al.*, 2009). Other interventions were based on the importance of group interactions (Jensen & Wheaton, 1997; Johnson *et al.*, 1992; Harlan, 1993) with the aim of supporting established relationships or enabling new social ties to form.

Some of the studies referred to a specific concept of the self, whereas others did not. The concepts used varied across studies, with some viewing the self as something which might be socially established or expressed (Cohen-Mansfield *et al.*, 2006; Massimi *et al.*, 2008) and some seeing it as being dependent on memory functioning (Johnson *et al.*, 1992; Massimi *et al.*, 2008; Romero & Wenz, 2001). Thus, it is clear that definitions of self and identity vary across studies, while in some cases no definition of the self is outlined. It is therefore important to note that while all of the interventions are based on self or identity, they may be referring to differing concepts, which makes it difficult to integrate the outcome of the studies and draw strong conclusions.

From a research perspective, the design of the studies was generally weak, with most exhibiting problematic design issues that to some extent limit the conclusions that can be drawn. Examples of such difficulties include the lack of a control group, a lack of clarity regarding how participants were assigned to groups, and no outcome data on which to base any conclusions.

The studies also showed considerable heterogeneity with respect to participant characteristics. The number of participants ranged from a single case (Massimi *et al.*, 2008) to over 90 (Cohen-Mansfield *et al.*, 2006), although some interventions involved ongoing therapy groups and therefore did not disclose the exact number of participants (Harlan, 1993; Johnson *et al.*, 1992). Some interventions involved participants with moderate to severe dementia while others included participants in the earlier stages of dementia. Some studies characterized the severity of dementia using the Mini Mental State Evaluation (Folstein, Folstein, & McHugh, 1975), but few included information about the range of severity within the sample, and some gave no explicit information about dementia severity. Without this information it is not possible to determine whether these various approaches to supporting the self are more or less suitable for people with dementia who are at different stages of severity.

Characteristics of the interventions varied greatly. Some were group-based (Harlan, 1993; Jensen & Wheaton, 1997; Johnson *et al.*, 1992), whereas the others were conducted with individuals, and one using a combined group and individual treatment approach (Romero & Wenz,). In many of the interventions, participants received the same treatment, whereas in a minority of interventions the content was tailored to the individuals (Cohen-Mansfield *et al.*, 2006; Romero & Wenz, 2001). The setting for the intervention also varied, from a four-week residential stay (Romero & Wenz, 2001) to being conducted in residential homes, special care units, or in the participant's own home. Equally, there were differences in the length and intensity of interventions, ranging from 40 minutes on a single day (Yasuda *et al.*, 2009) to 6 months of weekly sessions (Jensen & Wheaton, 1997). From the existing data, it is difficult to assess whether any of these approaches were more beneficial than others.

Unfortunately, not all of the interventions were monitored using formal outcome measures. In some, progress was determined by the impression of the therapist involved in delivering the intervention (e.g. Harlan, 1993; Jensen & Wheaton, 1997). Other interventions were evaluated using standardized measures, although not necessarily measures designed to capture features of the self. Measures that were used to reflect the self/identity included the Self Identity in Dementia Questionnaire (Cohen-Mansfield *et al.*, 2006), and the Self Image Profile–Adult (Butler & Gasson, 2004). Other measures were also used to assess well-being; for example, mood, and behavior and cognitive functioning. With such a variety of outcomes, it is not possible to integrate the results of the various interventions.

There are various ways in which future evaluations of treatments targeting the self could be improved. Future studies need to explicate which aspect of the self, if any, will be targeted, and the theoretical framework on which the intervention is based. Design issues such as a lack of control group or a lack of pre- and post-intervention measures also need to be taken into consideration. It would be helpful to establish the relationships between key variables (e.g. aspects of the self and identity, memory, and well-being) before devising further interventions.

Another important consideration when designing treatments to support the self is to think about how any findings or successful interventions might be put into practice. For example, studies must consider whether the intervention would be suitable for people with dementia living at home, or in a residential or nursing home, and whether the resources would be available to conduct the intervention; for example, in terms of staff, time and finances. Also, while delivering any treatment, it is important to monitor the impact of the intervention on individuals by recording improvements or any detrimental effects, bearing in mind that individuals may react very differently to interventions in spite of being similar in other respects. These factors play a major role in determining how interventions or treatments are applied in practice, and so must also be strongly considered in the design of further research studies in this area.

Research on how the family might help to maintain the identity of a relative with dementia is extremely limited, although organizations such as the Alzheimer's Society emphasize the importance of helping to support the person's identity (e.g., on websites and in factsheets). However, several suggestions could be drawn from the interventions described above. For example, it might be possible for relatives to help an individual with dementia to create a "life story" book using photographs (as in Haight *et al.*, 2006), or to make familiar music easily accessible (e.g., Sherratt *et al.*, 2004). It could also be beneficial to help the family member maintain roles that they previously fulfilled, such as cooking or gardening (e.g. Cohen-Mansfield *et al.*, 2006). Further research should focus on developing guidelines concerning how to help maintain the identity of a family member with dementia with the aim of supporting well-being.

Conclusion

This chapter has discussed the various concepts concerning the self that have been applied when working with people with dementia, as well as interventions that have been developed with the aim of supporting the self. It is clear that the diverse definitions of "the self" have led to the development of a wide variety of interventions with differing underlying assumptions, and thus it is challenging to draw strong conclusions regarding exactly what type of treatment is effective in supporting the self in people with dementia. A related difficulty is finding ways in which the self or identity in dementia can be measured or quantified. There are very few current methods that have been employed across different studies, adding to the challenge in integrating the outcomes of existing interventions and drawing strong conclusions. These issues highlight considerations for future work concerning the self.

While some of the existing studies focused specifically on improvements in identity (Cohen-Mansfield *et al.*, 2006; Massimi *et al.*, 2008), most reported changes in terms of aspects of well-being. It is, however, encouraging that interventions aiming to support self or identity have resulted in positive changes in well-being, for example in mood (e.g. Haight *et al.*, 2006; Romero & Wenz, 2001), in pleasure, and in interest (e.g. Cohen-Mansfield *et al.*, 2006), and a decrease in agitation and anxiety (e.g. Irish *et al.*, 2006). This

suggests that it would be valuable to conduct further studies into the self in people with dementia, with the aim of understanding more about the experience of the self, as well as its relationship with aspects of well-being. Such knowledge would provide a sound basis for developing further psychosocial interventions to support the self, taking into consideration the limitations of existing studies described in this chapter. This research is required to enhance current practices in dementia care and to improve the quality of life for those living with dementia, as well as their carers, in various settings.

References

Addis, D. R., & Tippett, L. J. (2004). Memory of myself: Autobiographical memory and identity in Alzheimer's disease. *Memory*, 12, 56–74. doi: 10.1080/09658210244000423

Beard, R. L. (2004). In their voices: Identity preservation and experiences of Alzheimer's disease. *Journal of Aging Studies*, 18, 415–428. doi: 10.1016/j.jaging.2004.06.005

Biringer, F., & Anderson, J. R. (1992). Self-recognition in Alzheimer's disease: A mirror and video study. *Journal of Gerontology: Psychological Sciences*, 47(6), 385–388. Retrieved from http://psychsocgerontology.oxfordjournals.org/

Bologna, S. M., & Camp, C. J. (1995). Self-recognition in Alzheimer's disease: Evidence of an explicit/implicit dissociation. *Clinical Gerontologist*, 15, 51–54. Retrieved from http://www.tandfonline.com/toc/wcli20/current

Brown, J. W. (1976). Consciousness and pathology of language. In R. W. Rieber (Ed.), *Neuropsychology of Language – Essays in Honor of Eric Lenneberg* (pp. 72-93). London: Plenum Press.

Butler, R. J., & Gasson, S.L. (2004). *The Self Image Profile for Adults*. Oxford: Harcourt Assessment.

Caddell, L.S., & Clare, L. (2010). The impact of dementia on self and identity: A systematic review. *Clinical Psychology Review*, 30(1), 113–126. doi: 10.1016/j.cpr.2009.10.003

Caddell, L. S., & Clare, L. (2011a). I'm still the same person: The impact of early-stage dementia on identity. *Dementia*, 10(3), 379–398. doi: 10.1177/1471301211408255

Caddell, L. S., & Clare, L. (2011b). Interventions supporting self and identity in people with dementia: A systematic review. *Aging and Mental Health*, 15(7), 797–810. doi: 10.1080/13607863.2011.575352

Caddell, L. S., & Clare, L. (2012). Identity, mood and quality of life in early-stage dementia. *International Psychogeriatrics*, 24(8), 1306–1315. doi: http://dx.doi.org/10.1017/S104161021100278X

Caddell, L. S., & Clare, L. (2013). How does identity relate to cognition and functional abilities in early-stage dementia? *Aging, Neuropsychology and Cognition*, 20(1), 1–21. doi: 10.1080/13825585.2012.656575

Clare, L. (2003). Managing threats to self: Awareness in early-stage Alzheimer's disease. *Social Science and Medicine*, 57, 1017–1029. doi: 10.1016/S0277-9536(02)00476-8

Clarke, A., Hanson, E. J., & Ross, H. (2003). Seeing the person behind the patient: Enhancing the care of older people using a biographical approach. *Journal of Clinical Nursing*, 12, 697–706. Retrieved from http://www.wiley.com/bw/journal.asp?ref=0962-1067

Cohen, A., & Eisdorfer, C. (1986). *The Loss of Self*. New York, NY: Norton.

Cohen-Mansfield, J., Golander, H., & Arnheim, G. (2000). Self-identity in older persons suffering from dementia: Preliminary results. *Social Science and Medicine*, 51, 381–394. Retrieved from http://journals.elsevier.com/02779536/social-science-and-medicine/

Cohen-Mansfield, J. A., Parpura-Gill, A., & Golander, H. (2006). Utilisation of self-identity roles for designing interventions for persons with dementia. *Journal of Gerontology: Psychological Sciences*, 61B, 202–212. Retrieved from http://psychsocgerontology.oxfordjournals.org/

Dementia UK. (2007). *The Full Report*. Retrieved June 20, 2011, from http://alzheimers.org.uk/site/scripts/download_info.php?fileID=2

Farthing, G. W. (1992). *The Psychology of Consciousness*. Englewood Cliffs, NJ: Prentice Hall.

Fazio, S. (2008). *The Enduring Self in People with Alzheimer's: Getting to the Heart of Individualized Care*. Baltimore, MD: Health Professions Press.

Fazio, S., & Mitchell, D. B. (2009). Persistence of self in individuals with Alzheimer's disease. *Dementia*, 8(1), 39–59. doi: 10.1177/1471301208099044

Folstein, M. F., Folstein, S. E., & McHugh, P. R. (1975). Mini-Mental State: A practical method of grading the cognitive state of patients for the clinician. *Journal of Psychiatric Research*, 12, 189. Retrieved from http://www.elsevier.com/wps/find/journaldescription.cws_home/241/description

Fontana, A., & Smith, R. W. (1989). Alzheimer's disease victims: The 'unbecoming' of self and the normalization of competence. *Sociological Perspectives*, 32(1), 35–46. Retrieved from http://ucpressjournals.com/journal.asp?j=sop

George, L. K. (1998). Self and identity in later life: Protecting and enhancing the self. *Journal of Aging and Identity*, 3(3), 133–152. doi: 10.1023/A:1022863632210

Gillies, B., & Johnston, G. (2004). Identity loss and maintenance: Commonality of experience in cancer and dementia. *European Journal of Cancer Care*, 13, 436–442. doi: 10.1111/j.1365-2354.2004.00550.x

Grewal, R. P. (1994). Self-recognition in dementia of the Alzheimer type. *Perceptual and Motor Skills*, 79(2), 1009–1010. Retrieved from http://www.amsciepub.com/loi/pms

Groves, W. C., Brandt, J., Steinberg, M., *et al.* (2000). Vascular dementia and Alzheimer's disease: Is there a difference? A comparison of symptoms by disease duration. *The Journal of Neuropsychiatry and Clinical Neurosciences*, 12, 305–315. doi: 10.1176/appi.neuropsych.12.3.305

Haight, B. K., Gibson, F., & Michel, Y. (2006). The Northern Ireland life review/life storybook project for people with dementia. *Alzheimer's and Dementia*, 2, 56–58. doi: 10.1016/j.jalz.2005.12.003

Harlan, J. E. (1993). The therapeutic value of art for persons with Alzheimer's disease and related disorders. *Loss, Grief & Care*, 6(4), 99–106. Retrieved from http://www.informaworld.com/smpp/title~content=t904385074~db=all

Harrison, C. (1993). Personhood, dementia, and the integrity of a life. *Canadian Journal of Aging*, 12, 428–440. doi: 10.1017/S0714980800011983

Hehman, J. A., German, T. P., & Klein, S. B. (2005). Impaired self-recognition from recent photographs in a case of late-stage Alzheimer's disease. *Social Cognition*, 23(1), 118–123. doi: 10.1521/soco.23.1.118.59197

Hubbard, G., Cook, A., Tester, S., & Downs, M. (2002). Beyond words: Older people with dementia using and interpreting nonverbal behaviour. *Journal of Aging Studies*, 16, 155–167. doi: 10.1016/S0890-4065(02)00041-5

Irish, M., Cunningham, C. J., Walsh, J. B., *et al.* (2006). Investigating the enhancing effect of music on autobiographical memory in mild Alzheimer's disease. *Dementia and Geriatric Cognitive Disorders*, 22, 108–120. doi: 10.1159/000093487

James, W. (1950). *The Principles of Psychology*. New York, NY: Dover.

Jensen, S. M., & Wheaton, I.L. (1997). Multiple pathways to self: A multisensory art experience. *Art Therapy: Journal of the American Art Therapy Association*, 14, 178–186. Retrieved from http://www.arttherapyjournal.org/index.html

Johnson, C., Lahey, P. P., & Shore, A. (1992). An exploration of creative arts therapeutic group work on an Alzheimer's unit. *The Arts in Psychotherapy*, 19, 269–277. Retrieved from http://www.sciencedirect.com/science/journal/01974556

Kitwood, T. (1997). *Dementia Reconsidered: The Person Comes First*. Buckingham: Open University Press.

Klein, S. B., Cosmides, L., & Costabile, K. A. (2003). Preserved knowledge of self in a case of Alzheimer's dementia. *Social Cognition*, 21, 157–165. doi: 10.1521/soco.21.2.157.21317

Kontos, P. C. (2004). Ethnographic reflections on selfhood, embodiment and Alzheimer's disease. *Ageing and Society*, 24, 829–849. doi: 10.1017/S0144686X04002375

Li, R., & Orleans, M. (2002). Personhood in a world of forgetfulness: An ethnography of the self-process among Alzheimer's patients. *Journal of Aging and Identity*, 7(4), 227–244. doi: 10.1023/A:1020709504186

Massimi, M., Berry, E., Browne, G., *et al.* (2008). An exploratory case study of the impact of ambient biographical displays on identity in a patient with Alzheimer's disease. *Neuropsychological Rehabilitation*, 18, 742–765. doi: 0.1080/09602010802130924

Mead, G. H. (1934). *Mind, Self and Society*. Chicago, IL: University of Chicago Press.

Mills, M. A. (1997). Narrative identity and dementia: A study of emotion and narrative in older people with dementia. *Ageing and Society*, 17, 673–698. doi: 10.1017/50144686X97006673

Morin, A. (2006). Levels of consciousness and self-awareness: A comparison and integration of various neurocognitive views. *Consciousness and Cognition*, 15, 358–371. doi: 10.1016/j.concog.2005.09.006

National Institute for Health and Clinical Excellence. (2011). Dementia: Supporting people with dementia and their carers in health and social care. Retrieved from http://guidance.nice.org.uk/CG42/NICEGuidance/pdf/English

Neisser, U. (1988). Five kinds of self-knowledge. *Philosophical Psychology*, 1(1), 35–59. doi: 10.1080/09515088808572924

Neisser, U. (1997). Concepts and self-concepts. In U. Neisser, & D. A. Jopling (Eds.), *The Conceptual Self in Context*. Cambridge: Cambridge University Press.

Newen, A., & Vogeley, K. (2003). Self-representation: Searching for a neural signature of self-consciousness. *Consciousness and Cognition*, 12, 529–543. doi: 10.1016/S1053-8100(03)00090-1

Rankin, K. P., Baldwin, E., Pace-Savitsky, C., Kramer, J. H., & Miller, B. L. (2005). Self awareness and personality change in dementia. *Journal of Neurology and Neurosurgical Psychiatry*, 76, 632–639. doi: 10.1136/jnnp.2004.042879

Robertson, A. (1991). The politics of Alzheimer's disease: A case study in apocalyptic demography. In M. Minkler & C. L. Estes (Eds.), *The Political and Moral Economy of Growing Old*. Amityville, NY: Baywood Publishing Company.

Romero, B., & Wenz, M. (2001). Self-maintenance therapy in Alzheimer's disease. *Neuropsychological Rehabilitation*, 11, 333–355. doi: 10.1080/09602010143000040

Ronch, J. L. (1996). Assessment of quality of life: Preservation of the self. *International Psychogeriatrics*, 8(2), 267–275. Retrieved from http://journals.cambridge.org/action/displayJournal?jid=IPG

Ruby, P., Collette, F., D'Argembeau, A., *et al.* (2009). Perspective taking to assess self-personality: What's modified in Alzheimer's disease? *Neurobiology of Aging*, 30(10), 1636–1651. doi: 10.1016/j.neurobiolaging.2007.12.014

Ruby, P., Schmidt, C., Hogge, M., *et al.* (2007). Social mind representation: Where does it fail in frontotemporal dementia? *Journal of Cognitive Neuroscience*, 19(4), 671–683. doi: 10.1016/j.neurobiolaging.2007.12.014

Sabat, S. R., & Harre, R. (1992). The construction and deconstruction of self in Alzheimer's disease. *Ageing and Society*, 12, 443–461. doi: 10.1017/S0144686X00005262

Saunders, P. A. (1998). "My brain's on strike" – The construction of identity through memory accounts by dementia patients. *Research on Aging*, 20(1), 65–90. doi: 10.1177/0164027598201005

Sherratt, K., Thornton, A., & Hatton, C. (2004). Music interventions for people with dementia: A review of the literature. *Aging and Mental Health*, 8(1), 3–12. doi: 10.1080/13607860310001613275

Small, J. A., Geldart, K., Gutman, G., & Scott, M. A. C. (1998). The discourse of self in dementia. *Ageing and Society*, 18, 291–316. Retrieved from http://journals.cambridge.org/action/displayJournal?jid=ASO

Tappen, R. M., Williams, C., Fishman, S., & Touhy, T. (1999). Persistence of self in advanced Alzheimer's disease. *Journal of Nursing Scholarship*, 31(2), 121–125. doi: 10.111/j.1547-5069.1999.tb00445.x

Tindall, L., & Manthorpe, J. (1997). Early onset dementia: A case of ill-timing? *Journal of Mental Health*, 6(3), 237–249. Retrieved from http://informahealthcare.com/jmh

Usita, P. M., Hyman, I. E., & Herman, K. C. (1998). Narrative intentions: Listening to life stories in Alzheimer's disease. *Journal of Aging Studies*, 12(2), 185–197. doi: 10.1016/S0890-4065(98)90014-7

Welsh Assembly Government. (2011). National Dementia Vision for Wales: Dementia Supportive Communities.

Yasuda, K., Kuwabara, K., Kuwahara, N., Abe, S., & Tetsutani, N. (2009). Effectiveness of personalised reminiscence photo videos for individuals with dementia. *Neuropsychological Rehabilitation*, 19(4), 603–619. doi: 10.1080/09602010802586216

The self in gender dysphoria: a developmental perspective

Kenneth J. Zucker and Doug P. VanderLaan

With this volume's focus on the "self," it is of note that the diagnosis of Gender Identity Disorder (GID) has been one of only three diagnoses in the DSM that has contained the term "identity" in it. In DSM-III (American Psychiatric Association, 1980), there was the more generic diagnosis of Identity Disorder. In the DSM-IV (American Psychiatric Association, 1994), it was renamed "Identity Problem" and given as an example of a V-code. In DSM-IV, another diagnosis, Dissociative Identity Disorder (DID), also contained the term identity in it. In DSM-5 (American Psychiatric Association, 2013), however, the GID diagnostic label was replaced with a new one, gender dysphoria (GD), thus removing the word identity.

Despite this change in diagnostic label, gender *identity* is certainly the key feature in understanding the core phenomenology of this condition. Accordingly, in this chapter, we will provide an overview of what we know about the place gender identity has in the development of the self, its role in understanding gender dysphoria, and some of the therapeutic approaches that have been considered in attempting to address the suffering ("dysphoria") that individuals experience with regard to their gendered sense of self.

Emergence of the gendered self

Gender as a binary social category (boy–girl, man–woman) is arguably one of the most salient parameters by which people organize and think about social life (Maccoby, 1988). In contemporary Western culture, some adolescents and adults identify as "agender" or "gender neutral," but, to identify as such, there needs to be an overarching gender category from which

to "de-identify." As one 15-year-old adolescent patient told us, "I don't want to be female. I don't want to be male. I want to be a tomato."

The capacity to self-label as a boy or as a girl emerges for most children by the age of 3 (Martin, Ruble, & Szkrybalo, 2002). Thus, gender may well be one of the first elements of a nascent identity that are salient to toddlers (see Lewis & Brooks-Gunn, 1979, pp. 234–237). Developmentalists, however, have pointed out that gender identity as a stable part of the self emerges only gradually and research on the concept of "gender constancy" (Kohlberg, 1966) has received much attention.

Following the emergence of the capacity to correctly identify oneself as a boy or as a girl, young children next develop an understanding of gender stability (e.g., that a girl will grow up to be a "Mommy," not a "Daddy"), and then an understanding of gender consistency (e.g., that surface alterations of gender cues, such as clothing, do not change one's gender). Developmental data show that it is only with the emergence of concrete operational thought, around the age of 5–7 years, that full gender constancy is achieved (for review, see Ruble, Martin, & Berenbaum, 2006, pp. 906–908; Tobin *et al.*, 2010).

In addition to the role that cognitive maturation plays in consolidating a stable gendered sense of self, it is important to consider the role of other influences, including biological and psychosocial factors. For example, the "organizational hypothesis" of sex differences in prenatal sex hormone exposure has been one of the most prominent theoretical models in accounting for sex differences in behavior (Berenbaum, Owen Blakemore, & Beltz, 2011; Wallen, 2009). Drawing on this theory, Swaab, Gooren, and Hofman (1992)

The Self in Understanding and Treating Psychological Disorders, ed. Michael Kyrios, Richard Moulding, Guy Doron, Sunil S. Bhar, Maja Nedeljkovic, and Mario Mikulincer. Published by Cambridge University Press. © Cambridge University Press, 2016.

asserted that gender identity is very difficult to change "probably because [it is] fixed in the brain" (p. 52).

Regarding psychosocial factors, one might consider the salience of socialization factors that come from parents, the peer group, the media, etc., in which expectations for "conformity" to sex-typed patterns of behavior occur to a greater or lesser degree (e.g., Lytton & Romney, 1991). Although parents vary considerably in their expectations for adherence to stereotypic gender role behaviors, most parents do not question, challenge or contest their child's gender identity as a boy or as a girl.

A related line of research on children's understanding of gender categories has been advanced by theorists interested in essentialist reasoning (Gelman, 2003). In the "switched-at-birth" task, preschoolers believe that animals raised by members of another species will retain their category identity across time and develop the physical and behavioral properties typical of their birth category, not the category of their environment (Gelman & Wellman, 1991; see also Taylor, 1996). In contrast, both older children and adults are more likely to believe the opposite – that infants would develop the behavioral properties associated with their environment of upbringing (see Taylor, Rhodes, & Gelman, 2009).

If young children are prone to psychological essentialism when it comes to gender (and other categories), how might this inform us about the gendered cognitions of young children with gender dysphoria? It is conceivable that a young child with marked cross-gender interests might conclude that he or she *must* (or, at least, might) be a member of the other gender, relying on associational explanations (e.g., "I like the color pink. Girls usually like the color pink. Therefore, I must be a girl"). Such children might also raise questions about their sexual anatomy: "If I like things that boys like and boys have a penis, then why don't I have a penis?" Given young children's reliance on psychological essentialism (with physical development strongly constrained by category membership), this may explain, in part, why anatomic dysphoria (expressions of dislike about one's sexual anatomy) is not as common a marker of GD until later in childhood and adolescence/adulthood (Zucker, 2010). With older gender-dysphoric children, however, it could be argued that, with a lessening of essentialist reasoning, there is a greater awareness of environmental influences on the gendered sense of self – a recognition that it is their pervasive cross-gendered interests that contribute to the feeling that they are more like a member of the other (and desired) gender.

A second aspect of the cognitive-developmental literature pertains to the observation that young children have rather rigid, if not obsessional, interests in engaging in stereotypical sex-typed behavior: for girls, Halim *et al.* (2014) dubbed this the "pink frilly dress" phenomenon. Halim *et al.* argued that this gender rigidity was part of the young child's effort to master gender categories and to securely (affectively) place oneself in the "right" category. It is of note that parents of such children do not particularly encourage the rigidity, but they also do not discourage it and there is the assumption that such rigidity will wane over developmental time and that there will be a concomitant increase in flexibility in elements of surface expression of gender role behavior.

Phenomenology of gender dysphoria

Children and adolescents with GD show an array of sex-typed behaviors that suggest a strong identification with the opposite sex (Zucker, 2010). In many respects, GD is a deeply phenomenological and subjective condition. Children and adolescents develop a felt sense of gender identity in a sociocultural context, in an iterative matching process, in which they have the opportunity to observe and learn how boys and girls/men and women are categorized and behave (Fausto-Sterling, Garcia Coll, & Lamarre, 2012; Martin *et al.*, 2002; Ruble *et al.*, 2006). In adolescents and adults, the DSM 5 diagnostic criteria do not include behavioral indicators that are as concrete as they are for children; those given are more abstract (e.g., Criterion A6 reads as "A strong conviction that one has the typical feelings and reactions of the other gender … or some alternative gender different from one's assigned gender").

For the purpose of this volume, we want to highlight what is arguably the most important parameter of GD, namely, the strong desire to be of the other gender. Some children, however, go beyond the mere desire to be of the other gender: they declare that they "are" the other gender. In contrast to children, however, adolescents and adults "know" that they "are" of a biological sex that does not match their felt gender and, in this respect, appear to differ from young children who may well not have a firm understanding of this fact. Thus, in DSM-5, the diagnostic criterion reads somewhat differently for children than it does for adolescents/adults ("A strong desire to be of the other gender or an insistence that one is the other gender … or some alternative gender different from one's assigned gender" vs. "A strong desire to be of the other gender … or some alternative gender different from one's assigned gender").

Assessment of gender identity in children with gender dysphoria

Zucker *et al.* (1999) administered Slaby and Frey's (1975) Gender Constancy Interview to 206 children referred clinically for gender identity concerns and 95 control children (M age, 6.6 years; range, 3–12). When asked the question "Are you a boy or a girl?" only 6.8% of the gender-referred children answered the question "incorrectly" (e.g., a biological male stating that he was a girl, not a boy). Although this was significantly higher than the 1.1% of the control children who also answered the question incorrectly (Cohen's *d* = .21), it is apparent that not many gender-referred children "mislabeled" their gender identity. The differences between the two groups were, however, stronger for the developmentally more complicated questions pertaining to gender stability (over time) and gender consistency (across situations). For these two questions, the percentage of gender-referred children who answered them incorrectly was 20.4% and 65.5%, respectively, compared to 8.4% and 45.3% for the control children (Cohen's *d* = .28 and .38, respectively).

When asked about the desire to be of the other gender, using an item on the Gender Identity Interview for Children (Wallien *et al.*, 2009; Zucker *et al.*, 1993) that reads "In your mind, do you ever think that you would like to be a (for natal males, girl; for natal females, boy)?", Wallien *et al.* found that 65.5% of the gender-referred children answered sometimes or yes, compared to only 13.3% of control children. Thus, it is clear that the desire or wish to be of the other gender is much more common than a literal mislabeling of one's gender in relation to natal sex.

Zucker *et al.* (1999) suggested that children with GD may have a "developmental lag" in gender constancy acquisition. Because the children in the study of Zucker *et al.* had a mean age between 6 and 7 years at the time of assessment, it is possible that some of the gender-referred children who correctly self-labeled their gender may not have done so earlier in development and at a rate higher than that of the control children.

If early gender identity "mislabeling" is a contributing factor that organizes the cross-gender identification among children with GD, the question then is why children with GD might be more prone to such mislabeling. One possibility is that children with GD are not provided with sufficient external input (e.g., by parents) that facilitates the development of correct gender self-labeling. For example, the parents of a 4-year-old boy that we evaluated noted that, when he was 2, he would insist that he was a girl. They chose never to "correct" him as they worried that this would make matters "worse." Thus, for a period of over 2 years, he would frequently state that he was a girl but with no parental input that might suggest alternatives (e.g., "Well, you are a boy who likes to do things that girls like").

As children with GD begin to express and display various surface markers of cross-gender identification, such as cross-dressing or enactment of cross-gender roles in fantasy play, this could have a feedback effect on gender identity self-labeling, as noted earlier with regard to associational influences in the psychological essentialism literature. Thus, Zucker *et al.* (1999) suggested that there is some type of causal interface between the child's extensive cross-gender behavior and delayed gender constancy development. Regarding the phenotypic cue of hair style, one 4-year-old boy remarked that he "sometimes" got "mixed up" about whether he was a boy or a girl when "my mommy lets my hair grow real long and she forgets to get me a haircut."

Assessment of gender identity in adolescents and adults with gender dysphoria

In adolescents and adults, assessment of gender dysphoria includes an evaluation of the desire to be of the other gender. For example, the 27-item dimensional measure of gender dysphoria, the Gender Identity/Gender Dysphoria Questionnaire for Adolescents and Adults (GIDYQ), contains the item "In the past 12 months, have you had the wish or desire to be a woman?" (male version) or "In the past 12 months, have you had the wish or desire to be a man?" (female version), rated, like all of the other items, on a five-point response scale ranging from never to always.

Virtually all patients who are referred clinically for gender identity concerns endorse this item, compared to almost none of the controls. The GIDYQ has shown a strong one-factor solution containing all 27 items and, using a cut-off score of <3.00 to indicate caseness, yields very high sensitivity and specificity rates (Deogracias *et al.*, 2007; Singh *et al.*, 2010; Zucker *et al.*, 2012). Yet, as noted earlier, adolescents and adults with GD clearly do not really show any gross mislabeling of their gender in relation to biological sex. The phenomenological issue is the incongruence between one's felt gender and somatic sex, which is emphasized in the DSM-5: "A marked incongruence between one's experienced/expressed gender and assigned gender …" and which is captured by the term gender dysphoria (cf. Fisk, 1973). From a developmental perspective, it becomes important to understand the factors that might contribute to gender dysphoria in adolescence and adulthood in which the (negative) affect surrounding gender is more salient than any type of cognitive gender identity "confusion."

One developmental scenario concerns those adolescents/adults who have an "early-onset" history of cross-gender identification, i.e., a history of cross-gender behavior, including the desire to be of the other gender, that extends back to early childhood. For many of these patients, they will recall that, as they got older, they felt more and more "different" from same-sex peers, feeling that they had little in common with them in terms of shared interests, etc. With the onset of puberty and the development of secondary sex characteristics, the incongruence between their felt gender and somatic sex intensifies and such individuals are unable to attribute any positive affect or valuation of a gender identity that is congruent with their birth sex. When this occurs, many adolescents will begin a formal social transition to live as the desired gender and to seek out biomedical treatments for the phenotypic markers of biological sex that can be altered.

Is gender dysphoria stable?

When a child presents to a clinician with a behavior pattern that corresponds to the DSM-5 diagnosis of GD, many parents want information about long-term developmental trajectories. Will their child continue to feel gender-dysphoric and, eventually, seek out biomedical treatment (hormonal treatment and sex reassignment surgery) and "formally" transition to living in the desired gender? Will their child's GD "desist" and will they thus become more comfortable with a gender identity that matches their birth sex?

Between 1968 and 2012, there have been 10 follow-up studies. The early reports relied primarily on clinical interview data or information provided by informants, such as parents (see Zucker & Bradley, 1995, pp. 285–287). The four most recent follow-up studies used standardized clinical interviews and psychometric measures (Drummond, Bradley, Badali-Peterson, & Zucker, 2008; Green, 1987; Singh, 2012; Wallien & Cohen-Kettenis, 2008). In nine samples that included boys (total $N = 297$), the persistence of GD ranged from 0% to 20.3%. In three samples that included girls (total $N = 45$), the persistence of GD ranged from 0% to 50.0%. The most notable variation was between two follow-up samples of girls (12% in Drummond *et al.* vs. 50% in Wallien and Cohen-Kettenis), but the sample sizes were sufficiently small that it would be imprudent to overinterpret the meaning of this variation. From these studies, it could be argued that, with the exception of the female data from Wallien and Cohen-Kettenis, the percentage of children where the GD persists into late adolescence or early adulthood is on the low side. The persistence rate is certainly much lower than what one finds in GD patients who are evaluated for the first time in adolescence and certainly for adults (for review, see Zucker *et al.*, 2011). In general, the follow-up studies suggest that a cross-gender identity in childhood is not overwhelmingly stable.

Regarding children with GD, then, we need to understand why, for the majority, gender dysphoria appears to remit by adolescence, if not earlier. One explanation is that of "false positives": the children did not really have a cross-gender identity to begin with; rather, they simply displayed marked gender-variant surface behaviors. A second possible explanation concerns referral bias. Green (1974) argued that children with GD who are referred for clinical assessment (and then, in some cases, therapy) may come from families in which there is more concern than is the case for adolescents and adults, the majority of whom did not receive a clinical evaluation and treatment during childhood.

The concepts of developmental malleability and plasticity deserve consideration here. It is possible, for example, that gender identity shows relative malleability during childhood, with a gradual narrowing of plasticity as the gendered sense of self consolidates as one approaches adolescence. As noted above, some support for this idea comes from follow-up studies of adolescents with GD, who appear to show a much higher rate of GD persistence as they are followed into young adulthood.

One contextual issue is that these samples entered clinic-based prospective studies during historical periods when the predominant therapeutic guidelines were to somehow try and help a child feel more comfortable with a gender identity that matched his or her birth sex or to at least not "encourage" a cross-gender identity (Zucker, Wood, Singh, & Bradley, 2012). This has changed rather dramatically in the past few years. For example, there is now what one could call the "early gender-transition movement" or subculture in which some clinicians and some parents view a child's early cross-gender identification as a fixed, unalterable, and essential part of the child's sense of self (Herthel & Jennings, 2014). Accordingly, some clinicians recommend that a young child begin a social transition to the desired gender long before puberty – in some cases, as early as the preschool years (see Byne *et al.*, 2012; Saeger, 2006; Schwartzapfel, 2013; Vanderburgh, 2009) and some parents implement this approach on their own. Indeed, there is now some empirical evidence that children who have made a gendered social transition in childhood (prior to puberty) show a much higher rate of GD persistence, compared to the other follow-up studies, suggesting that this type of "intervention" affects the developmental trajectory (Steensma, McGuire, Kreukels, Beekman, & Cohen-Kettenis, 2013).

It has long been recognized, particularly for natal males, that gender dysphoria sometimes does not express itself until around the time of puberty, if not much later, i.e., well into adulthood. Late-onset males with gender dysphoria typically do not have a strong history of cross-gender identification in childhood. In our own clinic, we see a fair number of adolescent males with GD who fit well into the late-onset subgroup and, for these youth, parents can serve as important informants. These parents almost never recall that the adolescent had engaged in pervasive gender non-conforming behavior in childhood, much less expressing a consistent desire to be of the other gender (Zucker *et al.*, 2012). In many respects, these male youth were stereotypically masculine. Some of these youth have had significant other clinical problems in childhood and the psychiatric records of these youth never identify concerns about gender identity. Late-onset males with GD often have a co-occurring history of transvestic disorder or autogynephilia (sexual arousal associated with the thought or image of oneself as a woman; American Psychiatric Association, 2013). One prominent theory regarding late-onset males with gender dysphoria is that it is the autogynephilic sexual arousal that

organizes the patient's felt sense of self as a woman, a kind of "paraphilic" gender identity (for review, see Blanchard, 2005; Lawrence, 2010, 2013).[1]

If these patients had a "typical" male gender identity in childhood, they pose a challenge to classical development accounts of gender identity development. The natural history suggests that there is a marked transformation of the gendered self between childhood and adolescence, which traditional theories of gender development would be hard-pressed to explain. It has, however, been argued that some of these patients did, in fact, feel like they were female in childhood, but did not express it for fear of social censure (Veale, Lomax, & Clarke, 2010). However, the social censure idea has relied on retrospective accounts of adult patients, which may well be subject to recall bias, and our own data from our adolescent patients and their parents do not provide much support for the hypothesis.

Treatment of gender dysphoria

A developmental perspective is critical in thinking about best-practice treatment for people with gender dysphoria (Zucker *et al.*, 2012). If, for example, a cross-gendered or "transgendered" self has consolidated by the time of adolescence and certainly by adulthood, one should be very cautious in offering treatment designed to change a person's gender identity, even if the person desires it. Thus, from a therapeutic perspective, the clinician needs to make a judgment regarding how fixed or stable a person's gender identity is. If for adolescents and adults, the conclusion is that the cross-gendered identity is fixed and stable, then the best-practice treatment approach would be to support the person's social migration to the desired gender role and concomitant biomedical treatment.

If, however, the gendered sense of self is judged to still be in flux, then it is reasonable to consider an array of psychosocial treatments, including treatments that might facilitate a gender identity that is more congruent with the patient's birth sex. Below, we provide some vignettes in which a consideration of various issues for which gendered self-representations might be explored from a psychotherapeutic point of view.

Gender identity self-labeling

As noted earlier, some young children with GD appear to misclassify their gender in relation to their birth sex or to be confused about it.

Kim was a 7-year-old natal male with an IQ of 102. A few months prior to the assessment, Kim, with his mother's support, had transitioned socially from the male gender role to the female gender role (the parents were separated and the father had only minimal involvement in Kim's life). Kim's gender-neutral name, hairstyle, and clothing style easily allowed "her" to be perceived by children and adults who did not know "his" biological sex as a girl. Yet, it was unclear to us if Kim had completely consolidated a female gender identity. There were hints that Kim was still confused about it. For example, on the Gender Identity Interview for Children (Zucker et al., 1993), when asked "Are you a boy or a girl?", Kim answered "boy and girl … both …" When asked "When you grow up will you be a Daddy or a Mommy?", Kim answered "Daddy," but when asked "Could you ever grow up to be a Mommy?", Kim said "Yes." On the Rorschach test, Kim had several "Unusual Verbalizations" (Exner, 1990) coded as Incongruous Combinations (e.g., a "wolf–bat" or "two elephant people"), suggestive of an underlying confusion. During the assessment, Kim's mother reported that she asked him "So, do you want to be a boy or a girl?" and Kim's response was "What do you want me to be?" We suggested to Kim's mother that Kim might benefit from individual play therapy in which Kim would have a safe space to figure out what he (or she?) wanted to be, but she elected not to enroll Kim in therapy.[2]

Cognitive representations of gender

In cognitive social psychology, there is an important literature on in-group vs. out-group preferences, i.e., the propensity to evaluate more favorably one's own group vs. the "other" (e.g., with regard to ethnicity, religion, country, etc.; Tajfel, 1982; Turner, 1978). Regarding gender, it is of interest that girls show a stronger in-group bias than do boys (Powlishta, 1995; Susskind & Hodges, 2007). That is, they are more likely to allocate positive traits than negative traits to girls and more likely to allocate negative traits than positive traits to boys. This is, perhaps, the one instance in which girls are more gender stereotyped than boys are.

Leroux (2008) assessed in-group vs. out-group bias in children with GD. Leroux found that girls with GD were, like control girls, more likely to view girls as way more positive than boys, which struck us as a rather counter-intuitive finding. However, boys with GD, like clinical control boys, were less likely to show an in-group bias favoring boys than were non-clinical

Table 22.1 Gender representations of an 8-year-old boy with gender dysphoria.[1]

About girls
• Because they are nice
• Because they are good
• Because they never get in trouble
• Because they look pretty
• Gooder (*sic*) toys
• Father and mother are nice to girls
• Girls don't have to do anything

About boys
• Um … uh … they don't play nicely
• All they care about is playing with Army men
• Only care about doing the work
• No time to play
• And they don't look good

[1] The child was asked "Tell me the 'good' things about girls (boys)" and "Tell me the 'bad' things about girls (boys)." No "bad" things were identified for girls and no "good" things were identified for boys.

control boys. From a clinical perspective, it is common to observe that children with GD have very positive, if not idealized, representations of the other sex and more negative, if not devalued, representations of their own sex. Table 22.1 provides an example of this based on a clinical interview of an 8-year-old boy with GD. It can be seen that "girlness" was valued and "boyness" was devalued.

From a therapeutic perspective, one could explore ways in which this type of good vs. bad dichotomy could be reduced, resulting in more flexible gender-schematic representations. Thus, for example, if one provided exemplars that boys can play nicely or that boys like to play with a number of things, not just Army men, would it help this youngster see that there are various ways in which one can "be" a boy? Along similar lines, if one provided exemplars that not all girls are nice or that fathers and mothers can also be nice to boys, would it help this youngster have a less idealized representation of girls? If so, would this lessen this youngster's feeling that he should be a girl?

There is some evidence that many children with GD show very focused and intense cross-gendered interests (VanderLaan et al., 2015b). As noted earlier, these surface behaviors can have a feedback effect on a child's gendered sense of self, particularly if they are continually reinforced. The importance of the flexibility–rigidity dimension may also be a critical factor in understanding why there appears to be an over-representation of gender dysphoria among children and adolescents with an autism spectrum disorder (ASD; de Vries, Noens, Cohen-Kettenis, van Berckelaer-Onnes, & Doreleijers, 2010). It is well-established that patients with an ASD have circumscribed, focused, and obsessional interests. Gender may be a particularly potent fixed and focused obsession, especially if it is reinforced in the social environment, regardless of the risk factors that might predispose towards it (VanderLaan, Leef, Wood, Hughes, & Zucker, 2015a).

Is there a true gendered self?

In the therapeutic literature on gender dysphoria, it is sometimes argued that any attempt (even with young children) to use psychotherapeutic methods to align gender identity with their birth sex is akin, in the Winnicottian sense, to promoting a false self (Winnicott, 1955). It is certainly the case that adults with gender dysphoria will report trying to live in a gender role congruent with birth sex as a result of social pressures (e.g., from a spouse, because of religious beliefs, etc.). In this respect, there may well be merit to the argument that such maneuvers likely promote a "false" self. From a developmental perspective, however, the issue may be much more complicated and requires psychotherapeutic exploration in order to help a patient sort out what is the best adaptation *vis-à-vis* gender.

Fiona was a 17-year-old natal female with an IQ of 93. Fiona never felt that she fit in with other girls, but did not report a childhood history of wanting to be a boy. At the time of assessment, she presented with a "goth" appearance and was "experienced" by the clinicians who evaluated her to be an adolescent girl. She was sexually attracted to girls, but was largely asexual. She did not identify as a lesbian because she felt that she was a "guy in the wrong body." She had had a long and stormy relationship with her parents. She was quite immature. Her parents provided little in the way of maturity demands. Her parents were quite opposed to Fiona's desire to be a boy. The parents reported that Fiona often fluctuated between presenting as a feminine girl (in terms of hairstyle and clothing style) and taking on the more "goth" presentation. The parents showed us various pictures of Fiona after she would ask her mother to purchase her "girly" clothes. Fiona would counter that she would only do this to appease her parents. Psychotherapy was recommended

to explore further Fiona's fluctuating presentation of gender in order to understand better what her "true self" really was.

As illustrated in Kim's case described above, one could argue that the boundary between Kim's gendered sense of self and the mother's own desires were not clear (cf. Stoller, 1975). Clinical experience with many such youngsters suggests that this is a common and important issue to examine. Consider these comments from the mothers of several boys with GD:

Mother 1:	"I know what he is feeling because it is like I am inside of him."
Mother 2:	"He knows exactly what I am feeling. We are like twins."
Mother 3:	"I can finish his thoughts. He can finish mine."
Mother 4:	"When I am sick, he always asks me if I am ok. He will make me a cup of tea, rub my back, and brush my hair."

In these instances, one can ask: where does empathy end and enmeshment begin (see Owen-Anderson, 2006)?

The gendered self and the sexual identity self in adolescence

Sexual orientation is an important parameter to assess among adolescents with GD (Zucker, 2006). Consider a female adolescent who has transitioned to the cross-gender role and is sexually attracted to females. If one uses birth sex as the referent point, one could say that this adolescent is homosexual. If one uses gender identity as the referent point, one could say that this adolescent is heterosexual. In both cases, one could say that the adolescent has a "gynephilic" sexual orientation. Female adolescents with GD who have a childhood history of cross-gender identification ("early-onset") are almost always sexually attracted to females.

In clinical practice, it is common for such females to report that they have vacillated in their self-identity as either lesbian or as transgendered. In essence, they report struggling or thinking about which "category" works better for them. On this point, an important study by Lee (2001) found that the developmental histories of "butch lesbians" and female-to-male transsexuals showed many similarities and it was difficult to predict, on an individual basis, which "group" these females would wind up in.

The gendered self and identity diffusion in adolescence

In adults with gender dysphoria, a considerable literature has accumulated regarding the co-occurrence of personality disorders (Lawrence & Zucker, 2014). Four decades ago, Lothstein (1983) argued that, in female-to-male transsexuals, borderline personality disorder was present in all cases. This was clearly an overstatement and certainly not confirmed by many other studies. However, when a personality disorder is present, a case formulation needs to consider whether it functions as a predisposing factor to GD, is a "consequence" of the stress some individuals experience from having GD, or if it is simply related to generic risk factors for a personality disorder common to all people. In borderline personality disorder, an unstable sense of self is a key part of the clinical picture. In DSM-3, for example, Criterion A4 was "[I]dentity disturbance as manifested by uncertainty about several issues relating to identity, such as self-image, *gender identity* … (e.g., 'Who am I? …')" (our emphasis). In DSM-5, Criterion A3 is "Identity disturbance: markedly and persistently unstable self-image or sense of self." For adolescents with GD, one should certainly screen for the presence of personality disorders and consider the extent to which the GD might be conceptualized as a symptom of a more generic struggle with identity.

Annie was a 16-year-old natal female with an IQ of 104. At the age of 13, Annie had several inpatient admissions because of depression and self-harming behavior and, prior to that, had a fairly long outpatient history of oppositional behavior. Annie grew up in a family in which there was substantial marital discord, leading to a parental separation. Annie's mother was a fundamentalist Christian and her religious beliefs played a central role in the family's life. The gender developmental history did not suggest any indication of childhood cross-gender identification. The background psychiatric reports from when Annie was a child and when she was admitted to hospital did not give any indication that she was struggling with her gender identity. From our own assessment, it was apparent that Annie's gender dysphoria was "late-onset," i.e., she did not start to feel distressed about being a female until she was 14 years of age. Nonetheless, at the time of assessment, Annie was presenting in the male gender role and had adopted the preferred name of Zack. Zack was an active participant in a support group for LGBT youth and indicated no desire to be seen in any kind of therapy. Zack expressed an interest in starting on either hormonal blockers or cross-sex hormone therapy (testosterone) and so a referral to an endocrinologist was made. For reasons that were not clear, Zack cancelled his appointment with the endocrinologist. When Zack was 19, we called the family residence, asking to speak with Zack as we were interested in knowing how the past couple of years had gone. Zack did not want to speak with us, but said that we could talk to his mother. Zack's mother reported that he attended first-year university in the male gender role but had not initiated hormonal treatment. However, at the beginning of second-year university, his mother said that Zack returned to living in the female gender role. Although Zack's mother had been quite troubled by the gender dysphoria and did not "support" the gender transition, she was still distraught. When asked why, she said that Annie had now fully rejected the family's religious heritage and had embraced the Muslim faith and wore a burka full-time at university: "This is even worse than wanting to be a man." This left us wondering if our original assessment had missed a more generic struggle with identity, of which the gender identity issue was just one particular manifestation.

Summary

This chapter has examined the gendered self, with an emphasis on its developmental aspects. Gender identity, in its nascent stage, appears quite early in development, and is a stable component of the self in most people. For individuals who experience gender dysphoria, however, the data show that there is probably more malleability in gender identity in younger children than in both adolescents and adults. Thus, for at least some people, gender identity as a core part of the self may be more fluid than previously thought. Key developmental issues were identified that may be appropriate targets for therapeutic intervention, in which a focus on the self may serve as the mechanism of change.

Notes

1   Late-onset females with gender dysphoria are not the precise parallel of late-onset males. For example, some late-onset females do have a history of marked cross-gender behavior in childhood, but many do not (Zucker *et al.*, 2012) and thus they also appear to challenge traditional accounts of gender identity development. They also do not appear to have a history of transvestic disorder or autoandrophilia (sexual arousal associated with the thought or image of oneself as a man).

2   Saketopoulou's (2014) 6-year-old natal male patient, who had transitioned to the female gender role prior to treatment, through "her" drawings of an "ostricken" (a chicken–ostrich), provides another example of an Incongruous Combination.

References

American Psychiatric Association. (1980). *Diagnostic and Statistical Manual of Mental Disorders* (3rd ed.). Washington, DC: American Psychiatric Association.

American Psychiatric Association. (1994). *Diagnostic and Statistical Manual of Mental Disorders* (4th ed.). Washington, DC: American Psychiatric Association.

American Psychiatric Association. (2013). *Diagnostic and Statistical Manual of Mental Disorders* (5th ed.). Arlington, VA: American Psychiatric Association.

Berenbaum, S. A., Owen Blakemore, J. E., & Beltz, A. M. (2011). A role for biology in gender-related behavior. *Sex Roles, 64*, 804–825.

Blanchard, R. (2005). Early history of the concept of autogynephilia. *Archives of Sexual Behavior, 34*, 439–446.

Byne, W., Bradley, S. J., Coleman, E., *et al.* (2012). Report of the American Psychiatric Association Task Force on Treatment of Gender Identity Disorder. *Archives of Sexual Behavior, 41*, 759–796.

de Vries, A. L. C., Noens, I. L., Cohen-Kettenis, P. T., van Berckelaer-Onnes, I. A., & Doreleijers, T. A. H. (2010). Autism spectrum disorders in gender dysphoric children and adolescents. *Journal of Autism and Developmental Disorders, 40*, 930–936.

Deogracias, J. J., Johnson, L. L., Meyer-Bahlburg, H. F. L., *et al.* (2007). The Gender Identity/Gender Dysphoria Questionnaire for Adolescents and Adults. *Journal of Sex Research, 44*, 370–379.

Drummond, K. D., Bradley, S. J., Badali-Peterson, M., & Zucker, K. J. (2008). A follow-up study of girls with gender identity disorder. *Developmental Psychology, 44*, 34–45.

Exner, J. E. (1990). *A Rorschach Workbook for the Comprehensive System* (3rd ed.). Asheville, NC: Rorschach Workshops.

Fausto-Sterling, A., Garcia Coll, C., & Lamarre, M. (2012). Sexing the baby: Part 2: Applying dynamic systems theory to the emergences of sex-related differences in infants and toddlers. *Social Science & Medicine, 74*, 1693–1702.

Fisk, N. (1973). Gender dysphoria syndrome (the how, what, and why of a disease). In D. Laub & P. Gandy (Eds.), *Proceedings of the Second Interdisciplinary Symposium on Gender Dysphoria Syndrome* (pp. 7–14). Palo Alto, CA: Stanford University Press.

Gelman, S. A. (2003). *The Essential Child: Origins of Essentialism in Everyday Thought*. Oxford: Oxford University Press.

Gelman, S. A., & Wellman, H. M. (1991). Insides and essences: Early understanding of the nonobvious. *Cognition, 23*, 183–209.

Green, R. (1974). *Sexual Identity Conflict in Children and Adults*. New York, NY: Basic Books.

Green, R. (1987). *The "Sissy Boy Syndrome" and the Development of Homosexuality*. New Haven, CT: Yale University Press.

Halim, N. L., Ruble, D. N., Tamis-LeMonda, C. S., *et al.* (2014). Pink frilly dresses and the avoidance of all things "girly": Children's appearance rigidity and cognitive theories of gender development. *Developmental Psychology, 50*, 1091–1101.

Herthel, J., & Jennings, J. (2014). *I am Jazz*. New York, NY: Penguin Group.

Kohlberg, L. (1966). A cognitive-developmental analysis of children's sex-role concepts and attitudes. In E. E. Maccoby (Ed.), *The Development of Sex Differences* (pp. 82–173). Stanford, CA: Stanford University Press.

Lawrence, A. A. (2010). Sexual orientation versus age of onset as bases for typologies (subtypes) for gender identity disorder in adolescents and adults. *Archives of Sexual Behavior, 39*, 514–545.

Lawrence, A. A. (2013). *Men Trapped in Men's Bodies: Narratives of Autogynephilic Transsexualism*. New York, NY: Springer.

Lawrence, A. A., & Zucker, K. J. (2014). Gender dysphoria. In D. C. Beidel, B. C. Frueh, & M. Hersen (Eds.), *Adult Psychopathology and Diagnosis* (7th ed., pp. 603–639). Hoboken, NJ: John Wiley & Sons.

Lee, T. (2001). Trans(re)lations: Lesbian and female to male transsexual accounts of identity. *Women's Studies International Forum, 24*, 347–377.

Leroux, A. (2008). *Do children with gender identity disorder have an in-group or an out-group gender-based bias?* Unpublished Master's thesis, Ontario Institute for Studies in Education of the University of Toronto, Toronto, Ontario.

Lewis, M., & Brooks-Gunn, J. (1979). *Social Cognition and the Acquisition of Self*. New York, NY: Plenum Press.

Lothstein, L. M. (1983). *Female-to-Male Transsexualism: Historical, Clinical, and Theoretical Issues*. Boston, MA: Routledge & Kegan Paul.

Lytton, H., & Romney, D. M. (1991). Parents' differential socialization of boys and girls: A meta-analysis. *Psychological Bulletin, 109*, 267–296.

Maccoby, E. E. (1988). Gender as a social category. *Developmental Psychology, 24*, 755–765.

Martin, C. L., Ruble, D. N., & Szkrybalo, J. (2002). Cognitive theories of early gender development. *Psychological Bulletin, 128*, 903–933.

Owen-Anderson, A. (2006). *"I know what he is feeling because it is like I am inside of him." Examining sensory sensitivities, empathy, and expressed emotion in boys with gender identity disorder and their mothers: A comparison to clinical control boys and community control boys and girls*. Unpublished doctoral dissertation, Ontario Institute for Studies in Education of the University of Toronto, Toronto, Ontario.

Powlishta, K. K. (1995b). Gender bias in children's perceptions of personality traits. *Sex Roles*, 32, 17–28.

Ruble, D. N., Martin, C. L., & Berenbaum, S. A. (2006). Gender development. In W. Damon & R. M. Lerner (series eds.) and N. Eisenberg (vol. ed.), *Handbook of Child Psychology* (6th ed.). *Vol. 3: Social, Emotional, and Personality Development* (pp. 858–932). New York, NY: Wiley.

Saeger, K. (2006). Finding our way: Guiding a young transgender child. *Journal of GLBT Family Studies*, 2, 207–245.

Saketopoulou, A. (2014). Mourning the body as bedrock: Developmental considerations in treating transsexual patients analytically. *International Journal of Psychoanalysis*, 62, 773–806.

Schwartzapfel, B. (2013, March). Born this way? *The American Prospect*. Retrieved from http://prospect.org/article/born-way

Singh, D. (2012). *A follow-up study of boys with gender identity disorder*. Unpublished doctoral dissertation, Ontario Institute for Studies in Education of the University of Toronto, Toronto, Ontario.

Singh, D., Deogracias, J. J., Johnson, L. L., *et al.* (2010). The Gender Identity/Gender Dysphoria Questionnaire for Adolescents and Adults: Further validity evidence. *Journal of Sex Research*, 47, 49–58.

Slaby, R. G., & Frey, K. S. (1975). Development of gender constancy and selective attention to same-sex models. *Child Development*, 46, 849–856.

Steensma, T. D., McGuire, J. K., Kreukels, B. P. C., Beekman, A. J., & Cohen-Kettenis, P. T. (2013). Factors associated with desistence and persistence of childhood gender dysphoria: A quantitative follow-up study. *Journal of the American Academy of Child and Adolescent Psychiatry*, 52, 582–590.

Stoller, R. J. (1975). *Sex and Gender* (Vol. II). *The Transsexual Experiment*. London: Hogarth Press.

Susskind, J. E., & Hodges, C. (2007). Decoupling children's gender-based in-group positivity from out-group negativity. *Sex Roles*, 56, 707–716.

Swaab, D. F., Gooren, L. J. G., & Hofman, M. A. (1992). Gender and sexual orientation in relation to hypothalamic structures. *Hormone Research*, 38(Suppl. 2), 51–61.

Tajfel, H. (1982). Social psychology of intergroup relations. *Annual Review of Psychology*, 33, 1–39.

Taylor, M. G. (1996). The development of children's beliefs about social and biological aspects of gender differences. *Child Development*, 67, 1555–1571.

Taylor, M. G., Rhodes, M., & Gelman, S. A. (2009). Boys will be boys; cows will be cows: Children's essentialist reasoning about gender categories and animal species. *Child Development*, 80, 461–481.

Tobin, D. D., Menon, M., Menon, M., *et al.* (2010). The intrapsychics of gender: A model of self-socialization. *Psychological Review*, 117, 601–622.

Turner, J. C. (1978). Social comparison, similarity and ingroup favoritism. In H. Tajfel (Ed.), *Differentiation Between Social Groups: Studies in the Social Psychology of Intergroup Relations* (pp. 235–250). Oxford: Academic Press.

Vanderburgh, R. (2009). Appropriate therapeutic care for families with pre-pubescent transgender/gender-dissonant children. *Child and Adolescent Social Work Journal*, 26, 135–154.

VanderLaan, D. P., Leef, J. H., Wood, H., Hughes, K., & Zucker, K. J. (2015a). Autism spectrum disorder risk factors and autistic traits in gender dysphoric children. *Journal of Autism and Developmental Disorders*, 45, 1742–1750.

VanderLaan, D. P., Postema, L., Wood, H., *et al.* (2015b). Do children with gender dysphoria have intense/obsessional interests? *Journal of Sex Research*, 52, 213–219.

Veale, J. F., Lomax, T. C., & Clarke, D. E. (2010). The identity-defence theory model of gender-variant development. *International Journal of Transgenderism*, 12, 125–138.

Wallen, K. (2009). The organizational hypothesis: Reflections on the 50th anniversary of the publication of Phoenix, Goy, Gerall, and Young (1959). *Hormones and Behavior*, 55, 561–565.

Wallien, M. S. C., & Cohen-Kettenis, P. T. (2008). Psychosexual outcome of gender dysphoric children. *Journal of the American Academy of Child and Adolescent Psychiatry*, 47, 1413–1423.

Wallien, M. S. C., Quilty, L. C., Steensma, T. D., *et al.* (2009). Cross-national replication of the Gender Identity Interview for Children. *Journal of Personality Assessment*, 91, 545–552.

Winnicott, D. W. (1955). Meta-psychological and clinical aspects of regression with the psycho-analytical set-up. *International Journal of Psychoanalysis*, 36, 16–26.

Zucker, K. J. (2006). Gender identity disorder. In D. A. Wolfe & E. J. Mash (Eds.), *Behavioral and Emotional Disorders in Adolescents: Nature, Assessment, and Treatment* (pp. 535–562). New York, NY: Guilford Press.

Zucker, K. J. (2010). The DSM diagnostic criteria for gender identity disorder in children. *Archives of Sexual Behavior*, 39, 477–498.

Zucker, K. J., & Bradley, S. J. (1995). *Gender Identity Disorder and Psychosexual Problems in Children and Adolescents*. New York, NY: Guilford Press.

Zucker, K. J., Bradley, S. J., Kuksis, M., *et al.* (1999). Gender constancy judgments in children with gender identity disorder: Evidence for a developmental lag. *Archives of Sexual Behavior*, 28, 475–502.

Zucker, K. J., Bradley, S. J., Lowry Sullivan, C. B., *et al.* (1993). A gender identity interview for children. *Journal of Personality Assessment*, 61, 443–456.

Zucker, K. J., Bradley, S. J., Owen-Anderson, A., *et al.* (2011). Puberty-blocking hormonal therapy for adolescents with gender identity disorder: A descriptive clinical study. *Journal of Gay & Lesbian Mental Health*, 15, 58–82.

Zucker, K. J., Bradley, S. J., Owen-Anderson, A., *et al.* (2012). Demographics, behavior problems, and psychosexual characteristics of adolescents with gender identity disorder or transvestic fetishism. *Journal of Sex & Marital Therapy*, 38, 151–189.

Zucker, K. J., Wood, H., Singh, D., & Bradley, S. J. (2012). A developmental, biopsychosocial model for the treatment of children with gender identity disorder. *Journal of Homosexuality*, 59, 369–397.

Chapter

23

Future directions in examining the self in psychological disorders

Michael Kyrios, Richard Moulding, Sunil S. Bhar, Guy Doron,
Maja Nedeljkovic, and Mario Mikulincer

As has been demonstrated throughout this book, the concept of the "self" opens up many opportunities for advancing our understanding of human psychological functioning and dysfunction. It is also apparent that the use of this concept gives us multiple options to facilitate developments in the treatment of disorder and, perhaps, could improve the efficacy and effectiveness of therapy for a broad range of psychological conditions. Despite such potential advantages, numerous issues have been identified, inclusive of the disparities in the definition and operationalization of the term "self" itself, and also in discrepant foci on aspects of the self (Katzko, 2003).

Starting with issues relating to the definition and operationalization of the "self," researchers have recently provided a simple characterization:

> … the term self often refers to a warm sense or a warm feeling that something is "about me" or "about us." Reflecting on oneself…requires that there is an "I" that can consider an object that is "me." The term self includes both the actor who thinks ("I am thinking") and the object of thinking ("about me").
>
> (Oyserman, Elmore, & Smith, 2012, p. 71)

However, the "self" remains a fuzzy concept. Leary and Tangney (2012) identified five distinct ways in which the self has been used by researchers (self as the total person, self as personality, self as experiencing subject, self as beliefs about oneself, self as executive agent). Their review of the literature reveals 66 self-related constructs, processes, or phenomena, although this is likely to be an underestimate, and they acknowledge that there is little research exploring their interrelationships. Despite such "conceptual morass" (Leary & Tangney, 2012, p. 5), the notion of the "self" has shown itself to have great persistence for a range of reasons including its

utility, its face validity, its ability to be integrated with other frameworks (e.g., cognitive, psychoanalytic, social), and because of the opportunities it allows for empirical investigation.

The usage of "self" varies depending on one's preferred psychological paradigm. The psychoanalytic approach focuses on internal structures and the dynamics between them, but there is variation even within this approach from Freud's traditional egopsychology through to interpersonal object relations theory and beyond (Fosshage, 2009; Guntrip, 1977; Kohut, 1971, 1977). The cognitive approach, which has been influential most recently in the clinical domain, has also embraced the self. Self-concepts are considered to be cognitive structures incorporating content, attitudes, evaluative judgments and attentional processes that aim to facilitate goal achievement and self-protection (Oyserman & Markus, 1998).

Throughout this volume, we have seen a number of approaches to understanding the role of self in psychological disorders. In some instances, authors have emphasized that the self is part of the core phenomena of the disorder (e.g., ipseity in schizophrenia). Other times, the self is considered an etiological underpinning of the clinical phenomena (e.g., moral self in OCD). Other authors see the self as part of both core phenomena and processes that maintains the disorder (e.g., self processing in social anxiety). In some instances, a bidirectional relationship with symptoms has been emphasized (e.g., disruptions in attachment and the capacity to mentalize in depression and its subsequent impact on mentalizing). In most cases, however, authors have highlighted the complex transactional relationships between ruptures in self and symptoms of disorder.

The Self in Understanding and Treating Psychological Disorders, ed. Michael Kyrios, Richard Moulding, Guy Doron, Sunil S. Bhar, Maja Nedeljkovic, and Mario Mikulincer. Published by Cambridge University Press. © Cambridge University Press, 2016.

A key theme throughout a number of chapters is that the self is not a static construct and that the experience of self is not a property of the individual, but, as Liotti and Farina (Chapter 17) put it, "an emergent, intersubjective property of human relatedness" (p. 175). All authors have emphasized general aspects of the self that require targeting in treatment, as well as the need for ongoing research to better identify aspects of the self that are related to specific disorders and that require targeting in treatment. Calls for theoretical integration, using the self and related concepts such as attachment as central tenets, have been made throughout the book in order to better understand psychological processes underpinning specific disorders. Moreover, paying greater attention to the self as a therapeutic target has been proposed across the board as a way forward in improving therapeutic outcomes and in decreasing relapse and vulnerability to disorder.

What is the direction that the study of self should proceed to in the future? Given such diverse perspectives, how can a common language about the self be reached? Can the construct of self, as understood through a psychoanalytic perspective, be at all similar to the notion as understood through cognitive and social perspectives? Throughout this book, we have seen that the self as understood by proponents of different theoretical orientations may appear to reflect radically differing constructs. Yet, can there be a common theme or an overarching narrative that encompasses such divergent perspectives on this thing called "self"? If so, would a consensus in depicting the self be useful for research or for psychotherapy?

In our opinion, such endeavors towards defining self are worthwhile. The task of reaching a consensus definition brings with it the potential for an integrative approach to the construct that is inclusive of various theoretical perspectives, and that is clarifying of whether differences in the definition are substantial or simply semantic. With such inclusivity, cross-theory collaborative efforts in research are more likely. Researchers from various orientations may be more likely to work together if there can be some agreement about the construct under study. The self no longer needs to be a divisive concept between different theoretical camps, but conversely could become a construct that brings such camps together. The consensus definition of self could also be theoretically clarifying, as differences in language will need to be distinguished from differences in inferences about the self. For example, when the self is

described as "compartmentalized," "conflicted," and/or "complex," are such descriptions simply semantically different, but alluding to the same multifaceted properties of self-concept? Such debates will – in our opinion – serve to clarify what is common but potentially described differently by researchers of the self.

In sum, we need a clearer operationalization of the "self"; and further, perhaps what is needed is a consensus language around terms such as self-concept, self-esteem, self-structure, self-integration, and so forth. The Common Language for Psychotherapy initiative may be a place to start in bridging across diverse theoretical orientations to reach a common language in psychotherapy and psychological research in relation to the self.

Turning to the perspective of a practicing clinician, a number of questions need to be considered. How can a clinician seek leverage in the notion of self-concept in therapy – and in what ways does this already occur within various schools of therapy? From various theoretical standpoints and paradigms, the self already occupies a central position in the formulation of disorders, yet how do therapists tailor their treatment strategies and techniques around such self-based formulations? To what extent is treatment within these perspectives informed by an understanding of the self-concept of the patient? Do therapists have the skills and training required to accommodate such formulations? These are issues for further research and consideration.

At a more "macro" level, an obvious future direction is the development of evidence-based preventative, early intervention, treatment, or relapse-prevention programs that target self-construals, presuming we are correct that such construals make individuals vulnerable to psychological disorder, resistant to treatment, or prone to relapse. As self-narratives are potentially redemptive, in that they are useful for buffering against distress, they have importance for prevention, treatment outcomes, and relapse prevention across disorders. Therapists can address attachment insecurities to assuage damaged or irreconcilable self-concepts, emphasizing their potential importance in therapeutic alliance and engagement, and in motivational and treatment processes. Specifically considering self-concept as a therapeutic target for focused psychological techniques could be an important way forward in augmenting current treatments, in the hope of achieving improved outcomes; therapy for social anxiety disorder is a prototypical example where self-processing techniques have already led to improved outcomes. Consideration of self-construals would also be useful in case formulations, as therapists can incorporate developmental, functional, and symptomatic information to develop treatment plans. All this is consistent with the bidirectional need to integrate our understanding of phenomena and theory within a scientist–practitioner framework (Salkovskis, 2002). Understanding symptoms or related phenomena from the emerging theoretical and empirical literature on the self appears to have enormous potential across the range of disorders.

What is interesting, however, is that despite several examples of specificity in some self-disorder associations, interventions have several components that are shared, for example, these include reparenting, rescripting, reflecting on and making sense of one's experiences (i.e., mentalizing), creating narratives that link maladaptive beliefs to their external sources and origins rather than reflections of reality, etc. The commonality of these therapeutic strategies could be explained by an attachment framework and the therapeutic alliance in psychotherapy. Alternatively, given the importance of specific models of disorder in evidence-based treatment, targeting disorder-specific aspects of self could inform further development in treatment. Irrespective, the proposed ruptures in self-structures that are at the heart of disorder hold important implications more generally for scientist-practitioners, whatever their psychotherapeutic orientation.

Additionally, it is notable to state that most authors have come from the clinical arena. Given that the focus of this book has been on psychopathology, this is not surprising. However, research and theoretical work on the self is actually primarily conducted by social and cognitive psychologists. This is not atypical of the way in which clinical researchers, in search of ways to augment their existing models, integrate alternative frameworks from allied areas of psychology that have face validity or potential utility, rather than solely on the basis of true and comprehensive theoretical discourse. The advantages of clinicians using such constructs is that they are easily able to translate them into the clinical arena in a manner that is meaningful to practitioners and clinical researchers. However, often this development is then recast – the resulting revised models are considered to be theoretically derived in their own right, rather than pragmatically derived. As such, there is a potential disadvantage to clinical researchers using self-constructs in that they run the risk of omitting important theoretical nuances

that cognitive and social psychologists hold in understanding their methodology and the results (and of course, *conflicting* results) within their research field. That is not to say that the clinical and social or cognitive psychological fields are anathema to each other. There is a growing effort in psychology to integrate clinical and both social and cognitive psychology constructs and methodologies; indeed journals such as the *Journal of Social and Clinical Psychology* explicitly aim to bridge this gap. This book also represents a step towards integration and it is hoped it will spur future research also incorporating true collaboration and the development of a "shared language" between clinical and social or cognitive psychologists investigating the "self." Conversely, it could also be argued that a focus on specific self constructs has emerged from an understanding of clinical phenomena and that a clinical perspective can advance understanding of the self.

With respect to future research, a number of additional options can be identified. Longitudinal research in psychopathology tracking the development of self processes and construals against the emergence of symptoms reflective of specific disorders would provide useful data for the etiological association between self and psychopathology. In addition, the impact of developmental processes, such as parenting and attachment patterns, on the emergence of the self would be of particular utility in understanding psychopathology; indeed, attachment research – spanning from a background in biological, developmental, and psychodynamic theory but incorporating cognitive and affective theoretical formulations – could serve as a focal point for integrative work on the self. Similarly, experimental psychopathology would also help elucidate etiological associations between self and symptoms. It is entirely possible that self construals as measured in adult research are the result of psychopathology which tends to emerge in adolescence or early adulthood or even, in many cases, childhood.

Furthermore, considering our overarching discussion of the organization of the self, we believe that research needs to move away from being one-dimensional – focusing just on the beliefs held about self – to being two-dimensional – focusing on both the structure of the self-concept and the cohesion of such self-beliefs. Ironically, such an approach may imply moving "back to the future" – incorporating notions such as those from theoretician/clinician George Kelly's Personal Construct Theory (1966/2003). Within the "Fragmentation Corollary," Kelly noted that individuals' belief systems are so large that a "person may successively employ a variety of construction subsystems which are inferentially incompatible with each other" (p. 13); as one's self-system comprises one's most developed belief system, its structure and consistency bears the greatest opportunity for inconsistency and fragmentation. Clearly, then, what one thinks of one aspect of self needs to be studied in the context of other competing beliefs one has about oneself. We need research methods to capture both foci. Another useful distinction is between *physical* and *psychological* aspects of the self, as was explicated with regards to a number of disorders (e.g., autism, bipolar disorder, chronic fatigue syndrome). This distinction can, however, be applied across a number of disorders where physiological aspects of, for example, anxiety are likely to impact upon constructions of self and other cognitive functions. In addition, research using implicit measures is also instructive, because it goes beyond the explicit declarative statements consciously made about self to study more automatic processes, and potentially taps into alternative ways that such knowledge about self is stored. However, as noted above, given the complex theoretical underpinning of implicit vs. explicit views of self, and the numerous contradictions and complications of research and theory in the area (e.g., see Hughes, Barnes-Holmes, & Vahey, 2012; Nosek, Hawkins, & Frazier, 2011), explicit involvement of social psychologists would be welcomed to assist such endeavors. Similarly, of course, work from cognitive scientists and cognitive neuroscientists will also give shape to this discourse about self, as exemplified by work in this book with respect to psychotic disorders and autism.

In conclusion, we can see that a large challenge awaits us as theoreticians and clinicians. However, we believe that the work in this book highlights the enormous advances we are making in our knowledge and use of techniques regarding the "self" in the understanding and treatment of psychological disorders. We remain optimistic about the future of work in this field, given the relative youth of this work, and considering further the relatively recent emergence of psychology itself as a science when compared to its philosophical roots. We hope this important task is taken up with vigour, and hope that our enthusiasm is infectious, particularly when we are looking forward to the next generations of researchers and practitioners moving into the field.

References

Fosshage, J. L. (2009). Some key features in the evolution of self psychology and psychoanalysis. *Self and Systems: Annals of the New York Academy of Sciences*, 1159, 1–18. doi: 10.1111/j.1749-6632.2008.04346.x

Guntrip, H. (1977). *Psychoanalytic Theory, Therapy, And The Self*. New York, NY: Basic Books.

Katzko, M. W. (2003). Unity versus multiplicity: A conceptual analysis of the term "self" and its use in personality theories. *Journal of Personality*, 71(1), 83–114. doi: 10.1111/1467–6494.t01-1-00004.

Kelly, G. A. (2003). A brief introduction to Personal Construct Theory. In F. Fransella (Ed.), *International Handbook of Personal Construct Theory*. Chichester: Wiley.

Kohut, H. (1971). *The Analysis of the Self*. New York, NY: International Universities Press.

Kohut, H. (1977). *The Restoration of the Self*. New York, NY: International Universities Press

Leary, M. R. & Tangney, J. P. (2012). The Self as an organizing construct in the behavioral and social sciences. In M. R. Leary & J. P. Tangney (Eds.), *Handbook of Self and Identity* (2nd ed., pp. 1–18). New York, NY: Guilford.

Hughes, S., Barnes-Holmes, D., & Vahey, N. (2012). Holding on to our functional roots when exploring new intellectual islands: A voyage through implicit cognition research. *Journal of Contextual Behavioral Science*, 1(1), 17–38.

Nosek, B. A., Hawkins, C. B., & Frazier, R. S. (2011). Implicit social cognition: From measures to mechanisms. *Trends in Cognitive Sciences*, 15(4), 152–159.

Oyserman, D., Elmore, K., & Smith, G. (2012). Self, self-concept, and identity. In M. R. Leary & J. P. Tangney (Eds.), *Handbook of Self and Identity* (2nd ed., pp. 69–104). New York, NY: Guilford.

Oyserman, D., & Markus, H. R. (1998). Self as social representation. In S. U. Flick (Ed.), *The Psychology of the Social* (pp. 107–125). New York, NY: Cambridge University Press.

Salkovskis, P. M. (2002). Empirically grounded clinical interventions: Cognitive-behavioural therapy progresses through a multi-dimensional approach to clinical science. *Behavioural and Cognitive Psychotherapy*, 30, 3–9.

Index